Hypertension

METHODS IN MOLECULAR MEDICINE™

John M. Walker, SERIES EDITOR

METHODS IN MOLECULAR MEDICINE™

Hypertension

Methods and Protocols

Edited by

Jérôme P. Fennell

Moyne Institute for Preventive Medicine,
Trinity College, Dublin, Ireland

Andrew H. Baker

Division of Cardiovascular and Medical Sciences,
BHF Glasgow Cardiovascular Research Centre,
University of Glasgow, Glasgow, UK

HUMANA PRESS ❋ TOTOWA, NEW JERSEY

© 2005 Humana Press Inc.
999 Riverview Drive, Suite 208
Totowa, New Jersey 07512

www.humanapress.com

This publication is printed on acid-free paper. ∞
ANSI Z39.48-1984 (American Standards Institute) Permanence of Paper for Printed Library Materials.

For additional copies, pricing for bulk purchases, and/or information about other Humana titles, contact Humana at the above address or at any of the following numbers: Tel.: 973-256-1699; Fax: 973-256-8341; E-mail: humana@humanapr.com; or visit our Website: www.humanapress.com.

Production Editor: Mark J. Breaugh
Cover design by Patricia F. Cleary
Cover illustration: Figure 1 from Chapter 7, "A Guide to Wire Myography," by Angela Spiers and Neal Padmanabhan.

Printed in the United States of America. 10 9 8 7 6 5 4 3 2 1

eISBN 1-59259-850-1
ISSN 1543-1894

Library of Congress Cataloging in Publication Data

Hypertension : methods and protocols / edited by Jérôme P. Fennell, Andrew H. Baker.
    p. ; cm. -- (Methods in molecular medicine, ISSN 1543-1894 ; 108)
  Includes bibliographical references and index.
  ISBN 1-58829-323-8 (alk. paper)
    1. Hypertension--Molecular aspects--Laboratory manuals. I. Fennell, Jérôme P. II. Baker, Andrew H. III. Series.
  [DNLM: 1. Hypertension--genetics. 2. Clinical protocols. 3. Genetic Techniques. 4. Hypertension--therapy. 5. Models, Animal. WG 340 H99582 2005]
  RC685.H8H855 2005
  616.1'32--dc22

2004054260

Preface

Hypertension is thought to affect about one quarter of the population in the western world. Worldwide, the numbers of patients will continue to increase as less affluent countries follow this trend and adopt first world dietary habits and lifestyles. Hypertension is known to increase the risk of stroke, myocardial infarction, renal failure, and cardiac failure, and treatment is known to reduce these risks. We still do not have a complete understanding of essential hypertension, let alone a cure. Since the clinical importance of hypertension became fully appreciated in the last century, research in the field has continued to accelerate. New methods in molecular biology have arrived at an exponentially accelerating rate since the seminal discoveries of nucleotide sequencing and recombinant DNA technology of the 1970s. Modern molecular biology provides a bridge of understanding from the chemical through to the clinical. The availability of such new information as that derived from the Human Genome project and the accessibility of that information via the Internet have revolutionized medical research. The application and availability of new molecular techniques and knowledge mean that our understanding of the pathogenesis of hypertension and the potential for improved clinical intervention have never been greater. We hope that the process detailed in *Hypertension: Methods and Protocols* will help researchers to develop a greater understanding of hypertension and uncover new potential targets for antihypertensive therapy.

Hypertension: Methods and Protocols provides many new and essential methods that span the entire spectrum of modern molecular biology. The authors offer an elite collection of knowledge and experience assembled from the four corners of the world. The accessible format of the protocols makes them easy to perform, even by beginners in the field. The breadth of protocols provided will attract experienced scientists interested in pursuing new avenues of research in hypertension.

The first part deals with animal models of hypertension and describes methods of producing congenic, consomic, transgenic, and knockout models of hypertension. The final chapter in this section describes a method for the telemetric measurement of blood pressure in such animals.

Free radical-mediated damage plays an important role in many chronic diseases, including hypertension. The second part of this book describes methods of assessing the role of free radicals in hypertension that are applicable to all forms of endothelial dysfunction. The quantitative method of chemiluminescence and the qualitative method of dihydroethidine staining combined with wire myography assessment provide methods of assessing hypertension and other forms of endothelial dysfunction at both a molecular and a physiological level.

As our molecular understanding improved, the emphasis in hypertension research moved from rare monogenetic disorders to understanding the complex contribution of genetics to essential hypertension. Much work has gone into the pursuit of the genes associated with hypertension. Part III contains several methods to aid in the genetic dissection of hypertension, such as the candidate gene approach, genome wide scans, SNP analysis, and microarray analysis. One of the most promising aspects of human genetic research is the search for SNPs associated with hypertension. Several methods of SNP analysis, such as Taqman, WAVE, SSCP, and mass spectrometry, are provided. Genotyping may allow stratification of patients according to risk, but will also guide therapy one day. Pharmacogenetics and pharmacogenomics will become increasingly important and are also discussed. Functional genomics using microarray analysis will lead to the discovery of new genetic pathways, and thus to greater insights into the genetic input in hypertension and the patients' likely response to treatment.

Part IV describes two very different protein techniques. The first chapter looks at the analysis of a small number of related yet relevant amino acids. The roles of arginine and ADMA have become increasingly associated with endothelial dysfunction and hypertension. The HPLC analysis of ADMA and other arginine analogs is discussed. The second chapter discusses a proteomics procedure for the large-scale analysis of protein expression. Proteomics holds great promise for the field of cardiovascular biology; benefits will include the identification of marker proteins, dissection of signaling pathways affected by the underlying perturbation, and drug-target identification and validation. This chapter focuses on a few examples of how the powerful combination of two-dimensional gel electrophoresis, bioinformatics, and mass spectrometric analysis can be applied to the study of hypertension.

Gene transfer of specific genetic material to either overexpress or inhibit gene expression is a useful scientific tool and a potential source for the future long-term treatment of hypertension. The last decade has shown many exciting developments in this field, so Part V includes a comprehensive section on gene transfer. Several nonviral methods are described including nonviral techniques using polymers, liposomes, and antisense agents. Post-transcriptional inhibition using siRNA is also described. One of the most popular viral vectors used in hypertension research is the adenoviral vector; therefore two chapters of adenoviral methods are presented: one describing the generation of large-capacity, sustained-expression vectors and another describing the practical application of adenoviral vectors to reduce blood pressure in an animal model using superoxide dismutase gene transfer. The liver and spleen absorb the vast majority of systemically injected viral vectors, reducing their effectiveness. The possibility of selectively targeting vectors to the endothelium of the systemic vasculature or other target organs would have major implications. Selectively targeted vectors would improve the efficacy of gene transfer, thereby reducing the viral dose required and improving the safety profile. The chapter on in vivo biopanning using phage display describes a remarkable technique for isolating targeting peptides, which could enable in vivo organ- or tissue-specific binding of gene transfer vectors.

Stem cells research may have the potential to supply replacement cells for the cells damaged by hypertensive remodeling or from the complications of hypertension, such as myocardial infarction. These previously unimaginable prospects may soon be reality. Part VI describes a practical method for the derivation of cardiomyocytes from embryonic stem cells.

In recent years a veritable avalanche of accessible technology and information has become available though the Internet. The information technology revolution has been of enormous benefit to molecular biology research and promises even more. Embryonic areas of research—such as microarrays, proteomics, and pharmacogenomics — would simply not exist without the help of modern IT systems. Although many chapters contain relevant IT information, Part VII is dedicated solely to bioinformatics, with an excellent introduction to bioinformatic resources for pharmacogenomics and a more practical chapter describing the application of *in silico* strategies to identify nuclear matrix attachment regions.

I would like to thank my family, Dr. Catherine Cleary, and Dr. William Fennell for their patience, advice, and support. This work would not have been possible without the contributions of our series editor John M. Walker and of course our publisher, Humana Press. Finally I would especially like to thank my coeditor, Andrew H. Baker for his extensive efforts and guidance in this project.

Jérôme P. Fennell
Andrew H. Baker

Contents

Contributors

JAIME WENDT ANDRAE • *Human and Molecular Genetics Center, Medical College of Wisconsin, Milwaukee, WI*

MICHAEL BADER • *Max Delbrück Center for Molecular Medicine (MDC), Berlin-Buch, Germany*

ANDREW H. BAKER • *Division of Cardiovascular and Medical Sciences, BHF Glasgow Cardiovascular Research Centre, University of Glasgow, Glasgow, UK*

IAN M. BIRD • *Department of Obstetrics and Gynecology, University Wisconsin, Madison, WI*

KENNETH R. BOHELER • *National Institute on Aging, NIH, Baltimore, MD*

NICHOLAS J. R. BRAIN • *BHF Glasgow Cardiovascular Research Centre, University of Glasgow, Glasgow, UK*

MARK J. CAULFIELD • *The Genome Centre and Clinical Pharmacology, The William Harvey Research Institute, Barts and The London, Charterhouse Square, London, UK*

LAWRENCE CHAN • *Department of Molecular & Cellular Biology and Medicine, Division of Endorcrinology and Metabolism, Baylor College of Medicine, Houston, TX*

KEITH M. CHANNON • *Department of Cardiovascular Medicine, John Radcliffe Hospital, University of Oxford, Oxford, UK*

YI CHU • *Cardiovascular Center, Department of Internal Medicine, University of Iowa, Carver College of Medicine, Iowa City, IA*

RAINER CRAMER • *Ludwig Institute for Cancer Research and Department of Biochemistry and Molecular Biology, Royal Free and University College London Medical School, London, UK*

DAVID G. CRIDER • *National Institute on Aging, NIH, Baltimore, MD*

GEORGE N. DEMARTINO • *Department of Physiology, The University of Texas Southwestern University, Dallas, TX*

LAURA DENBY • *BHF Glasgow Cardiovascular Research Centre, University of Glasgow, Glasgow, UK*

FILOMENA DE NIGRIS • *Department of Pharmacological Sciences, University of Salerno, Italy*

ANNA F. DOMINICZAK • *BHF Glasgow Cardiovascular Research Centre, University of Glasgow, Glasgow, UK*

YANBIN DONG • *Georgia Prevention Institute, Medical College of Georgia, Augusta, GA*

ELIZABETH DONOHOE • *National Centre for Medical Genetics, Our Lady's Hospital for Sick Children, Crumlin, Dublin, Republic of Ireland*

PETER A. DORIS • *The University of Texas, Institute of Molecular Medicine, Research Center for Human Genetics, Houston, TX*

SORIN DRAGHICI • *Department of Computer Sciences, Center for Scientific Computing, Wayne State University, Detroit, MI*

LIVIUS V. D'USCIO • *Departments of Anesthesiology and Molecular Pharmacology & Experimental Therapeutics, Mayo Clinic and Foundation, Rochester, MN*

ROSALIND FABUNMI • *American Heart Association, Greenville Avenue, Dallas, TX*

JÉRÔME P. FENNELL • *Moyne Institute for Preventive Medicine, Trinity College, Dublin, Ireland*

MYRIAM FORNAGE • *The University of Texas, Institute of Molecular Medicine, Research Center for Human Genetics, Houston, TX*

PIERS GALLNEY • *Ludwig Institute for Cancer Research, Royal Free and University College London Medical School, London, UK*

ROBERT GOODRICH • *Department of Obstetrics and Gynecology, Center for Molecular Medicine and Genetics, Wayne State University, Detroit, MI*

DELYTH GRAHAM • *BHF Glasgow Cardiovascular Research Centre, University of Glasgow, Glasgow, UK*

TOMASZ J. GUZIK • *Departments of Pharmacology and Internal Medicine, Jagiellonian University, Cracow, Poland*

CLAIRE HASTIE • *Ludwig Institute for Cancer Research, Royal Free and University College London Medical School, London, UK*

ZANNA HYVÖNEN • *Department of Pharmaceutics, University of Kuopio, Kuopio, Finland*

HOWARD J. JACOB • *Human and Molecular Genetics Center, Medical College of Wisconsin, Milwaukee, WI*

ZVONIMIR S. KATUSIC • *Departments of Anesthesiology and Molecular Pharmacology & Experimental Therapeutics, Mayo Clinic and Foundation, Rochester, MN*

KATHLEEN KENNEDY • *Human and Molecular Genetics Center, Medical College of Wisconsin, Milwaukee, WI*

BIRGITTA KIMURA • *Department of Anthropology, University of Florida, Gainesville, FL*

KLAAS KRAMER • *Department of Safety and Environmental Affairs (DVM), Free University, Amsterdam, The Netherlands; and International Microsurgical Training Centre, Lelystad, The Netherlands*

STEPHEN A. KRAWETZ • *Departments of Obstetrics and Gynecology and Computer Sciences, Center for Molecular Medicine and Genetics, Center for Scientific Computing, Wayne State University, Detroit, MI*

ALEXANDER KRIVOKHARCHENKO • *Max Delbrück Center for Molecular Medicine (MDC) Berlin-Buch, Germany*

KLAUS LINDPAINTNER • *Roche Genetics, F. Hoffmann-La Roche, Ltd, Basel, Switzerland*

ZHANDONG LIU • *Department of Computer Sciences, Wayne State University, Detroit, MI*

VICTOR A. MALTSEV • *National Institute on Aging, NIH, Baltimore, MD*

MARTIN W. MCBRIDE • *BHF Glasgow Cardiovascular Research Centre, University of Glasgow, Glasgow, UK*

CHARLES A. MEIN • *The Genome Centre and Clinical Pharmacology, The William Harvey Research Institute, Barts and The London, Charterhouse Square, London, UK*

CAROL MORENO • *Human and Molecular Genetics Center, Medical College of Wisconsin, Milwaukee, WI*

PATRICIA B. MUNROE • *The Genome Centre and Clinical Pharmacology, The William Harvey Research Institute, Barts and The London, Charterhouse Square, London, UK*

SOREN NAABY-HANSEN • *Ludwig Institute for Cancer Research and Department of Biochemistry and Molecular Biology, Royal Free and University College London Medical School, London, UK*

SHOTA NAKAMURA • *Department of Cardiovascular Medicine, Kumamoto University School of Medicine, Honjo, Kumamoto, Japan*

CLAUDIO NAPOLI • *Department of Medicine and Division of Clinical Pathology, University of Naples, Italy; Evans Department of Medicine and Whitaker Cardiovascular Institute, Boston University, Boston, MA*

CAMPBELL G. NICOL • *BHF Glasgow Cardiovascular Research Centre, University of Glasgow, Glasgow, UK*

TIMOTHY O'BRIEN • *Department of Medicine, Clinical Science Institute, University College Hospital, Galway, Ireland*

HISAO OGAWA • *Department of Cardiovascular Medicine, Kumamoto University School of Medicine, Honjo, Kumamoto, Japan*

KAZUHIRO OKA • *Departments of Molecular and Cellular Biology, Medicine, and Neurology, Baylor College of Medicine, Houston, TX*

G. CHARLES OSTERMEIER • *Department of Obstetrics and Gynecology, Center for Molecular Medicine and Genetics, Wayne State University, Detroit, MI*

NEAL PADMANABHAN • *Division of Cardiovascular and Medical Sciences, University of Glasgow, Glasgow, UK*

TIMOTHY E. PETERSON • *Departments of Anesthesiology and Molecular Pharmacology & Experimental Therapeutics, Mayo Clinic and Foundation, Rochester, MN*

M. IAN PHILLIPS • *Department of Physiology & Internal Medicine, University of South Florida, Tampa, FL*

ELENA POPOVA • *Max Delbrück Center for Molecular Medicine (MDC) Berlin-Buch, Germany*

RENÉ REMIE • *Solvay Pharmaceuticals, Weesp, The Netherlands; and International Microsurgical Training Centre (IMTC), Lelystad, The Netherlands*

MARIKA RUPONEN • *Department of Pharmaceutics, University of Kuopio, Kuopio, Finland*

SABYASACHI SEN • *Department of Medicine, St. Elizabeth's Medical Center, Boston, MA*

VINCENZO SICA • *Division of Clinical Pathology, University of Naples, Italy*

ANGELA SPIERS • *Division of Cardiovascular and Medical Sciences, University of Glasgow, Glasgow, UK*

PADRAIG M. STRAPPE • *Department of Medicine, Clinical Science Institute, University College Hospital, Galway, Ireland*

YELENA TARASOVA • *National Institute on Aging, NIH, Baltimore, MD*

TOM TEERLINK • *Department of Clinical Chemistry, VU University Medical Center, Amsterdam, The Netherlands*

ARTO URTTI • *Department of Pharmaceutics, University of Kuopio, Kuopio, Finland*

GAYATHRI D. WARNASURIYA • *Ludwig Institute for Cancer Research, Royal Free and University College London Medical School, London, UK*

CEZARY WÓJCIK • *Department of Physiology, The University of Texas Southwestern University, Dallas, TX*

LORRAINE M. WORK • *BHF Glasgow Cardiovascular Research Centre, University of Glasgow, Glasgow, UK*

QING YAN • *MedImmune Inc., Mountain View, CA*

SEPPO YLÄ-HERTTUALA • *Department of Medicine and Gene Therapy Unit, Kuopio University Hospital, Kuopio, Finland*

MICHIHIRO YOSHIMURA • *Department of Cardiovascular Medicine, Graduate School of Medical Sciences, Kumamoto University School of Medicine, Honjo, Kumamoto, Japan*

MICHELA ZANETTI • *Department of Clinical, Morphological, and Technological Sciences, UCO di Clinica Medica, University of Trieste, Italy*

HAIDONG ZHU • *Georgia Prevention Institute, Medical College of Georgia, Augusta, GA*

I

Models of Hypertension

1

Congenic/Consomic Models of Hypertension

Delyth Graham, Martin W. McBride, Nicholas J. R. Brain, and Anna F. Dominiczak

Summary

Human essential hypertension is a complex, multifactorial, quantitative trait under polygenic control. Despite major recent advances in genome sequencing and statistical tools, the genetic dissection of essential hypertension still provides a formidable challenge. Genetic models of essential hypertension such as the spontaneously hypertensive stroke-prone rat (SHRSP) provide the scientist with genetic homogeneity, not possible within a human population, to aid the search for causative genes. The principal strategy in the rat has been the identification of quantitative trait loci (QTL) responsible for blood-pressure regulation by genome-wide scanning. In this chapter we focus on congenic and consomic breeding strategies for the confirmation of QTL and the genetic dissection of the implicated regions.

Key Words: Genotyping; polymerase chain reaction; microsatellite markers; quantitative trait locus (QTL); congenic; consomic, hypertension; stroke-prone spontaneously hypertensive rat (SHRSP); Wistar Kyoto rat (WKY).

1. Introduction

An important approach to the study of multifactorial, polygenic diseases such as essential hypertension is the use of appropriate inbred animal models. Major advantages of inbred animal models include genetic homogeneity and the complete control of environmental influences. Most important, the ability to produce specific intercrosses between normotensive and hypertensive strains represents a powerful experimental tool for performing linkage analyses far beyond the scope of human studies *(1)*.

Many hypertensive rat strains have been produced over the past 30 yr, ranging from the spontaneously hypertensive rat (SHR) and stroke-prone spontaneously hypertensive rat (SHRSP) to strains in which high dietary salt is necessary to induce hypertension, such as the Dahl salt-sensitive and Sabra

From: *Methods in Molecular Medicine, Vol. 108: Hypertension: Methods and Protocols*
Edited by: J. P. Fennell and A. H. Baker © Humana Press Inc., Totowa, NJ

rats. These models also exhibit end-organ damage phenotypes similar to those seen in human essential hypertension, including left ventricular hypertrophy, stroke, and renal failure *(2–4)*. Most inbred rat strains have been derived from Wistar-related stocks and others from Sprague-Dawley; however, as these strains have a common origin, there is relatively little genetic diversity. The exception is the fawn hooded rat, which may have a more distant origin *(5)*.

The major strategy in the search for causative genes underlying complex polygenic traits such as hypertension has been the identification of quantitative trait loci (QTL) in F2 segregating populations (i.e., the genome-wide scan or linkage analysis) *(6)*. A QTL defines a large chromosomal region (approx 20–30 cM) containing one or more loci controlling a quantitative trait. Numerous linkage analysis studies in experimental crosses between hypertensive and normotensive reference rat strains have been carried out over the past 10 yr, which have identified QTL for blood pressure on every rat chromosome *(6,7)*. Since rodent QTL regions are too large to test functionally all putative candidate genes, the identification of a blood pressure QTL can be considered as only the first step toward causative gene identification *(8)*. Further strategies include production of consomic or congenic strains and substrains to confirm the existence of the QTL and to allow genetic dissection of the implicated region *(9)*.

A congenic/consomic strain is one in which part of the genome of one rat strain is selectively transferred to another by backcrossing a donor rat strain to a recipient strain with appropriate selection. In the case of consomic strains (chromosome substitution), a whole chromosome is transferred *(10,11)*, whereas in the case of congenic strain, a defined chromosomal segment (the differential segment) is transferred. It should be noted that congenic strains contain not only the selected differential locus, but also an associated length of the surrounding donor chromosome. Consomic strains have proved to be invaluable in the study of the nonrecombining Y chromosome effect on hypertension *(11–13)*. Furthermore, a large panel of consomic rat strains has recently been developed *(14)*, in which each autosome has been individually replaced. Consomic panels can be used to determine the chromosomal location of genes contributing to particular phenotypes and to generate congenic strains for positional cloning rapidly.

Classically, the congenic strain breeding procedure involves serially backcrossing the donor strain to the recipient, while selecting progeny carrying the desired QTL region in each generation of backcrossing (**Fig. 1**). According to Mendelian laws, between 8 and 10 backcrosses are required to dilute the donor genome into >99% that of the recipient. Brother–sister mating can then "fix" the desired introgressed segment as homozygous and the congenic strain can then be phenotyped. A variety of rat congenic strains has been produced in this

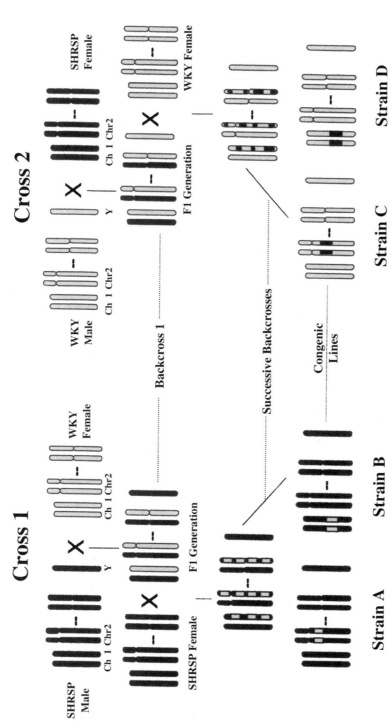

Fig. 1. Construction of reciprocal congenic strains using SHRSP and WKY parental strains. Cross 1, WKY chromosomal regions introgressed into SHRSP background (strains A and B). Cross 2, SHRSP chromosomal regions introgressed into WKY background (strains C and D).

manner. In order to ensure transfer of entire QTL, original congenic strains tend to have large chromosomal regions introgressed, therefore smaller substrains (minimal congenics) are required to reduce the size and hence the implicated region. In some cases there may be more than one QTL present in any given region, therefore, several substrains are necessary to dissect the implicated region *(15)*. Substrains are constructed by crossing the original congenic strain with the recipient stain and brother–sister mating the resultant heterozygous offspring. Recombination events occurring at meiosis allow for the production of progeny with smaller introgressed regions that can be selected by genotyping densely spaced polymorphic markers *(16)*.

The traditional breeding strategy takes approx 3–4 yr to produce a congenic strain *(17)*. This time can be shortened by utilizing a marker-assisted "speed" congenic breeding strategy, previously tested in the mouse *(18)*. Jeffs et al. *(19)* were the first to show that this strategy can also be successful in the rat. Lander and Schork *(20)* proposed that screening of polymorphic genetic markers covering the entire background of the genome could be used to select male offspring with least donor alleles in their background. In this way, the next round of breeding using the "best" male could dramatically reduce the time taken to clear the background of the recipient strain (**Fig. 2**). It has been calculated that by four backcross generations, donor genome contamination would be less than 1% if 60 background markers, spaced on average 25 cM apart, were used for screening 16 males at each generation. This speed congenic approach therefore reduces the average time required to produce strains to approx 2 yr *(19)*.

In this chapter we describe the methodology for a speed congenic/consomic breeding strategy and high-throughput fluorescent genotyping using the stroke-prone spontaneously hypertensive rat (SHRSP) and the normotensive Wistar-Kyoto (WKY) strain.

2. Materials

2.1. Genomic DNA Isolation (Animal Tail Tip)

1. 0.5 *M* EDTA (pH 8.0): Sterilization by autoclaving.
2. Nuclei lysis solution: (Promega, cat. no. A7943).
3. Protein precipitation solution: (Promega, cat. no. A7953).
4. 20 mg/mL Proteinase K.
5. Isopropanol.
6. 70% Ethanol.
7. Benchtop microcentrifuge.
8. Whirli mixer (e.g., FSA Laboratory Supplies)
9. Hybridization oven.
10. Sterile pipet tips.

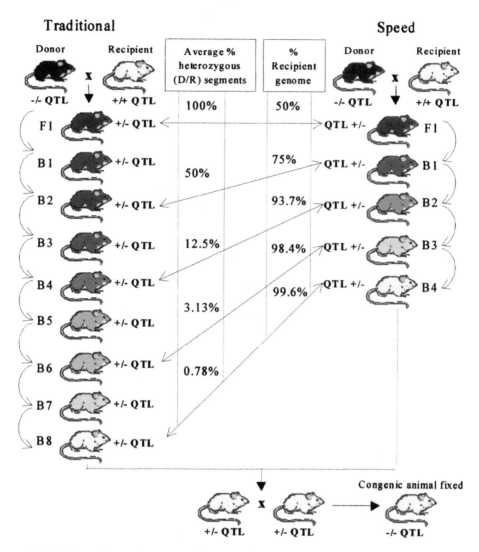

Fig. 2. Congenic strain construction, illustrating differences between the traditional and marker-assisted speed congenic approach. The arrows indicate the backcross at which background heterozygosity is theoretically the same. Decreasing shades of gray to white represent the serial dilution of the donor genome in the genetic background. D, donor strain alleles; R, recipient strain alleles; B, backcross; F1, first filial generation.

2.2. Quantification of Genomic DNA

1. UV/visible Spectrophotometer (e.g., Pharmacia Biotech Ultrospec 2000).
2. Quartz cuvets.
3. Parafilm.

2.3. Polymerase Chain Reaction

1. Deep 96-well plate.
2. Thermo-fast 96-well skirted polymerase chain reaction (PCR) plates (ABgene cat. no. AB-0800).
3. PCR plate with adhesive cover.
4. 1 m*M* dNTPs stocks.
5. 10X Hotstar *Taq* DNA polymerase buffer (Qiagen, UK) (*see* **Note 1**).
6. Forward and reverse primers (20 pmol/μL conc.).
7. 0.5 U/μL Hotstar *Taq* DNA polymerase (Qiagen, UK).
8. Thermal Cycler hot lid PCR machine (e.g., MJ Research PTC-225 Peltier).
9. Multichannel electric pipet.

2.4. PCR Pooling

1. Thermo-fast 96-well skirted PCR plates (ABgene cat. no. AB-0800).
2. Multichannel electric pipet.

2.5. Casting Gels for the ABI Prism 377XL

1. Powder-free gloves (*see* **Note 2**).
2. 50% Long Ranger gel solution (Cambrex Corporation, NJ).
3. Ultrapure urea.
4. Bio-Rad AG 501-X8 (D) deionizing resin.
5. Deionized water.
6. 50-mL Measuring cylinder.
7. 10% w/v Ammonium persulfate.
8. Whatman cellulose filters.
9. 10X TBE: 0.89 M Tris-borate pH 8.3, 20 m*M* Na$_2$EDTA.
10. TEMED (*N,N,N',N'*- tetramethylehtylenediamine, Sigma 7024).
11. 60-mL syringe.
12. Bubble catcher.
13. Bulldog clips.

3. Methods

3.1. Marker-Assisted "Speed" Congenic Strategy

1. Congenic strains are constructed using a speed congenic (or marker-assisted) strategy whereby various segments of the rat chromosome of interest are introgressed from the normotensive WKY strain to the genetic background of the SHRSP, and in the reciprocal direction from SHRSP to the genetic background of the WKY.

2. Reciprocal F1 generations are produced by crossing WKY and SHRSP (one breeding pair per cross is sufficient). Resulting male F1 hybrids are mated to the desired recipient strain (WKY or SHRSP) females (*see* **Note 3**).
3. Microsatellite markers throughout the chromosomal region of interest, and additional markers broadly spanning the remaining genome, are genotyped (*see* **Subheading 3.3.**) in the offspring from this first backcross (*see* **Note 4**). Those males identified as heterozygous for marker alleles within the chromosomal region of interest, but with most homozygosity for recipient alleles throughout the remaining genome, are selected as "best" males for breeding (*see* **Note 5**). These best males are mated with recipient strain females to produce a second backcross generation and the offspring are genotyped.
4. Procedure is repeated by backcrossing "best" male offspring until all donor alleles in the genetic background (indicated by the background markers) are eradicated (*see* **Note 6**). Approximately four to five backcross generations are required to achieve recipient strain homozygosity in all background markers. The differential chromosomal region is then fixed and made homozygous by crossing appropriate males and females.
5. Fixed congenic strains are maintained by brother–sister mating.
6. Confirmation of successful QTL capture by phenotypic measurement within a congenic strain is followed by congenic substrain (or minimal congenic) production with smaller donor regions. This strategy dissects the introgressed region, allowing further localization of the QTL.
7. Congenic substrain production is undertaken by backcrossing congenic males to recipient females to yield rats heterozygous within the original introgressed segment, while maintaining recipient strain homozygosity in the remaining genome.
8. Resulting heterozygous F1 rats are intercrossed and the offspring genotyped to identify appropriate males and females with smaller regions of donor allele homozygosity. These smaller regions are fixed and the new substrains maintained by brother-sister mating.
9. Linked databases for management of genotyping data and breeding protocols were designed and implemented in-house (Microsoft Access 2000).

3.2. Marker-Assisted "Speed" Consomic Strategy

An identical speed breeding strategy can be applied to consomic strain production. In this case the entire chromosome of interest is introgressed from donor into the recipient strain. For production of Y-chromosome consomic strains, slight modifications to the breeding strategy are required, as follows:

1. The Y chromosome contains a large nonrecombining region; therefore the origin of the male F1 progenitor will determine the Y chromosome in all resulting F1 hybrid males.
2. Microsatellite markers broadly spanning all of the autosomes are genotyped (*see* **Subheading 3.3.**) in the offspring from a first backcross generation. "Best" males for backcrossing to recipient strain females are chosen on the basis of least heterozygosity throughout the autosomal background.

3. Backcrossing is continued until all donor alleles in the genetic background (indicated by background markers) are eradicated.
4. Y-chromosome consomic strains can be fixed and maintained by backcrossing to recipient strain females.

3.3. High-Throughput Fluorescent Genotyping

3.3.1. Genomic DNA Isolation From Animal Tail Tip

1. Briefly anaesthetize the animal with halothane/oxygen, remove a 4-mm tip from the tail, and immediately cauterize wound (*see* **Note 7**).
2. Prepare the tail tip samples for digestion; add 120 μL of 0.5 *M* EDTA to 500 μL of nuclei lysis solution for each sample into an appropriate-sized tube.
3. Chill the mix on ice for 5 min.
4. Add 600 μL of the prepared mix to each tail tip sample and add 17.5 μL of 20 mg/mL proteinase K solution. Incubate the samples in a rotating hybridization oven at 37°C overnight (*see* **Note 8**).
5. Allow the samples to cool to room temperature.
6. Add 200 μL of protein precipitation solution to each of the samples and mix by vortex for 20 s.
7. Chill the samples on ice for 5 min.
8. Centrifuge the samples for 4 min at 13,000*g* (full speed in Eppendorf centrifuge) at room temperature (*see* **Note 9**).
9. Transfer the supernatant to a fresh 1.5-mL Eppendorf.
10. Add 600 μL of room-temperature isopropanol and mix by inversion (*see* **Note 10**).
11. Centrifuge the sample for 2 min at 13,000*g* at room temperature.
12. Carefully decant the supernatant and ensure that there is a white pellet visible and it is not disturbed.
13. Wash the DNA pellet by adding 1 mL of 70% ethanol.
14. Centrifuge the sample for 1 min at 13,000*g* at room temperature.
15. Carefully remove the supernatant by pipet and invert the tube on a piece of absorbent paper. DNA pellet and then store the samples in a 4°C fridge overnight.

3.3.2. Quantification of Genomic DNA

1. Allow the spectrophotometer to self-calibrate.
2. Blank-correct by adding 1 mL of sterile water to a clean quartz cuvet and insert it into the main reading holder.
3. Replace the cuvet in the main reading holder. The absorbance reading should be zero.
4. Empty the cuvet and wash thoroughly with distilled water.
5. Add 995 μL of sterile water to the cuvet.
6. Add 5 μL of sample DNA to the cuvet and mix well by inversion (cover the cuvet opening with parafilm and mix). This reading will give a reading for the 1/200 dilution factor for the DNA.
7. Insert the cuvet into the main reading holder and press Run.

8. Record the OD_{260} concentration value given on the machine.
9. To obtain the 260/280 ratio value, press the down arrow key (*see* **Note 11**).
10. Add a further 5 μL of the sample DNA to the cuvet (mix as before) and repeat as before. This value will give a reading for the 1/100 dilution factor for the DNA.
11. Empty the contents and wash the cuvet with distilled water and repeat the procedure for each sample.
12. Make DNA stocks of 20 ng/μL.

3.3.3. Polymorphic Fluorescent Microsatellite Markers

Polymorphic microsatellite markers are synthesized with a fluorescent molecule (either TET, FAM, and HEX available from ABI) at the 5' end of the forward primer. Microsatellite markers of a similar size are synthesized with different color fluorophores. This allows greatest flexibility when considering pooling strategies (*see* **Subheading 3.3.5.**).

3.3.4. Polymerase Chain Reaction

1. Prepare deep-well plate of 20 ng/μL DNA stock: Add the calculated volume of DNA to a sterile deep-well plate and make the volume up to a total of 500 μL with sterile water. This will provide the template DNA for future PCR procedures.
2. Label thermo-fast 96-well plates with the appropriate primer used for PCR and date.
3. Transfer 5 μL of the previously prepared 20-ng/μL DNA template with a multichannel pipet.
4. Prepare a PCR master mix (*see* **Note 12**). Per sample:
   a. 2.0 μL 10X Hotstar *Taq* buffer.
   b. 4.0 μL dNTPs (1-m*M* stock).
   c. 0.5 μL each of forward and reverse primer (20 pmol/μL stock).
   d. 6.96 μL sterile water.
   e. 0.04 μL Hotstar *Taq* enzyme (*see* **Note 13**).
5. Add 15 μL of the prepared master mix to the samples in each well.
6. Firmly place an adhesive cover on the prepared PCR plate and seal tightly.
7. Place the plate in a PCR machine and tighten the lid (*see* **Note 14**).
8. Standard themocycler PCR conditions:
   a. 95°C for 15 min (1X).
   b. 95°C for 1 min.
   c. 55°C 1 min.
   d. 72°C for 2 min (35X).

3.3.5. PCR Pooling

Pooling of PCR products before loading samples on to the acrylamide gel reduces the number of lanes required for genotyping and is a key step for high-throughput genotyping. Pooling involves mixing between 5 and 10 PCR amplicons from a number of microsatellite amplification reactions into a single tube. Dilutions of this pooled mixture are then loaded onto the acrylamide gel. The only requirement is that microsatellite markers with similar PCR product sizes are either synthesized with different fluorophores or placed in different pools.

3.3.6. Casting Polyacrylamide Gels for the ABI Prism 377XL

1. To a 100-mL beaker add: 18.0 g of urea, 5.0 mL of Long Ranger 50% stock gel solution, 0.5 g (approx) Bod-Rad AG 501-X8 (D) resin, a stirrer bar, and deionized water up to approx 45 mL. Leave the gel solution to stir for 15 min.
2. Set the cassette on a flat surface with the laser shutter, and therefore the bottom of the gel, closest to you and place the back plate into the cassette so that the etched writing is on the bottom surface (back-to-front as you look at it). Take care to avoid touching the bottom 3 in of the plate, as this is the read region. Pull the plate toward you until it rests on the metal pins.
3. Position the spacers so that the cutouts are at the top of the gel and facing inward.
4. Position the front plate on top of the spacers with the straight edge at the bottom of the gel cassette.
5. Verify that the plates and spacers are aligned and that the cassette is square and then secure all but the bottom and top clips on each side of the cassette.
6. Position the clear plastic top clamp at the top of the plates and clip it into place.
7. Take the gel injection device, pull the black handles up, and position it on the bottom of the gel plates. Push the handles down, thus pulling the gel injector onto the bottom of the plates. Twist the bottom clips on the cassette so that they fit over the gel injector.
8. Take the assembled cassette through to the sequencer along with the comb.
9. Pour the gel solution into a clean 50-mL measuring cylinder and make up the volume to 45 mL with deionized water. Pour it back into the beaker and take the beaker, 10X TBE, P5000 with tip, and the Whatman filters through to the filter unit.
10. Assemble the filter unit with a cellulose filter in place. The filters are packed with the filtration surface uppermost. Connect to the water pump and turn on the water. Check that water is not flashing back into the filter unit!
11. Pipet 5 mL of 10X TBE into the filter, allow this to go through, and then add the gel solution. Once the gel solution has been added, screw the lid onto the unit and stand it on the shelf next to the dH$_2$O still. Leave to degas.
12. Make up at least 260 μL of 10% w/v APS.
13. Pour the degassed gel solution back into the beaker, and rinse the filter unit. Add 250 μL of 10% APS, 25 μL TEMED, and stir carefully with a 60-mL syringe. Draw the solution into the syringe, screw the syringe into the gel injection device, and push the solution into the plates, tapping them to maintain a smooth interface as you do.
14. Any bubbles greater than 2 cm from the spacers will affect the loading of samples. These should be removed using a bubble catcher.

15. Wet the comb with gel solution and push it into the top of the plates. Check that no bubbles have been caught and clamp together with three bulldog clips.
16. Leave the gel for at least 1 h to polymerize.

3.3.7. Washing Gel Plates

1. Lay the cassette flat, and unclip the top buffer tank and plates from the cassette. Wash the cassette.
2. Use a plastic wedge to split the plates and remove the gel by laying a sheet of tissue on the plate and lifting it off (*see* **Note 15**).
3. Wash all components with hot tap water only (*see* **Note 16**), using the sponge and plastic tray under the bench. Plates should only be washed in the plastic tray.
4. Rinse all components with distilled water and leave to dry on tissue or in the rack. Stand the plates upside down so that all residual water runs away from the read region.

3.3.8. Genotyping

An ABI 377 DNA sequencer is used with appropriate Genotyper software to identify DNA fragments of differing sizes with laser signals. Polyacrylamide gels are run and software facilitates semiautomated calling of genotypes.

4. Notes

1. Hotstar enzyme is required to avoid spurious priming and extension events at low temperature.
2. Use powder-free gloves for this procedure to minimize fluorescent contamination.
3. To ensure the correct origin of the Y chromosome in the fixed congenic strain, male F1 hybrids having a SHRSP father should be backcrossed to SHRSP recipient strain females, and likewise male F1 hybrids having a WKY father should be backcrossed to WKY recipient strain females.
4. To reduce costs and minimize rat numbers, all females generated by backcrossing can be culled at weaning.
5. Using multiple breeding pairs or trios can increase the speed of identification of suitable backcross F1 males. However, space limitations and cost of maintenance must be considered.
6. Computer simulations have indicated that a relatively modest selection effort (60 background markers, 25-cM marker spacing, 16 males per generation) would typically reduce unlinked donor genome contamination to <1% by four backcross generations (*21,22*).
7. Do not remove any more than 4 mm, as this can affect DNA yields and quality.
8. Alternatively, incubation may be done for 3 h at 55°C with hourly vortex.
9. The white tight pellet will contain the precipitated protein. If no pellet is seen at this stage, then the sample was not cooled to room temperature before the addition of the protein precipitation solution. As a solution, cool the sample to room temperature, vortex for 20 s briefly, spin again, and proceed as normal.

10. At this stage, white thread-like DNA strands should be visible.
11. The ratio value given on the spectrophotometer gives an indication of the quality of the DNA extracted. The normal value for quality DNA is 1:800.
12. The PCR preparation should be done on ice. Once the dNTPs have been defrosted, use and discard the remainder. Repeated freeze–thawing of dNTPs is not good for successful PCR.
13. We use a hot-start enzyme that reduces the number of stutter peaks, aiding accurate genotyping. This is one-tenth the recommended amount of *Taq* polymerase, but in our hands this is sufficient for successful PCR, while keeping costs down.
14. The PCR reaction is mineral oil-free. To ensure the PCR sample does not evaporate, the hot lid must be tightened firmly.
15. Do not pull the spacers out before splitting the plates, as this tears them; and do not twist the wedge to split the plates, just push it in until the plates split.
16. Wash plates with hot water only; never use any detergent, as this increases background fluorescence.

References

1. McBride, M. W., Charchar, F. J., Graham, D., et al. (2004) Functional genomics in rodent models of hypertension. *J. Physiol.* **554,** 56–63.
2. Yamori, Y., Mori, C., Nishio, T., et al. (1979) Cardiac hypertrophy in early hypertension. *Am. J. Cardiol.* **44,** 964–969.
3. Conrad, C. H., Brooks, W. W., Robinson, K. G., Bing, O. H. (1991) Impaired myocardial function in spontaneously hypertensive rats with heart failure. *Am. J. Physiol.* **260,** H136–H145.
4. Jeffs, B., Clark, J. S., Anderson, N., et al. (1997) Sensitivity to cerebral ischemic insult in a rat model of stroke is determined by a single genetic locus. *Nat. Genet.* **16,** 364–367.
5. Lindsey, J. R. (1979) In *The Laboratory Rat. Biology and Diseases* (Barker, H. J., Lindsey, J. R., eds.), Academic, New York, Historical foundations, pp. 1–36.
6. Rapp, J. P. (2000) Genetic analysis of inherited hypertension in the rat. *Physiol. Rev.* **80,** 135–172.
7. Kwitek-Black, A. E. and Jacob, H. J. (2001) The use of designer rats in the genetic dissection of hypertension. *Curr. Hypertens. Rep.* **3,** 12–18.
8. Dominiczak, A. F., Clark, J. S., Jeffs, B., et al. (1998) Genetics of experimental hypertension. *J. Hypertens.* **16,** 1859–1869.
9. Garrett, M. R. and Rapp, J. P. (2002) Multiple blood pressure QTLs on rat chromosome 2 defined by congenic Dahl rats. *Mammal. Genome* **13,** 41–44.
10. Nadeau, J. H., Singer, J. B., Matin, A., and Lander, E. S. (2000) Analysing complex genetic traits with chromosome substitution strains. *Nat. Genet.* **24,** 221–225.
11. Negrin, C. D., McBride, M. W., Carswell, H. V. O., et al. (2001) Reciprocal consomic strains to evaluate Y chromosome effects. *Hypertension* **37,** 391–397.
12. Ely, D. L., Daneshvar, H., Turner, M. E., Johnson, M. L., and Salisbury, R. L.

(1993) The hypertensive Y chromosome elevates blood pressure in F11 normotensive rats. *Hypertension* **21,** 1071–1075.

13. Charchar, F. J., Tomaszewski, M., Strahorn, P., Champagne, B., and Dominiczak, A. F. (2003) Y is there a risk being male? *Trends Endocrinol. Metab.* **14,** 163–168.

14. Cowley, A. W. (2003) Genomics and homeostasis. *Am. J. Physiol. Regul. Integr. Comp. Physiol.* **284,** R611–R627.

15. Garett, M. R. and Rapp, J. P. (2003) Defining the blood pressure QTL on chromosome 7 in Dahl rats by a 177kb congenic segment containing Cyb11b1. *Mammal. Genome* **14,** 268–273.

16. Meng, H., Garrett, M. R., Dene, H., and Rapp, J. P. (2003) Localisation of a blood pressure QTL to a 2.4 cM interval on rat chromosome 9 using congenic strains. *Genomics* **81,** 210–220.

17. Frantz, S. A., Kaiser, M., Gardiner, S., et al. (1998) Successful isolation of a rat chromosome 1 blood pressure QTL in reciprocal congenic strain. *Hypertens.* **32,** 639–646.

18. Morel, L., Yu, Y., Blenman, K. R., Caldwell, R. A. and Wakeland, E. K. (1996) Production of congenic mouse strains carrying genomic intervals containing SLE-susceptibility genes derived from the SLE-prone NZM2410 strain. *Mammal. Genome* **7,** 335–339.

19. Jeffs, B., Negrin, C. D., Graham, D., et al. (2000) Applicability of a speed congenic strategy to dissect blood pressure QTL on rat chromosome 2. *Hypertens.* **35,** 179–187.

20. Lander, E. S. and Schork, N. J. (1994) Genetic dissection of complex traits. *Science* **265,** 2037–2048.

21. Wakeland, E., Morel, L., Achey, K., Yui, M., and Longmate, J. (1997) Speed congenics: a classic technique in the fast lane (relatively speaking). *Immunol. Today* **18,** 472–477.

22. Markel, P., Shu, P., Ebeling, C., et al. (1997) Theoretical and empirical issues for marker-assisted breeding of congenic mouse strains. *Nat. Genet.* **17,** 280–284.

2

Mouse Knockout Models of Hypertension

Michael Bader

Summary

Gene-targeting technology allows the planned alteration of any gene in the mouse genome and has been very successfully employed to study the function of numerous gene products in a complete animal. The method includes the design of a suitable targeting construct, its transfection into pluripotential embryonic stem cells, selection for cells in which one allele of the endogenous gene has been exchanged for the construct by homologous recombination, and the transfer of these cells into host blastocysts. The blastocysts are then transferred into the uterus of a pseudopregnant foster mother giving birth to chimeras, which are bred to yield heterozygous and finally homozygous mutant mice for the targeted gene.

Key Words: Embryonic stem cells; homologous recombination; gene targeting; knockout mouse; electroporation; double selection; gancyclovir; functional genomics; Chimera; pseudopregnancy.

1. Introduction

The genomes of humans and mice have been completely sequenced and about 30,000 genes have been detected in both organisms *(1–3)*. The challenge is now to elucidate the function of all these genes. The most powerful way to perform such "functional genomics" is gene targeting, allowing the targeted overexpression, deletion, or mutation of a gene product in a mouse and thereby studying its function in the context of all other unaffected genes. During the 15 yr in which this technology has been available, several thousand genes have been knocked out, i.e., they have been functionally ablated by gene targeting. Among these are numerous genes important for blood pressure regulation and the pathogenesis of hypertension (for review, *see* **refs**. *4* and *5)*. More than 80% of all genes remain to be characterized by this technology.

Besides the complete ablation of a gene, gene targeting also allows the introduction of subtle mutations into a gene and the conditional, i.e., tissue- or time-dependent knockout of a gene. The technologies developed for these pur-

From: *Methods in Molecular Medicine, Vol. 108: Hypertension: Methods and Protocols*
Edited by: J. P. Fennell and A. H. Baker © Humana Press Inc., Totowa, NJ

poses will not be described in this chapter. The reader is referred to recent reviews in this field *(6–8)*. This chapter will focus on the classical knockout technique, allowing the complete ablation of a gene.

Gene targeting technique is based on two lines of research that were developed in the early 1980s and converged a few years later *(9)*. At this time, Martin Evans had developed cell lines from the inner cell mass of mouse blastocysts that were immortal and pluripotent, i.e., they could differentiate into all tissues of a developing embryo in vitro and gave rise to teratocarcinomas when injected into adult mice. Moreover, when these so-called embryonic stem (ES) cells were introduced into recipient blastocysts, they took part in embryonic development and a chimeric mouse was born, in which ES cells had populated all tissues including the germline. Consequently, in the offspring of these mice, one haploid genome of some animals was entirely derived from the ES cells. Thus, genetic alterations in ES cells could be transferred into the genome of a living animal after two mouse generations.

In parallel, the groups of Oliver Smithies and Mario Capecchi had independently developed systems to introduce mutations in genes in cultured cells by exploiting the phenomenon of homologous recombination. Cells use this process during meiosis to exchange genetic material between homologous chromosomes. For this, the two homologous chromosomes recognize each other by a not yet fully understood process and align. Then, pieces of homologous DNA are exchanged between the chromosomes by double crossover of the DNA strands. Capecchi and Smithies found that they only had to introduce several kilobases of chromosomal DNA into cells to allow this process to happen. These relatively short DNA fragments also aligned with their homologous region on the cellular chromosome, and by double crossover parts in the center of the homology region on the introduced DNA could be exchanged and ended up in the chromosome. Thus, they could freely decide how to change a gene of interest by putting a mutation into the central part of the homology region and letting the homologous recombination machinery introduce this mutation into the chromosome. However, there was a major drawback. This process was very inefficient: it occurred in only about one of 1000 transfected cells. Thus, it was not practicable, although not impossible *(10)*, to use classical transgenic technology, i.e., the microinjection of such DNA constructs into fertilized oocytes (*see* Chapter 3) in order to introduce targeted mutations into the mouse genome.

But the ES cells just described by Martin Evans opened up a way to do this with relative ease, because they allowed a selection step, in which millions of cells were used as starting material and after which a few survivors carried the intended genetic alteration. These surviving clones could then be used to inject

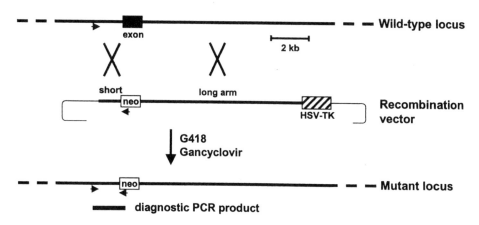

Fig. 1. Gene targeting by double selection technique. Two fragments of the gene of interest (thick lines) are cloned into a plasmid vector (thin lines) together with a neomycin resistance (neo) and a Herpes simplex virus thymidine kinase gene (HSV-TK). The linearized construct is transfected into ES cells and the cells are selected by G418 (a neomycin analog) and Gancyclovir (which kills HSV-TK expressing cells). Cells that have inserted the construct in their genome by homologous recombination have lost the *TK* gene and survive double selection.

blastocysts and to develop mice carrying the targeted mutation in all cells of the body via an intermediate chimeric step. The double-selection technique developed by Capecchi *(11)* is still the most widely used method for gene targeting, and its principle will therefore be described below.

The targeting constructs contain a neomycin resistance (neo) gene in the center of the homology region and a Herpes simplex virus (HSV) thymidine kinase (TK) gene outside of this region (**Fig. 1**). The constructs are introduced into ES cells by electroporation. Most of the cells that take up the foreign DNA insert it randomly into their genome as in classical transgenic technology. In this case, the TK gene enters a chromosome and remains in the genome of the cell. In very few cells, homologous recombination happens and the neo gene is integrated into the gene of interest, but the TK gene gets lost in this process. Thus, correctly targeted ES cells survive the following double selection with neomycin (or G418) and gancyclovir, which is phosphorylated by HSV-TK in cells and used for DNA and RNA synthesis leading to chain termination and death of TK-expressing cells. In contrast, cells with random transgene integration express the TK gene and are sensitive to gancyclovir, and cells that remained untransfected also die under double selection, since they lack the neo gene. Thus, the only survivors are ES cells that carry the intended genotype, at least in theory. In practice, sometimes more than 90% of the surviving clones show random integration of the targeting construct, because of the fact that the TK gene can also be inactivated during random insertion into the genome by partial deletion, mutation, or by the silencing influence of neighboring DNA regions. Nevertheless, the efficiency is high enough to find clones with relative ease in which homologous recombination has occurred and which, therefore, carry the intended genetic alteration. Such clones are identified either by Southern blot detecting DNA fragments specific for the targeted locus, or more conveniently by polymerase chain reaction (PCR). To allow the efficient use of such a diagnostic PCR, the targeting constructs are mostly not symmetrically designed, i.e., the two fragments of homologous DNA flanking the neo gene are of different lengths. One "arm" is short (max 1000 bp) and the other arm is long (min 4 kb) (**Fig. 1**). For the diagnostic PCR, one primer is designed in the region on the gene of interest immediately upstream of the short arm but outside of the homology region on the targeting construct and another one on the neo gene. They are only able to give rise to a PCR fragment when their binding sites are brought close together during homologous recombination.

The positively identified clones are then used to generate gene-targeted mice by blastocyst injection and breeding of the resulting chimera (**Fig. 2**). In the majority of cases the experiment is still not finished when the first animals with the targeted mutation are born from the chimera, because they are mutated on only one allele. In these heterozygous mutants the intact allele is mostly dominant and the phenotype of the mutation is not obvious. Thus, these animals have to be bred, and after another mouse generation, homozygous "knockout" animals are born, which carry the targeted mutation on both homologous chromosomes and therefore exhibit the phenotype of the genetic ablation. Although this is not the subject of this chapter, the work needed to detect and describe this phenotype should not be underestimated. It mostly surpasses the time needed to generate the animal model and needs elaborate embryological and/or physiological methodology.

One major drawback of the gene targeting technology is its availability only for the mouse, whereas the rat would be the preferred animal model for cardiovascular research. This limitation is due to the lack of germline-competent ES cells for any other species besides the mouse. All attempts to establish such cells for rats have been unsuccessful (*12–14*). Furthermore, nuclear transfer technology, which allows generation of germline mutations in animals other than mice (*15,16*) has not yet been established in the rat (*17*). Only recently, random mutagenesis using ethylnitrosurea (ENU) followed by a facilitated yeast-based screen for mutations in a gene of interest has allowed for the first time the ablation of a specific gene in the rat (*18*). However, this technology requires the screening of hundreds of rats and creates animals with multiple

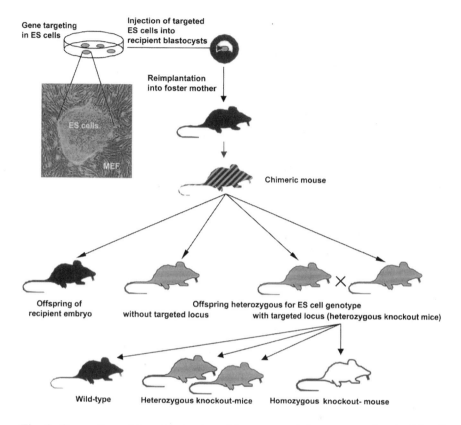

Fig. 2. Generation of knockout mice. After successful gene targeting in ES cells, which grow as three-dimensional clumps on mouse embryo fibroblasts (MEFs), the cells are injected into a host blastocyst, which is then transferred into the uterus of a pseudopregnant foster mother. The resulting chimeras are bred and, if the cells have populated the germline, give heterozygous knockout offspring. Interbreeding of those mice yields homozygous knockout mice.

additional mutations in the genome, with unpredictable influences on the phenotype. Antisense RNA *(19)* and recently also RNA interference *(20)* in combination with classical transgenic technology, has been employed successfully to blunt expression of genes in rats, but the general applicability of these methods is questionable. Thus, there is still the need to establish gene targeting technology in the preferred animal model for hypertension research, the rat.

2. Materials

2.1. Equipment

1. Tissue culture hood.

2. Tissue culture incubator at 37°C with 5% CO_2 and saturated-water atmosphere.
3. Inverted microscope, fitting into the tissue culture hood.
4. Inverted microscope with Nomarski optic, 10X and 40X objectives, and two micromanipulators on a vibration-free table.
5. Binocular microscope.
6. Pipet puller.
7. Microforge.
8. Electroporator.
9. Liquid nitrogen container.

2.2. Plastic Ware

1. Polystyrene tissue culture dishes: 10 cm (10 mL), 6 cm (4 mL), 12 well (each 2 mL), 24 well (each 1.5 mL), 96 well (each 0.5 mL).
2. Plastic centrifuge tubes: 50 mL, 15 mL.
3. Cryotubes: 2 mL.
4. Plastic pipets: 1 mL, 5 mL, 10 mL, 25 mL.
5. Electroporation cuvets: 0.4 cm.

2.3. Reagents and Solutions

1. 10X phosphate-buffered saline (PBS): 1.37 M NaCl, 26.8 mM KCl, 80.6 mM $Na_2HPO_4 \cdot 7H_2O$, 14.7 mM $KH_2PO_4 \cdot 2H_2O$, pH. 7.4 (store at 4°C).
2. Dulbecco's Modified Eagles Medium (DMEM) with high glucose (4.5 g/L), without sodium pyruvate (store at 4°C, replace after 3 wk, prewarm before use).
3. Fetal calf serum (FCS), ES-cell tested (store at –20°C, heat-inactivate the complement system at 56°C for 30 min before use) (*see* **Note 1**).
4. 100X Pen/Strep (50 U/mL penicillin, 50 U/mL streptomycin) (store at –20°C).
5. 100X L-Glutamine (200 mM) (store at –20°C).
6. 100X MEM nonessential amino acids (store at –20°C).
7. Leukemia-inhibiting factor (LIF, Esgro) (store at –20°C).
8. 100X β-Mercaptoethanol: 7 μL β-mercaptoethanol in 10 mL PBS (10 mM; prepare fresh).
9. Medium for mouse embryo fibroblasts (MEF) (store at 4°C, prewarm before use): DMEM, 10% FCS, 1X Pen/Strep, 1X glutamine.
10. Medium for ES cells (store at 4°C, prewarm before use): DMEM, 15% FCS, 1X Pen/Strep, 1X glutamine, 1X MEM nonessential amino acids, 1X β-mercaptoethanol, 10^3 U/mL LIF.
11. Freezing medium (store at 4°C): 40% DMEM, 50% FCS, 10% dimethyl sulfoxide (DMSO).
12. M16 and M2 medium (store at 4°C): M2 and M16 are media optimized for the culture of preimplantation embryos (commercially available, e.g., from Sigma). M16 is not suitable for long-term handling outside the CO_2 incubator because its pH is kept stable by 5% CO_2 in the atmosphere. M2 medium has a stable pH because of HEPES buffer.
13. Gelatine solution: 0.1% in 1X PBS (store at 4°C).

Table 1
Compositions of M16 and M2

Compound	M2	M16
NaCl	94.66 mM	94.66 mM
KCl	4.78 mM	4.78 mM
KH_2PO_4	1.19 mM	1.19 mM
$MgSO_4$	1.19 mM	1.19 mM
Na lactate	23.28 mM	23.28 mM
Glucose	5.56 mM	5.56 mM
$NaHCO_3$	4.15 mM	25.0 mM
Na pyruvate	0.33 mM	0.33 mM
$CaCl_2$	1.71 mM	1.71 mM
HEPES, pH 7.4	20.0 mM	—
Phenol red	1 mg/mL	1 mg/mL
BSA (Bovine Serum Albumin)	4 mg/mL	4 mg/mL

14. Capecchi buffer: 20 mM HEPES-Na, 137 mM NaCl, 5 mM KCl, 0.7 mM Na_2HPO_4, 6 mM glucose, 0.1 mM β-mercaptoethanol.
15. Trypsin/EDTA: 0.05% trypsin, 0.02% EDTA (store at 4°C for up to 2 wk).
16. Mitomycin solution: 1 mg/mL mitomycin C in 1X PBS (store at –20°C).
17. G418 (Geneticin) solution 100 mg/mL in H_2O (store at –20°C).
18. Gancyclovir (Cytovene, Syntex) solution: 200 μM in H_2O (store at –20°C).
19. Proteinase K solution: 10 mg/mL in H_2O (store at –20°C).
20. DNAse I solution: 10 mg/mL in H_2O (store at –20°C).
21. Anesthetic solution: 10% (v/v) ketamine, 0.02 % (v/v) xylazine, 0.9% (w/v) NaCl in H_2O (prepare fresh before use).

2.4. Animals

Male and female (21–23 d old) mice of the C57Bl/6 strain are necessary to get blastocysts, and females as well as vasectomized males of the outbred NMRI strain or F1 hybrids (e.g., C57Bl/6 X DBA) are used to generate foster mothers. All these strains are available from commercial breeders.

3. Methods

3.1. Design and Generation of Targeting Construct

3.1.1. Selection of Targeting Region

The first question that has to be addressed before a gene targeting experiment can be started is which part of the gene of interest should be affected. If functional deletion of the gene is intended, the functionally most important part of the gene should be selected. In rare cases, the decision is easy because the whole coding region of the gene resides on one exon, such as for most G protein-coupled receptors. However, in the majority of cases, genes comprise several exons and cover tens of kilobases of genomic DNA. Consequently, the researcher has to decide which exons should be deleted in order to inactivate the gene. For enzymes, exons coding for the active site might be selected, for receptors or transcription factors the ligand or the DNA-binding domains, respectively, might be targeted. Alternatively, one of the first exons of a gene may be deleted. Insertion of the neo cassette should lead to missplicing and thereby to a nonfunctional mRNA. In addition, most neo cassettes, if cloned in the same orientation as the arms, contain a transcriptional stop signal ([poly(A) site]) that should not only stop transcription from the promoter driving the neo gene but also target gene transcription (*see* **Note 2**). This strategy may fail if transcriptional read-through and alternative splicing of the gene leads to mRNAs with partial or even complete restoration of a functional protein coding sequence *(21)*. If possible, one of the first coding exons should therefore be selected, the length of which in base pairs cannot be divisible by three. Even if alternative splicing would lead to the restoration of a near-full-length mRNA, the coding frame would be shifted and no functional protein would be generated. The length of the deleted region ideally should be about 1 kb because the neo gene, which is inserted at this site by the targeting procedure, would then restore the length of the genomic region. However, deletions from a few bases up to several kilobases have also been achieved *(22)*.

3.1.2. Cloning of Genomic DNA Fragments

When the target region of the gene is selected, the next step is to clone the flanking genomic fragments necessary for the targeting construct. There are two options to do this. Classically, large DNA fragments are isolated from mouse genomic libraries, characterized by restriction mapping, and subfragments are cloned into the targeting vector. More flexible and convenient is the generation of the fragments by long-range PCR using commercially available kits from total genomic DNA. The completeness of the mouse genomic sequence in Genbank *(3)* allows the design of gene-specific primers, thereby determining the exact length and borders of the fragments and to include suitable restriction sites for the following cloning steps (*see* **Notes 3 and 4**). Two fragments flanking the region to be targeted need to be cloned or amplified by PCR; one should be short (around 1000 bp) and one should be long (4–10 kb) (**Fig. 1**). Thereby, the efficiency of homologous recombination increases with the size of the total homology region *(23,24)*. On the other hand, the efficiency of the long-range PCR decreases with the length of the amplified product, and the cloning of the long arm becomes more difficult the longer the fragments get. Therefore, a short arm of about 1 kb and a long arm of about 5 kb can be envisaged as suitable.

3.1.3. Cloning of Targeting Vector

These two arms are cloned into the targeting vector in the same orientation flanking a neomycin-resistance gene. The neo gene replaces the missing region of the target gene between the two arms. At the other end of the long arm the TK gene is inserted. Most laboratories generating knockout mice have basic targeting vectors with both selectable marker genes flanked by suitable multiple cloning sites. One essential feature of these vectors is that the expression of both marker genes is controlled by promoters active in undifferentiated ES cells, such as the HSV-TK promoter or the promoter for phosphoglycerokinase (PGK). When the construct is planned, it has to be ensured that the complete targeting vector can still be linearized by a restriction enzyme either at the beginning of the short arm or somewhere in the plasmid portion, because linear DNA has to be inserted into the ES cells for successful homologous recombination to take place. Linearization close to the TK gene is not recommended because it leads to an increased chance of mutation of this gene during random insertion and, thus, an augmentation of false clones surviving double selection. For the isolation of the fragments, genomic DNA from ES cells should be used because it has been shown that the targeting efficiency is markedly enhanced for isogenic DNA compared to DNA derived from other mouse strains *(24–26)*. The reasons for this are enigmatic because the exact mechanism of homologous recombination is still a matter of intensive research. A second construct should be prepared in parallel. It contains a longer short arm elongated at its 5' end by 50–200 bp and the neo gene but may lack the long arm and the TK gene. It is used as positive control for the diagnostic PCR to detect ES cell clones with a correctly targeted gene.

3.1.4. Establishment of Diagnostic PCR

The diagnostic PCR to detect correctly targeted ES cell clones must be established before the cells are transfected. The following two primers should be designed: A 5'-primer mapping in the region immediately upstream of the short arm on the gene of interest and the 3'-primer mapping on the neo gene (*see* **Note 5**). Thus, the primers will yield a PCR product only if the neo gene is inserted into the gene of interest by homologous recombination. The PCR is optimized for annealing temperature and magnesium concentration using serial dilutions of the elongated DNA construct mentioned in **Subheading 3.1.3.** (1 fg to 1 ng) together with 100 ng of genomic ES cell DNA. Only if the PCR gives a reproducible signal after 35 cycles down to 10 fg of the test construct, which mimics the situation in targeted ES cells clones, can the PCR be considered as sensitive and reliable enough.

3.2. Culture and Transfection of Embryonic Stem Cells

ES cells are particularly sensitive cells. They have special requirements for optimal growth and easily lose their capacity to contribute to the germline when the culture conditions are not optimal or when they are cultured for too many passages. Thus, experiments with ES cells should be started with cells of an early passage number (around 10) after establishment from blastocysts. The majority of ES cell lines have to be grown on feeder cells, mostly mitotically inactivated mouse embryo fibroblasts (MEFs), and need leukemia-inhibiting factor (LIF) in the medium to stay in the pluripotent state.

MEFs produce this factor, but because the secretion may be variable it should also be added to the medium. Undifferentiated ES cells on MEFs grow as three-dimensional clumps with irregularly round and borders shining brightly in the phase-contrast microscope (**Fig. 2**). Single cells are hardly visible in the clumps. If single cell borders are detectable or if flat cells appear at the edge of the colonies, the cells have started to differentiate and should not be used any more.

3.2.1. Isolation, Culture, and Mitotic Inactivation of MEFs

MEFs should be prepared from neomycin-resistant mice, best from heterozygous or homozygous knockouts regardless of which gene is altered in the animals, except for genes affecting very early embryonic development such as LIF.

1. Breed female and check for vaginal plug in the morning.
2. 13–15 d later, kill female, take uterus, and rinse twice with 1X PBS in 10-cm dishes in the tissue culture hood.
3. Take out embryos and remove head, liver, and heart.
4. Mince the remaining embryonic tissue with a razor blade or scalpel in 3 mL of 1X PBS per embryo.
5. Let tissue fragments precipitate in a 15-mL centrifuge tube at 4°C and remove supernatant.
6. Overlay with 1 mL trypsin/EDTA and leave at 4°C for 12–16 h.
7. Remove supernatant and incubate for 30 min at 37°C.
8. Add 10 mL of MEF medium and disaggregate cell clumps by pipeting with a 10-mL plastic pipet.
9. Distribute cells on one or two 10-cm dishes per embryo, add MEF medium to 10 mL, and put in incubator overnight.
10. The next day, wash cells three times with 1X PBS and add fresh MEF medium.
11. When MEF reach near confluency, remove MEF medium, wash twice with 1X PBS, add 2 mL of trypsin/EDTA solution, incubate at 37°C until cells detach (after about 3 min), add 2 mL of MEF medium to stop trypsin action (because of

trypsin inhibitors in the FCS component), dissociate and transfer the cells with a 10-mL pipet to a 15-mL centrifuge tube, and spin down at 120g for 3 min.

a. Splitting (1:4): Resuspend cell pellet in 4 mL MEF medium and pipet each 1 mL in cell culture dishes with 9 mL MEF. Trypsinization and splitting can be repeated twice before MEFs are used for mitomycin C treatment and ES cell culture.

b. For freezing, resuspend cell pellet in 1 mL of freezing medium, transfer into cryotubes, slowly freeze in a plastic container at –80°C overnight, and put for long-term storage in liquid nitrogen. For thawing, quickly warm up cryotube in 37°C, put contents in 15-mL centrifuge tube with 5 mL MEFs medium, spin down (120g, 3 min), resuspend pellet in 3 mL MEF medium, and transfer each 1 mL into 10-cm cell culture dishes with 9 mL of MEF medium.

12. For mitotic inactivation, remove MEF medium from near-confluent MEF, add 5 mL of MEF medium with 50 µL mitomycin C solution, incubate for 3 h at 37°C, remove medium, wash three times with 1X PBS, Trypsinize or freeze MEFs. Mitomycin C is cross-linked to DNA and thereby inhibits mitosis.

13. After splitting or thawing, count mitomycin-treated MEFs in haemocytometer and plate on gelatinized culture dishes or wells at a density of about 4×10^4 cells/cm^2. For gelatinization, cover bottom of dish or well with gelatine solution and incubate for at least 30 min at 37°C and afterwards wash twice with 1X PBS.

3.2.2. Culture of ES Cells

1. Thaw a vial of ES cells quickly in 37°C, put contents in 15-mL centrifuge tube with 5 mL ES medium, spin down (120g, 3 min), resuspend pellet in 3 mL ES medium, and transfer each into 10-cm cell culture dishes with MEFs 7 mL of ES medium. Change medium next day.

2. After 2–3 d, the cells need to be split. For this, replace medium 2 h before splitting, then remove the medium again, wash twice with 1X PBS, add 2 mL Trypsin/ EDTA solution, incubate at room temperature for 1–3 min, resuspend and dissociate cells with a 2-mL glass Pasteur pipet. Add suspension to 5 mL ES medium in centrifuge tube, spin down at 120g for 3 min, resuspend cell pellet in 2 mL of ES medium, plate on 5 to 10-cm dishes with MEFs and fill up ES medium to 10 mL. Repeat this splitting at least every 48 h.

3. Freezing of ES cells: Instead of replating the cells after trypsinization, transfer them into 15-mL centrifuge tube with 5 mL ES medium, spin down (120g, 3 min), resuspend pellet in 1 mL freezing medium, put in cryotubes, slowly freeze in a plastic container at –80°C overnight, and put for long-term storage in liquid nitrogen.

3.2.3. Transfection of ES Cells and Selection of Gene-Targeted Clones

1. Add fresh medium to a confluent 10-cm dish with ES cells and trypsinize 2–4 h later.

2. Spin down (120g, 3 min) cells and resuspend in Capecchi buffer, count in

hemocytometer.

3. Spin down again and resuspend at 1×10^7 cells in 0.4 mL Capecchi buffer, transfer into electroporation cuvet.

4. Add 20 µg linearized and purified gene-targeting construct in 20–50 µL sterile deionized water and mix with 2-mL plastic pipet.

5. Electroporate the cells at 240 mV and a capacitance of 500 µF, leave at room temperature for 10 min.

6. Add 1.5 mL ES medium to the cuvet, plate cells on three 10-cm dishes with neomycin-resistant MEFs in 10 mL ES medium.

7. 2 d later, change ES medium and start selection with 250 µg/mL G418.

8. 1 d later, change to ES medium with 250 µg/mL G418 and 2 µ*M* gancyclovir and change selection medium daily, because dead cells need to be removed quickly to avoid ES cell differentiation induced by cell debris (*see* **Note 6**).

9. Seven to ten days later, between 50 and several hundred ES cell colonies should be visible on each dish.

10. Prepare 96-well plate with MEFs on gelatine in ES cell medium.

11. Prepare 96-well plate with 50 µL trypsin/EDTA per well and 96 numbered PCR tubes.

12. Replace medium on colonies carefully with 5 mL of 1X PBS and put on microscope under the tissue culture hood.

13. Pick morphologically normal-looking clones with a plastic tip on a 20-µL pipet and transfer each into one well with trypsin/EDTA. To avoid too extended contact of the ES cells with trypsin and EDTA, stop after 12 clones, incubate 96-well plate for 2 min at 37°C, and stop the trypsin action by addition of 150 µL ES cell medium to each well (the serum in the medium contains a trypsin inhibitor). Resuspend cells of each well, put 100 µL of the suspension into the PCR tube with the corresponding number and 100 µL in the corresponding well with MEFs on the other 96-well plate, which is then returned directly to the incubator. Repeat the procedure for the next 12 clones until 96 clones are picked.

14. For DNA isolation and diagnostic PCR, spin down cells in PCR tubes (700*g*, 5 min), remove supernatant, add 20 µL H_2O and vortex. Then heat up to 90°C for 10 min, cool down to 55°C, add 2 µL proteinase K solution, centrifuge briefly and incubate for 55°C for 1 h (or 37°C over night). Finally, inactivate proteinase K at 90°C for 10 min, centrifuge (18,000*g*), transfer 5 µL of supernatant into a fresh PCR tube, and run a diagnostic PCR to detect correct targeting (*see* **Note 7**).

3.2.4. Generation and Breeding of Chimeras

1. For blastocyst isolation, 21–23 d old female C57Bl/6 mice are superovulated by injection at noon with five IU PMSG (pregnant mare's serum gonadotropin) and 46 h later with five IU hCG (human chorionic gonadotropin). They are then mated and the following morning the mice are checked for vaginal plugs.

2. 3 d later (3.5 d postcoitum), the mice are killed by cervical dislocation, the uterus is isolated, freed of fat tissue, and put into a Petri dish with 1X PBS. The two uterine horns are cut at the cervix and transferred into a dry 10-cm dish. After

ligation at the ovary side with forceps, 0.3 mL of M2 medium is flushed through each horn from the ovary side using a syringe with a G27 needle. Blastocysts are collected with a mouth pipet under a binocular microscope, transferred into M16 medium, and stored in a tissue culture incubator until use.

3. Micropipets are prepared from 1.5-mm borosilicate glass capillaries using a capillary puller, a microforge and a micropipet grinder (*see* **Note 8**). The holding pipet should have an inner diameter of 20–30 μm and an outer diameter of 100–150 μm and its tip should be smoothened by melting in the microforge. The injection capillary should have an outer diameter of 15–20 μm and an inner diameter slightly larger than the size of an ES cell. At the tip of the injection capillary a 45° bevel and a protruding needle should be generated by the use of the micropipet grinder and the microforge, respectively. Both pipets should be bent in the microforge to allow parallel movement of the tip relative to the surface of the injection chamber. The pipet is coated with 10% polyvinylpyrrolidone (PVP) in M2 medium immediately before use.

4. Pipet 200–500 ES cells into 30 μL of M2 medium covered with mineral oil on the bottom of the injection chamber on the inverted microscope with the micromanipulators. Add 20–30 blastocysts with the mouth pipet. Catch one blastocyst with the holding pipet and fix it with the inner cell mass near the opening of the holding pipet. Load 12–15 ES cells into the injection pipet and inject them into the cavity of the blastocyst (*see* **Note 9**). After removal of the pipet, the blastocyst will collapse. After injection, which should not take more than 30 min, transfer blastocysts into fresh M16 medium and incubate for 1–2 h in the tissue culture incubator.

5. For uterus transfer of blastocysts, induce pseudopregnancy in a female by mating with vasectomized male and check next morning for vaginal plug. Mostly, outbred (e.g., NMRI) or F1 hybrid (e.g., C57Bl/6XDBA) females are used as recipients. Two days later (d 2.5 postcoitum), anesthetize female by intraperitoneal injection of 17 μL per gram of body weight of anesthetic solution. Make an incision of 0.8 cm on the back on one side of the spine below the ribs, grasp the fat pad attached to the uterus with forceps and take out the uterus. Make a small hole into the uterus near the oviduct with a G27 needle. Load the mouth pipet with an air bubble followed by 15 blastocysts, and flush the blastocysts through the hole into the uterine lumen until the air bubble has reached the tip of the pipet; avoid releasing the air bubble into the uterus. Let the uterus slide back and close the wound with clips. Repeat on the other side.

6. Seventeen days later pups are born and, when the fur is visible a few days later, the degree of chimerism is deducible from the coat color. Because most ES cell lines have a male karyotype, male chimeras with high coat color chimerism have the highest chance of producing ES-cell-derived offspring, recognized by the pure agouti coat color. Fifty percent of these mice are heterozygous, i.e., they carry the mutation in one allele of the targeted gene. According to Mendel's laws, breeding of these mice will generate 25% homozygous knockout mice, with the mutation in both alleles recognized by PCR or Southern blot, which detects the

absence of the target region. If the offspring contains less than the expected 25% homozygous mice, prenatal or perinatal lethality must be assumed and an embryonic phenotype of the genetic alteration should be considered.

4. Notes

1. Different batches of FCS should be tested for plating efficiency and toxicity before use by plating 1000 ES cells in 6-cm dishes with MEF and LIF and both 10% and 30% FCS. After 7 d, count colonies and check for differentiation. There should be no less colonies with 30% FCS than with 10% FCS, and the colonies should look undifferentiated.
2. If the neo gene is inserted in the opposite orientation to the arms of the gene of interest in the targeting construct, it may completely inhibit target gene expression by a yet enigmatic mechanism *(27)*.
3. Avoid long stretches of repetitive DNA in the arms.
4. The generation of the homology regions by long-range PCR is suitable only for gene ablation experiments. If conditional gene targeting is intended, mutations induced by the thermostable polymerases, particularly in exons, may render the PCR products useless.
5. Sometimes several primer pairs have to be tested for the diagnostic PCR.
6. If medium becomes yellow, change it up to twice daily.
7. Before microinjection of positive clones, verify the correct genotype by Southern blot.
8. Alternatively, quite suitable pipets can be purchased from commercial suppliers
9. When the pipet is clogged, flush it with mineral oil and recoat with PVP solution.

Acknowledgments

The author would like to thank Vanessa Merino, Natasha Alenina, Cibele Campos Cardoso, Cécile Cayla, Tanja Schmidt, and Claudia Wilhelm for helpful discussions.

References

1. Venter, J. C., Adams, M. D., Myers, E. W., et al. (2001) The sequence of the human genome. *Science* **291,** 1304–1351.
2. Lander, E. S., Linton, L. M., Birren, B., et al. (2001) Initial sequencing and analysis of the human genome. *Nature* **409,** 860–921.
3. Waterston, R. H., Lindblad-Toh, K., Birney, E., et al. (2002) Initial sequencing and comparative analysis of the mouse genome. *Nature* **420,** 520–562.
4. Bader, M., Bohnemeier, H., Zollmann, F. S., Lockley-Jones, O. E., and Ganten, D. (2000) Transgenic animals in cardiovascular disease research. *Exp. Physiol.* **85,** 713–731.
5. Cvetkovic, B. and Sigmund, C. D. (2000) Understanding hypertension through genetic manipulation in mice. *Kidney Int.* **57,** 863–874.
6. Rajewsky, K., Gu, H., Kühn, R., et al. (1996) Conditional gene targeting. *J. Clin. Invest.* **98,** 600–603.

7. Lewandoski, M. (2001) Conditional control of gene expression in the mouse. *Nat. Rev. Genet.* **2,** 743–755.
8. Gossen, M. and Bujard, H. (2002) Studying gene function in eukaryotes by conditional gene inactivation. *Annu. Rev. Genet.* **36,** 153–173.
9. Evans, M. J., Smithies, O., and Capecchi, M. (2001) Mouse gene targeting. *Nat. Med.* **7,** 1081–1090.
10. Brinster, R. L., Braun, R. E., Lo, D., Avarbock, M. R., Oram, F., and Palmiter, R. D. (1989) Targeted correction of a major histocompatibility class II E alpha gene by DNA microinjected into mouse eggs. *Proc. Natl. Acad. Sci. USA* **86,** 7 087–7091.
11. Thomas, K. R. and Capecchi, M. R. (1987) Site-directed mutagenesis by gene targeting in mouse embryo-derived stem cells. *Cell* **51,** 503–512.
12. Brenin, D., Look, J., Bader, M., Hübner, N., Levan, G., and Iannaccone, P. (1997) Rat embryonic stem cells: a progress report. *Transplant. Proc.* **29,** 1761–1765.
13. Vassilieva, S., Guan, K., Pich, U., and Wobus, A. M. (2000) Establishment of SSEA-1- and Oct-4-expressing rat embryonic stem-like cell lines and effects of cytokines of the IL-6 family on clonal growth. *Exp. Cell Res.* **258,** 361–373.
14. Fändrich, F., Lin, X., Chai, G. X., et al. (2002) Preimplantation-stage stem cells induce allogeneic graft tolerance without supplementary host conditioning. *Nat. Med.* **8,** 171–178.
15. McCreath, K. J., Howcroft, J., Campbell, K. H., Colman, A., Schnieke, A. E., and Kind, A. J. (2000) Production of gene-targeted sheep by nuclear transfer from cultured somatic cells. *Nature* **405,** 1066–1069.
16. Phelps, C. J., Koike, C., Vaught, T. D., et al. (2003) Production of alpha 1,3-galactosyltransferase-deficient pigs. *Science* **299,** 411–414.
17. Iannaccone, P., Bader, M., and Galat, V. (2002) Cloning of rats. In *Principles of Cloning* (Cibelli, J., Lanza, R., Campbell, K., and West, M., eds.), Academic, San Diego, CA, pp. 403–415.
18. Zan, Y., Haag, J. D., Chen, K. S., et al. (2003) Production of knockout rats using ENU mutagenesis and a yeast-based screening assay. *Nat. Biotechnol.* **21,** 645–651.
19. Schinke, M., Baltatu, O., Böhm, M., et al. (1999) Blood pressure reduction and diabetes insipidus in transgenic rats deficient in brain angiotensinogen. *Proc. Natl. Acad. Sci. USA* **96,** 3975–3980.
20. Hasuwa, H., Kaseda, K., Einarsdottir, T., and Okabe, M. (2002) Small interfering RNA and gene silencing in transgenic mice and rats. *FEBS Lett.* **532,** 227–230.
21. Blendy, J. A., Kaestner, K. H., Schmid, W., Gass, P., and Schutz, G. (1996) Targeting of the CREB gene leads to up-regulation of a novel CREB mRNA isoform. *EMBO J.* **15,** 1098–1106.
22. Zhang, H., Hasty, P., and Bradley, A. (1994) Targeting frequency for deletion vectors in embryonic stem cells. *Mol. Cell Biol.* **14,** 2404–2410.
23. Hasty, P., Rivera-Perez, J., and Bradley, A. (1991) The length of homology required for gene targeting in embryonic stem cells. *Mol. Cell. Biol.* **11,** 5586–5591.

24. Deng, C. and Capecchi, M. R. (1992) Reexamination of gene targeting frequency as a function of the extent of homology between the targeting vector and the target locus. *Mol. Cell. Biol.* **12,** 3365–3371.

25. te Riele, H., Maandag, E. R., and Berns, A. (1992) Highly efficient gene targeting in embryonic stem cells through homologous recombination with isogenic DNA constructs. *Proc. Natl. Acad. Sci. USA* **89,** 5128–5132.

26. van Deursen, J. and Wieringa, B. (1992) Targeting of the creatine kinase M gene in embryonic stem cells using isogenic and nonisogenic vectors. *Nucl. Acids Res.* **20,** 3815–3820.

27. Morano, I., Chai, G. X., Baltas, L. G., et al. (2000) Smooth-muscle contraction without smooth-muscle myosin. *Nat. Cell Biol.* **2,** 371–375.

3

Production of Transgenic Models in Hypertension

Elena Popova, Michael Bader, and Alexander Krivokharchenko

Summary

This chapter describes the generation of transgenic mice and rats by microinjection of DNA constructs into the pronucleus of a zygote. The transgene DNA is randomly integrated as several tandem copies at one site into the genome and is transmitted to the offspring of the founder animal derived from the injected embryo, thereby creating a stable transgenic line. The technology includes the following steps: design and generation of the transgene construct, superovulation of donor animals, isolation of fertilized oocytes, microinjection of the transgene construct into one pronucleus of the zygotes, transfer of injected embryos into the oviduct of a foster mother, and identification of transgenic animals in the offspring.

Key Words: Transgenic rat; transgenic mouse; microinjection; superovulation; oviduct transfer; promoter; embryo culture; zygote; pronucleus; vasectomy; pseudopregnancy; genotyping.

1. Introduction

The technique to generate transgenic animal models by the integration of foreign DNA sequences into the genome of mammals was established more than 20 yr ago *(1–3)*. Most of the experiments since then have been performed in the mouse; however, the technology has been extended to other species such as the rat *(4,5)*. The development of transgenic technology in the rat was particularly important for hypertension research, for which the rat is the most common animal model. Because of the larger size compared to the mouse, this species is more accessible to microsurgical techniques, tissue sampling, and for the in vitro study of organ function. The technology for the production of transgenic rats is quite similar to the methodology used for the mouse. There are some peculiarities in rat transgenic technology that are described below. The efficiency of transgenic animal production depends on a lot of factors; the most important one is the skill of the scientist and others are discussed in this

From: *Methods in Molecular Medicine, Vol. 108: Hypertension: Methods and Protocols*
Edited by: J. P. Fennell and A. H. Baker © Humana Press Inc., Totowa, NJ

chapter. Published values range from 3% to 5% transgene-positive offspring (founder) per injected zygote for mice and from 0.2% to 2% for rats *(6–8)*.

The most commonly used technique for transgenesis is the microinjection of about 100 copies of a DNA construct into the pronucleus of a zygote. After microinjection, the transgene is integrated randomly into the genome mostly at a single site as tandem repeats of 1–100 copies by a yet enigmatic mechanism involving illegitimate recombination. Occasionally (<10% of the cases), the transgene integrates at two independent sites in the genome as indicated by the occurrence of more than 50% transgenic offspring born by the founder. The two sites need to be separated by controlled breeding yielding two independent transgenic lines. In about 10% of the cases, genes at the site of the transgene insertion are destroyed and unpredictable effects of this mutation might occur latest when the animals are bred to homozygosity concerning the transgene locus. However, because the integration never happens at the same chromosomal site, the generation of at least two distinct lines of transgenic animals with each construct avoids misinterpretation of the phenotype. Furthermore, generating several transgenic founders has additional advantages. First, it allows to cope with the fact that sometimes (about 20% of the cases) the transgene comes under the control of neighboring sequences on the chromosome, leading to unwanted tissue distribution of expression or complete silencing. There have been attempts to avoid this problem by coinjection of so-called insulator sequences together with the transgene which shield it from the influence of the chromosomal neighborhood *(9)*. However, in our hands, most transgenes were expressed in the intended tissues in nearly all lines generated, without the use of insulators. Second, some transgenic founders (about 10%) may not be fertile or may not transmit the transgene to their offspring, probably due to the inability to develop fully functional germ cells in the presence of the transgene.

This chapter describes the generation of transgenic mice and rats using the microinjection of DNA construct into the pronucleus of a zygote, with comparative analysis of details and differences between the two species in each step of this technology. This technology includes the following steps: design and generation of the transgene construct (**Fig. 1**), superovulation of donor animals, isolation of fertilized oocytes, microinjection of a small volume of solution containing the transgene construct into one pronucleus of the zygote (**Fig. 2**), transfer of injected embryos into a foster mother (**Fig. 3**), and identification of transgenic animals in the offspring (**Fig. 4**). This chapter does not describe systems that use the inducible expression of transgenes. For this the reader is referred to recent review articles *(10–12)*.

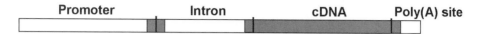

Fig. 1. Typical transgene DNA construct.

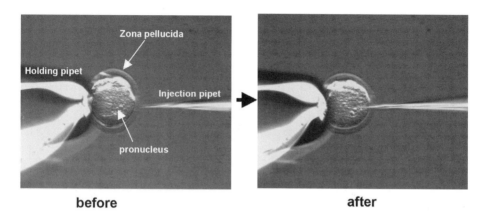

Fig. 2. Microinjected of DNA construct into one pronucleus of a zygote.

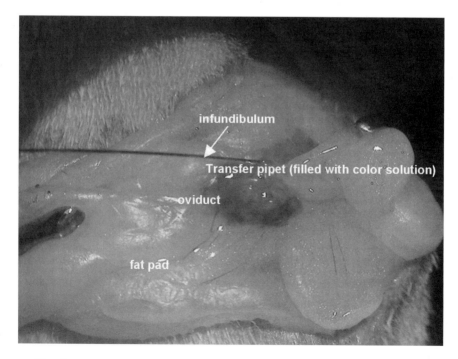

Fig. 3. Transfer of microinjected zygotes into the oviduct of a foster mother.

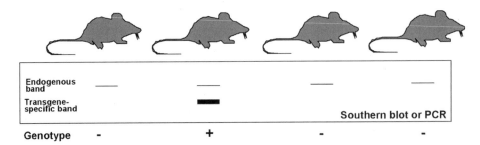

Fig. 4. Identification of transgene positive founder animals in the offspring by detecting the integration of the transgene into the genomic DNA with the use of a transgene specific PCR or Southern blot.

1.1. Selection of Strain

Choosing the right strain of mice for zygote isolation is important because the ease and efficiency of generating transgenic mice by pronuclear microinjection is highly strain-dependent. In general, the generation of transgenic mice and their subsequent breeding is more efficient when zygotes of hybrids are used for microinjection than with zygotes of inbred strains, because inbred mice generally have a relatively poor reproductive performance. F2-hybrid zygotes may be produced by mating between male and female mice from several different F1 hybrids: e.g., C57Bl/6J × SJL, C57Bl/6J × CBA/J, C3H/HeJ × C57Bl/6J, C3H/HeJ × DBA/2J, and C57Bl/6J × DBA/2J *(13)*. However, a defined inbred genetic background is preferable for genetic analyses such as the transfer of one allele of mouse gene into a strain carrying a different allele. To date the inbred strain most widely used is C57Bl/6J. However, two other mouse inbred strains, FVB/N *(14,15)* and SWR *(16)*, are convenient for transgenesis because of some characteristics of the embryos, including large prominent pronuclei, which facilitate microinjection of DNA, resistance to lysis, and good reproductive characteristics.

Establishment of transgenic rat production is a more recent development. Because of this, not many studies have been carried out using various rat strains for transgenic animal production in comparison to the mouse. Generally, outbred strains such a Sprague-Dawley (SD) and Wistar or F1 hybrids between two inbred strains can give a higher number of embryos and produce a higher litter size than inbred strains. In our lab, we have successfully worked with SD as outbred strain but also with Lewis (LEW), Wistar Kyoto (WKY), and stroke-prone spontaneously hypertensive rats (SHRSP) as representatives of inbred rat strains. Inbred Fischer rats have also been used for transgenesis.

1.2. Killing Mice and Rats

The recommended way of killing mice and young rats is cervical dislocation. This is quick and causes a minimum of distress for the animal. Other suitable methods, especially for older rats, include decapitation and ether overdosing.

1.3. Superovulation of Donor Animals (Mice and Rats)

Natural mating between mature animals can be used to supply the eggs for microinjection, but the yield is quite small, i.e., 10–15 ova per female depending on the strain used.

Therefore, superovulation is conducted in immature animals in order to provide a large number of ova for the microinjection. Generally, superovulation is induced by the injection of gonadotropic hormones such as pregnant mare's serum gonadotropin (PMSG) or follicle-stimulating hormone (FSH) followed by the injection of human chorionic gonadotropin (hCG). It has been reported that the efficiency of superovulation is dependent on the dose of the hormones, the route of administration, and the age and weight of the animals *(17)*. The most common method of superovulation in mice is intraperitoneal (ip) injection of five IU PMSG followed by ip injection of five IU hCG with 48–50 h of interval between the hormones.

Successful transgenic animal generation has been reported also after FSH treatment, and an FSH protocol for superovulation has been described for the production of large numbers of normally developed rat ova *(18)*. Recently, several groups successfully used a PMSG protocol to obtain a large number of ova in mice and rats for various manipulations. In our experience, PMSG (20 IU) or FSH together with hCG (30 IU) were equally effective, at least in immature SD rats, in terms of the efficiency of superovulation and the success of transgenic animal generation *(8)*. The easier use and the lower costs recommend PMSG for the production of transgenic rats. However, it is imperative to note that efficiency of superovulation may depend on season, strain of the animals, and quality of hormone preparations (*see* **Notes 1** and **2**).

1.4. Collection of Ova

On the following morning (d + 1) at 8:00–10:00 AM, each female should be checked for the presence of a copulatory plug (*see* **Note 3**). Animals are sacrificed at approximately 12 AM on d + 1 to collect fertilized eggs. In contrast to the mouse, a high proportion of ova from superovulated rats are unfertilized or abnormal. There is also a drastic difference in the number of isolated ova between individual rats, particularly when outbred strains are used.

2. Materials

The animals are kept at a temperature of $21 \pm 2°C$ in a 12-h light/dark cycle (lights on 6:00 AM–6:00 PM) with a humidity of $65 \pm 5\%$.

2.1. Superovulation

2.1.1. Induction of Superovulation by FSH Treatment (Using Minipumps)

1. FSH (NIH-FSH-P1; Vetrepharm, Ireland).
2. Osmotic minipumps (Alzet 2001).
3. 0.9% Saline.
4. Anesthetic (ether).
5. Animal shaver.
6. 70% Ethanol.
7. Large-toothed and blunt-ended forceps.
8. Surgical staples and spray.
9. Damp cotton buds.

2.1.2. Induction of Superovulation by PMSG Treatment (Single Injection)

1. PMSG; Intergonan (Intervet, Germany).
2. HCG (Sigma) or Ovogest (Intervet, Germany).
3. 0.9% Saline.
4. Syringe.

2.2. Collection of Ova

1. M16 medium (Sigma, USA). M16 is a modified Krebs-Ringer bicarbonate solution containing 94.66 mM NaCl, 4.78 mM KCl, 1.71 mM CaCl$_2$, 1.19 mM KH$_2$PO$_4$, 1.19 mM MgSO$_4$, 25.00 mM NaHCO$_3$, 23.28 mM sodium lactate, 0.33 mM sodium pyruvate, 5.56 mM glucose, 100 U/mL of penicillin G, 50 µg/mL of streptomycin sulfate, 10 µg/mL of phenol red.
2. M2 media (Sigma, USA). M2 is a modified Krebs-Ringer solution with some of the bicarbonate substituted with HEPES buffer to facilitate the survival of the embryos outside the incubator. M2 medium contains the same components as M16 but with 4.15 mM NaHCO$_3$ and 20.85 mM HEPES. Both M2 and M16 contain bovine serum albumin (BSA) (concentration of 4 mg/mL).
3. 35-mm sterile tissue-culture dishes.
4. Hyaluronidase (Sigma), 0.1% (w/v) in M2 medium.
5. 4-well sterile tissue-culture dishes (Nunc, Denmark).
6. Embryo transfer pipet and mouthpiece.
7. Stereomicroscope with understage illumination.
8. 37°C Incubator gassed with 5% CO$_2$.

2.3. Microinjection

1. Humidified CO$_2$ incubator (37°C) with atmosphere of 5% CO$_2$ and 95% air; or 5% O$_2$, 5% CO$_2$, and 90% N$_2$.

2. Transgene DNA solution at a concentration of approx 3 µg/mL.
3. Tris-EDTA buffer: 8–10 m*M* Tris-HCl, pH 7.4, containing 0.1–0.25 m*M* EDTA (*see* **Note 4**).
4. M2 medium (Sigma).
5. M16 medium (Sigma).
6. Glass tubing for microinjection pipet (outer diameter 1 mm, inner diameter 0.58 mm, filament diameter 0.133 mm) (e.g., Hilgenberg, Germany).
7. Pipet puller (e.g., Vertical Pipette Puller Model 750, David Kopf Instruments, Tujunga, CA).
8. Holding pipets (e.g., Biomedical Instruments, Germany).
9. Light paraffin oil (Sigma) (*see* **Note 5**).
10. Injection chamber or glass depression slide.
11. Micromanipulators: one for the holding pipet, which holds the zygote in place, and one for the microinjection pipet.
12. Inverted microscope with ×10 and ×40 objectives.
13. Microinjection system (manual or automatic).

2.4. Embryo Transfer

1. M2 medium.
2. Anesthetics: Ketavet (100 mg/mL Ketaminhydrochlorid; Pharmacia & Upjohn GmbH) and Rompun (2%; Xylazinhydrochlorid; Bayer AG, Leverkusen).
3. Dissection instruments: sharp, blunt, strong scissors, to open the outside skin; long-toothed forceps, to hold outside skin; sharp-pointed scissors, to separate the muscle from the skin and to make the incision in the muscle wall; fine-pointed forceps, to hold the muscle wall; small clip, to hold the fat pad in place.
4. Syringe loaded with adrenaline solution (Suprarenin; Hoechst AG; 1.0 mg/mL epinephrine [adrenaline]).
5. Small animal shavers.
6. Two microfine tweezers.
7. Cotton swabs.
8. "Mersilene" surgical suture (Ethicon, USA).
9. Wound clips.
10. Wound spray.
11. Surgical microscope with optional assistant's viewing head (e.g., Carl Zeiss, Germany).
12. Oviduct transfer pipets and mouthpiece for loading microinjected embryos into transfer pipet.
13. Antibiotics: Nebacetin (3250 I.E. neomycinsulfate, 250 I.E. bacitracin; Yamanouchi Pharma GmbH).
14. 70% Ethanol.

2.5. Identification of Transgenic Animals

1. Ear buffer: 100 m*M* Tris-HCl pH 8.5, 5 m*M* EDTA , 200 m*M* NaCl, 0.2% sodium dodecylsulfate (SDS).

2. Proteinase K: 10 mg/mL in H_2O (store at –20°C).
3. Stock RNAse A: 4 mg/mL in H_2O (store at –20°C).
4. 1X TE buffer: 10 mM Tris-HCl (pH 8.0), 1 mM EDTA.
5. TE/RNAse buffer: 20 µg/mL RNAse A in TE buffer (prepare fresh).
6. Lyses buffer: 50 mM Tris-HCl (pH 8.0), 100 mM NaCl, 100 mM EDTA, 1% SDS.

3. Methods

3.1. Superovulation

3.1.1. Filling and Implantation of Minimum and hCG Administration

Since purified FSH has a short half-life, it is administered as a continuous infusion via an Alzet model 2001 miniosmotic pump implanted subcutaneously (sc), delivering each hour approx 1 µL with 0.2 mg FSH to each female (*see* **Note 6**). The total amount of FSH delivered from the minipump during the whole experimental period is 10 mg per donor. The minipumps are prepared in the evening on d –3 (i.e., 3 d before mating), followed by an overnight stay at room temperature. It is also possible to allow the minipumps to equilibrate on d –2 with incubation for 1 h at 37°C before implantation. Prepared minipumps are implanted in rats at 8:00–10:00 AM on d –2. In contrast, simple injection is commonly used for induction of superovulation in mice.

1. Dissolve 20 mg of lyophilized hormone (Folltropin) in 2.1 mL of 0.9 % saline.
2. Introduce 100 µL of hormone solution into the minipump, using a small syringe (1.0 mL) with the supplied special needle; avoid air bubbles. Solutions should be at room temperature during filling.
3. After filling, the minipumps should be immersed in isotonic saline to promote the osmotic pumping action before implantation to the animal.
4. For implantation of the minipump, lightly anesthetize the rat with ether.
5. Shave a small area on the back of the neck and swab with spray.
6. Pinch the pelt with toothed forceps and make a small incision.
7. Insert blunt-ended forceps into the incision and work down to the left hind leg.
8. Insert the minipump into the pocket such that the top of the minipump is in an anterior position.
9. Close the wound with sterile surgical staples and spray the area.
10. 48–50 h After implantation of the minipump, the rats receive an ip injection of 30 IU hCG and mate with fertile males on the afternoon of d 0.

3.1.2. Administration of PMSG and hCG

Rats and mice receive PMSG by ip injection between 11 AM and 1 PM of d –2. Approximately 48–50 h after the beginning of gonadotropin treatment, animals are given hCG, also by ip injection.

To generate approx 100 viable mouse zygotes for microinjection 10 F1 hybrid females (12–14 g, 4–5 wk old) are used. To produce 100 fertilized rat oocytes we use 5–6 females (4 and 5 wk old). The total number and percentage of morphologically normal zygotes vary with strain and superovulation protocol.

1. Inject each animal ip with the following hormones:
     PMSG 100 µL of 50 IU/mL (5 IU/mouse)
     150 µL of 100 IU/mL PMSG (15 IU/rat)
     hCG 100 µL of 50 IU/mL (5 IU/mouse)
     300 µL of 100 IU/mL hCG (30 IU/rat)
2. After injection, place female with a male of the same strain on the afternoon of d 0.

3.2. Collection of Ova

1. At least 1 h before collecting ova, set up 35-mm tissue culture dishes and 4-well dishes containing M16 medium. Allow these to equilibrate in a 37°C incubator gassed with 5% CO_2.
2. At the same time, prepare tissue culture dishes containing M2 medium and leave at room temperature.
3. Kill the donor females.
4. Dissect each oviduct away from the fat pad and ovary.
5. Transfer the oviducts to a Petri dish containing M2 medium. Release ova from the ampullae of the oviduct under the microscope.
6. Remove the cumulus cells by placing the ova in M2 medium containing hyaluronidase (0.1% w/v) for 2–5 min. Their removal can be assisted by gently pipeting through a transfer pipet. The ova should not be in contact with the enzyme for any longer than the recommended period.
7. Wash the ova several times in M2 medium to remove hyaluronidase, and maintain in M16 culture medium at 37°C under 5% CO_2 until microinjection (*see* **Note 7**).

3.3. Design and Preparation of DNA for Microinjection

3.3.1. Design of DNA Construct

Most transgene constructs contain cDNAs of the protein to be overexpressed under the control of a promoter suitable for the intended tissue distribution of the transgene product. A schematic drawing of a typical transgene construct is shown in **Fig. 1**. **Table 1** summarizes promoters already used successfully in transgenic experiments to express genes in specific cell types important for cardiovascular regulation.

In order to increase the expression of the transgene *(19)*, an intron should be included in the construct, if the promoter does not already contain it such as some cardiac specific promoters do. Most commonly used for this purpose are the small intron of simian virus 40 (SV40) and the rabbit β-globin intron. In our experience, placement of the intron between promoter and cDNA is preferable to its insertion behind the cDNA. In our hands the use of the β-globin

Table 1
Promoters Commonly Used to Target Transgene Expression to Specific Cell Types Important for Hypertension Research

Promoter	Abbreviation	Cell type of highest activity	Reference
Myosin light chain 2	MLC-2	Cardiomyocytes	*28*
α-Cardiac myosin heavy chain	αMHC	Cardiomyocytes	*29*
tie2	tie2	Endothelial cells	*30*
SM22α	SM22α	Vascular smooth muscle cells	*31*
Smooth muscle α-actin	SMA	Smooth muscle cells	*32*
Smooth muscle myosin heavy chain	SM-MHC	Smooth muscle cells	*33*
Kidney androgen-responsive protein	KAP	Renal proximal tubular cells	*34*
Sodium chloride cotransporter	TSC	Renal distal tubular cells	*35*
Tamm Horsfall protein	THP	Renal tubular cells	*36*
Neuron-specific enolase	NSE	Neurons	*37*
Tubulin α-1	T-α1	Neurons	*38*
Ca^{2+}/calmodulin-dependent kinase II	CaMKII	Neurons	*39*
Glial fibrillary acidic protein	GFAP	Astrocytes	*40*

intron or of a promoter including introns generally resulted in better transgene expression than the use of the SV40 intron (*see* **Note 8**). To allow for correct transcriptional termination a polyadenylation [poly(A)] site should be included at the 3' end of the construct. Here, poly(A) sites of SV40 or bovine growth hormone are among the most frequently used. Note, that the construct must be released from vector sequences when completed; thus there should still be suitable restrictions sites left for this purpose (*see* **Note 9**).

3.3.2. Choice of Microinjection Buffer

A very important factor determining embryo survival is not only the injected DNA itself but the solution buffer of the DNA. There are many studies dealing with the optimal solution for dissolving DNA for microinjection. Researchers have even used water or 1X phosphate-buffered saline (PBS) for this purpose *(20,21)*. However, in most laboratories, including ours, Tris-EDTA buffer is used.

3.3.3. Purification of DNA-Construct for Microinjection

Success of microinjection depends on the method used for DNA preparation *(22)*. Vector-free DNA is isolated by restriction enzyme digestion followed by agar gel electrophoresis. Isolation of DNA from the agar gel by binding to glass beads followed by passage through a Sephadex G–50 column (QIAquick kit from Qiagen) and filtration through a 0.22-μm filter provides DNA of high quality.

The concentration of the DNA to be injected has been found to be a major criterion for embryo survival and efficiency of transgene integration *(6)*. A DNA concentration of 1 ng/μL was less detrimental to embryo survival than 10 ng/μL and lead to a higher rate of transgene integration than 0.1 ng/μL. A concentration of 3–5 ng/μL is most commonly used for the production of transgenic mice and rats.

1. Digest approx 20 μg of the DNA construct with restriction enzymes that will remove the plasmid sequences from the transgene.
2. Run the DNA on an agarose gel and elute the band containing the transgene to be injected. We have used a Qiaquick gel extraction kit from Qiagen. Any other phenol-free method that leaves little salt contamination is probably equivalent.
3. Repeat **step 2**.
4. Determine the DNA concentration by spectrophotometry.
5. Dilute the DNA to 1–5 ng/μL and check the concentration using comparative ethidium bromide staining with DNA standards of known concentration.
6. Filter the DNA solution through a small 0.22-μm Millipore filter attached to a syringe.

3.4. Microinjection

Despite some similarities, the methods for pronuclear microinjection (**Fig. 2**) of rat and mouse zygotes are quite different. As was shown by the majority of investigators, pronuclear microinjection in the rat is more difficult than in the mouse because of the morphological peculiarities of the zygotes. More precisely, the cytoplasmic membrane of rat zygotes is quite resistant to penetration, and the pronuclear membrane is very sticky. Because of this, it is necessary to penetrate with the pipet all the way through the rat zygote to the other side to pierce its membranes. That makes this procedure more difficult than in mice, and a large number of embryos undergo lysis after microinjection. In our experience, 10 to 50% of zygotes of the SD strain are destroyed by the injection. There is also a drastic difference in embryo survival rate between individual rats. In contrast, under optimal conditions in mice approx 80% of microinjected zygotes survive this manipulation.

1. Microinjection pipets are prepared from borosilicate glass capillaries with an internal glass filament, which are drawn out mechanically using the micropipet puller. Microinjection pipets are pulled when needed. Holding pipets can be purchased or produced in advance.
2. Place the distal end of the injection capillary into the DNA solution and allow the liquid to go up into the tip by capillary action.
3. Place 20–30 µL of M2 medium in the well of the slide and cover the medium with paraffin oil (*see* **Note 10**).
4. Place the slide on the stage of the microscope and then put the ova into this medium.
5. Using the micromanipulators, bring both the injection pipet filled with DNA solution and the holding pipet to the center of the field of view.
6. Focus on the large pronucleus and inject the DNA-construct using a pneumatic pump or a hand-operated syringe. Successful injection is indicated by swelling of the pierced pronucleus (*see* **Notes 11** and **12**).
7. Once all the zygotes in an injection chamber have been injected, return the survived embryos to M16 medium into the CO_2 incubator (*see* **Notes 13–15**).

3.5. Embryo Transfer

The last step in transgenic technology is the transfer of manipulated embryos into pseudopregnant recipients (**Fig. 3**). Fertilized oocytes, which survived the microinjection can be transferred on the day of the microinjection or following an overnight culture. Because of the well-established in vitro culture system for preimplantation mouse embryos, overnight culture of microinjected embryos is widely used for the selection of viable embryos before their transfer into foster mothers.

3.5.1. Choice of Animal Strains for Foster Mothers

Generally, the best recipients for transfer of microinjected zygotes are outbred mice, such as ICR, NMRI, CD-1, or SW, as well as F1 hybrid mice. The female should be at least 6 wk of age and weigh about 20 g.

A relatively limited number of rat strains has been described for the use as pseudopregnant recipients. Mostly used are animals of the outbred Wistar or SD strains, which have optimal reproductive and maternal characteristics and are relatively inexpensive and easy to handle. Females used as surrogate mothers need to be sexually mature (4 to 5 mo old) and approx 200 g in weight.

3.5.2. Vasectomized Males

Pseudopregnant foster mothers are produced by mating of mature females with vasectomized males. For this purpose, sexually mature males are sterilized by vasectomy or vasectomized males are purchased from a commercial animal breeder (*see* **Note 16**).

3.5.3. Synchronization of Transferred Embryos and Recipient

Microinjected embryos are transferred into the oviduct of pseudopregnant females on the day of microinjection (zygotes) or after overnight in vitro culture (2-cell stage). In our experience, the pregnancy rate of foster mothers used at d 1 of pseudopregnancy and survival rate to term was not different whether injected rat zygotes were transferred immediately after microinjection or after culture in M16 medium to the 2-cell stage (unpublished results). In contrast, it has been shown that transfer into a d 1 pseudopregnant female of microinjected rat zygotes cultured overnight resulted in lower pregnancy rates (27.8%) than when the transfer was performed immediately after microinjection (85.1%) *(7)*.

Taking into account most data available in the literature, it is preferable to perform the oviduct transfer of microinjected zygotes on the day of microinjection. It is optimal to transfer to each oviduct about 10–12 embryos to produce a normal litter size of 5–7 pups.

3.5.4. Procedure of Embryo Transfer

1. Mate female with vasectomized male, check copulatory plug next morning (*see* **Note 17**).
2. For mice the anesthetic mixture contains 0.1 mL Ketavet, 0.01 mL Rompun, and 0.9 mL physiological salt solution. Weigh the recipient and inject it ip with 0.01–0.012 mL of this mixture per gram of body weight. Rats are anesthetized with a mixture of Ketavet (1 mL/kg of body weight) and Rompun (0.2 mL/kg of body weight).
3. Place the animal on illuminated operation pad.
4. For mice, comb the hair away from the incision site, spray the back with ethanol, and make a cut in the skin. For rats, shave a square in the middle of the back, spray it with ethanol, make a cut in the skin from the center of the rat's back, and gently separate the skin from the muscle.
5. Make an incision in the muscle wall and pull up the large fat pad through the opening. The ovary, oviduct, and uterus will be pulled out as well.
6. Attach an artery clip to the fat pad.
7. Under the operating microscope, locate the oviduct beneath a transparent membrane (the bursa) and find an area of the membrane, preferably above the infundibulum (opening to the oviduct), that is free of capillaries.
8. Make a small incision in the bursa, and locate the infundibulum (*see* **Note 18**).
9. Load the embryos into an oviduct transfer pipet (M2 medium, air bubble, embryos, air bubble, M2 medium).
10. Place the transfer pipet inside the infundibulum and hold its in place while the embryos are transferred. In case of successful transfer you should be able to see the air bubbles in the oviduct.

11. Remove the pipet from the oviduct.
12. Gently place the fat pad back into the body cavity, stitch the wound, and repeat this procedure on the other side (*see* **Note 19**).
13. Operated animals are maintained under optimal husbandry conditions.

3.6. Identification of Transgenic Animals

Integration of the transgene into the recipient genome can be determined by transgene-specific polymerase chain reaction (PCR) or Southern blot with genomic DNA isolated from ear or tail biopsies of the offspring after weaning (Fig. 1). Tail biopsies are performed on a clean and disinfected work surface. Animals are toe-clipped and approximately 0.5 cm of their tail is snipped off and placed into a 1.5-mL microcentrifuge tube. DNA isolation is improved if the tail piece is cut into several smaller pieces. For an alternative method, *see* Chapter 1. Alternatively, the tissue released during earmarking of animals can be used for genomic DNA isolation. The tissue pieces can either be processed immediately or frozen at $-20°C$.

3.6.1. Isolation of Genomic DNA From Tail Pieces

1. Incubate the tail pieces in 700 µL of lysis buffer containing 35 µL proteinase K (10 mg/mL) at 55°C overnight with shaking.
2. In the morning, incubate samples on ice for 10 min, then mix with 300 µL of 6 *M* NaCl, and keep on ice for 5 min more.
3. After centrifugation (15,000*g*, 4°C, 10 min) transfer aqueous phase into a new tube and incubate for 15 min at 37°C with 5 µL of RNAse A (4 mg/mL).
4. Precipitate DNA by adding 1 mL of isopropanol followed by centrifugation (15,000*g*, 4°C, 15 min).
5. Wash pellet with 75% ethanol, dry, and resolve it in 100–200 µL of TE buffer. The concentration of extracted DNA is estimated by spectrophotometry. DNA is kept at $-20°C$.

3.6.2. Isolation of Genomic DNA From Ear Biopsies

1. Incubate ear biopsies for 2 h (or longer) in 100 µL of ear buffer containing 1 mg/mL proteinase K at 55°C with shaking.
2. After complete digestion of tissue, heat-inactivate proteinase K (95°C, 5 min), vortex samples, mix with 750 µL of TE/RNAse buffer, and freeze at $-20°C$. Use 2 µL of this DNA solution for the PCR to detect the transgene.

4. Notes

1. For each rat strain, it is better to test every lot of hormone before buying in bulk.
2. It is essential that the animals are maintained in optimal conditions and with a constant light–dark cycle.
3. In rats, the plug has often fallen out in the morning.
4. When preparing the injection buffer, use disposable plastic free of traces of detergents.

5. Paraffin oil used to prevent evaporation of the medium can be toxic to the embryos. Therefore it is advisable to test it by in vitro culturing of mouse zygotes until blastocyst stage in microdrops of medium under paraffin oil.

6. The procedure of miniosmotic pump implantation should be conducted in sterile surgical conditions and takes 2–3 min.

7. It is advisable to leave the zygotes in an incubator for several hours before microinjection.

8. Never flank a long cDNA (>300 bp) by two introns. This may result in the loss of the cDNA during splicing *(23)*.

9. Before microinjection, each transgene should be sequenced and tested for functionality in suitable cell culture systems, if possible.

10. Avoid releasing any air bubbles into the chamber, and the medium must be completely covered with paraffin oil to prevent evaporation.

11. For microinjection of rat zygotes, some researchers have used a piezoinjector or finger touching of the microscope stage (microvibration). This method of micropipet introduction made it possible to inject the DNA solution without detrimental effects on rat zygotes *(24,25)*.

12. Following injection, the injection pipet can be blocked and should be exchanged.

13. Zygotes are microinjected at room temperature or at 37°C using a warm plate. About 20–30 zygotes can be injected in 20–30 min depending on the technical skills of the investigator.

14. Culture media should previously be equilibrated with the gas phase and temperature in the CO_2 incubator for 2–3 h.

15. M16 medium may be used for short-time cultivation of injected rat zygotes (not more than overnight culture). For long-term culture of rat embryos, mR1ECM medium should be used *(26,27)*: 76.7 mM NaCl, 3.2 mM KCl, 2.0 mM CaCl$_2$, 0.5 mM MgCl$_2$, 25.0 mM NaHCO$_3$, 10 mM sodium lactate, 0.5 mM sodium pyruvate, 7.5 mM D-glucose, 1.0 mg/mL polyvinylalcohol (ave mol wt 30,000–70,000), 2% (v/v) mimimal essential medium (MEM), essential amino acid solution (Gibco, USA), 0.1 mM glutamine (Sigma), and 1% (v/v) MEM nonessential amino acid solution (Gibco). The osmolarity should be about 246 mOsmol and the pH about 7.4 after equilibration in incubator.

16. It is essential to check for successful vasectomy by mating each vasectomized male with a female for 2 wk. The female should have a copulatory plug but should not carry fertilized oocytes or become pregnant.

17. In rats the plug has often fallen out by the morning. Therefore it is imperative to check females for the presence of a copulatory plug at 8:00–9:00 AM. In contrast to the mouse, mature pseudopregnant rats often do not have a visible plug.

18. Rupture of the bursa membrane can lead to excessive bleeding, which may render the entrance to the infundibulum invisible. Bleeding can be stopped by either cauterization or topical application of adrenaline (Suprarenin).

19. A sterile surgical technique is essential for closure of the wound. It is advisable to administer antibiotics (Nebacetin) to the recipient female at the wound surface after surgery.

Acknowledgments

The authors thank Natasha Alenina, Tanja Chmidt, Larissa Vil'ianovitch, and Rosemarie Barnow for helpful discussions.

References

1. Harbers, K., Jähner, D., and Jaenisch, R. (1981) Microinjection of cloned retroviral genomes into mouse zygotes: integration and expression in the animal. *Nature* **293**, 540–542.
2. Wagner, E. F., Stewart, T. A., and Mintz, B. (1981) The human b-globin gene and a functional viral thymidine kinase gene in developing mice. *Proc. Natl. Acad. Sci. USA* **78**, 5016–5020.
3. Costantini, F. and Lacy, E. (1981) Introduction of a rabbit b-globin gene into the mouse germ line. *Nature* **294**, 92–94.
4. Mullins, J. J., Peters, J., and Ganten, D. (1990) Fulminant hypertension in transgenic rats harbouring the mouse Ren-2 gene. *Nature* **344**, 541–544.
5. Hammer, R. E., Maika, S. D., Richardson, J. A., Tang, J., and Taurog, J. D. (1990) Spontaneous inflammatory disease in transgenic rats expressing HLA-B27 and human b2m: An animal model of HLA-B27-associated human disorders. *Cell* **63**, 1099–1112.
6. Brinster, R. L., Chen, H. Y., Trumbauer, M. E., Yagle, M. K., and Palmiter, R. D. (1985) Factors affecting the efficiency of introducing foreign genes into mice by microinjecting eggs. *Proc. Natl. Acad. Sci. USA* **82**, 4438–4442.
7. Charreau, B., Tesson, L., Soulillou, J. P., Pourcel, C., and Anegon, I. (1996) Transgenesis in rats: technical aspects and models. *Transgenic Res.* **5**, 223–234.
8. Popova, E., Krivokharchenko, A., Ganten, D., and Bader, M. (2002) Comparison between PMSG and FSH induced superovulation for the generation of transgenic rats. *Mol. Reprod. Dev.* **63**, 177–182.
9. Zhan, H. C., Liu, D. P., and Liang, C. C. (2001) Insulator: from chromatin domain boundary to gene regulation. *Hum. Genet.* **109**, 471–478.
10. Gossen, M., Bonin, A. L., Freundlieb, S., and Bujard, H. (1994) Inducible gene expression systems for higher eukaryotic cells. *Curr. Opin. Biotechnol.* **5**, 516–520.
11. Ryding, A. D., Sharp, M. G., and Mullins, J. J. (2001) Conditional transgenic technologies. *J. Endocrinol.* **171**, 1–14.
12. Lewandoski, M. (2001) Conditional control of gene expression in the mouse. *Nat. Rev. Genet.* **2**, 743–755.
13. Hogan, B., Costantini, F., and Lacy, E. (1986) *Manipulating the Mouse Embryo.* Cold Spring Harbor Laboratory, Cold Spring Harbor, NY.
14. Taketo, M., Schroeder, A. C., Mobraaten, et al. (1991) FVB/N: an inbred mouse strain preferable for transgenic analyses. *Proc. Natl. Acad. Sci. USA* **88**, 2065–2069.
15. Auerbach, A. B., Norinsky, R., Ho, W., et al. (2003) Strain-dependent differences in the efficiency of transgenic mouse production. *Transgenic Res.* **12**, 59–69.
16. Osman, G. E., Jacobson, D. P., Li, S. W., Hood, L. E., Liggitt, H. D., and Ladiges, W. C. (1997) SWR: an inbred strain suitable for generating transgenic mice. *Lab. Anim. Sci.* **47**, 167–171.

17. Tain, C. F., Goh, V. H., and Ng, S. C. (2000) Effects of hyperstimulation with gonadotrophins and age of females on oocytes and their metaphase II status in rats. *Mol. Reprod. Dev.* **55,** 104–108.

18. Leveille, M. C. and Armstrong, D. T. (1989) Preimplantation embryo development and serum steroid levels in immature rats induced to ovulate or superovulate with pregnant mares serum gonadotropin injection or FSH infusion. *Gamete Res.* **23,** 127–138.

19. Brinster, R. L., Allen, J. M., Behringer, R. R., Gelinas, R. E., and Palmiter, R. D. (1988) Introns increase transcriptional efficiency in transgenic mice. *Proc. Natl. Acad. Sci. USA* **85,** 836–840.

20. Peura, T. T., Tolvanen, M., Hyttinen, J.-M., and Jänne, J. (1995) Effect of membrane piercing and the type of pronuclear injection fluid on development of in vitro produced bovine embryos. *Theriogenology* **43,** 1087–1096.

21. Nottle, M. B., Haskard, K. A., Verma, P. J., et al. (2001) Effect of DNA concentration on transgenesis rates in mice and pigs. *Transgenic Res.* **10,** 523–531.

22. Wall, R. J., Paleyanda, R. K., Foster, J. A., Powell, A., Rexroad, C., and Lubon, H. (2000) DNA preparation method can influence outcome of transgenic animal experiments. *Anim. Biotechnol.* **11,** 19–32.

23. Davisson, R. L., Nuutinen, N., Coleman, S. T., and Sigmund, C. D. (1996) Inappropriate splicing of a chimeric gene containing a large internal exon results in exon skipping in transgenic mice. *Nucl. Acids Res.* **24,** 4023–4028.

24. Takahashi, R., Hirabayashi, M., and Ueda, M. (1999) Production of transgenic rats using cryopreserved pronuclear-stage zygotes. *Transgenic Res.* **8,** 397–400.

25. Hirabayashi, M., Takahashi, R., Ito, K., et al. (2001) A comparative study on the integration of exogenous DNA into mouse, rat, rabbit, and pig genomes. *Exp. Anim.* **50,** 125–131.

26. Miyoshi K, Kono T, Niwa K. (1997) Stage-dependent development of rat 1-cell embryos in a chemically defined medium after fertilization in vivo and in vitro. *Biol. Reprod.* **56,** 180–185.

27. Krivokharchenko, A., Galat, V., Ganten, D., and Bader, M. (2002) In vitro formation of tetraploid rat blastocysts after fusion of two-cell embryos. *Mol. Reprod. Dev.* **61,** 460–465.

28. Lee, K., Ross, R., Rockman, H., et al. (1992) Myosin light chain-2 luciferase transgenic mice reveal distinct regulatory programs for cardiac and skeletal muscle-specific expression of a single contractile protein gene. *J. Biol. Chem.* **267,** 15,875–15,885.

29. Gulick, J., Subramaniam, A., Neumann, J., and Robbins, J. (1991) Isolation and characterization of the mouse cardiac myosin heavy chain gene promoter in transgenic mice. *J. Biol. Chem.* **266,** 9180–9185.

30. Korhonen, J., Lahtinen, I., Halmekyto, M., et al. (1995) Endothelial-specific gene expression directed by the tie gene promoter in vivo. *Blood* **86,** 1828–1835.

31. Li, L., Miano, J. M., Mercer, B., and Olson, E. N. (1996) Expression of the SM22alpha promoter in transgenic mice provides evidence for distinct transcriptional regulatory programs in vascular and visceral smooth muscle cells. *J. Cell Biol.* **132,** 849–859.

32. Wang, J., Niu, W., Nikiforov, Y., et al. (1997) Targeted overexpression of IGF-I evokes distinct patterns of organ remodeling in smooth muscle cell tissue beds of transgenic mice. *J. Clin. Invest.* **100,** 1425–1439.

33. Madsen, C. S., Regan, C. P., Hungerford, J. E., White, S. L., Manabe, I., and Owens, G. K. (1998) Smooth muscle-specific expression of the smooth muscle myosin heavy chain gene in transgenic mice requires 5'-flanking and first intronic DNA sequence. *Circ. Res.* **82,** 908–917.

34. Davisson, R. L., Ding, Y., Stec, D. E., Catterall, J. F., and Sigmund, C. D. (1999) Novel mechanism of hypertension revealed by cell-specific targeting of human angiotensinogen in transgenic mice. *Physiol. Genomics* **1,** 3–9.

35. Taniyama, Y., Sato, K., Sugawara, A., et al. (2001) Renal tubule-specific transcription and chromosomal localization of rat thiazide-sensitive Na-Cl cotransporter gene. *J. Biol. Chem.* **276,** 26260–26268.

36. Zhu, X., Cheng, J., Gao, J., et al. (2002) Isolation of mouse THP gene promoter and demonstration of its kidney-specific activity in transgenic mice. *Am. J. Physiol.* **282,** F608–F617.

37. Forss-Petter, S., Danielson, P. E., Catsicas, S., et al. (1990) Transgenic mice expressing b-galactosidase in mature neurons under neuron-specific enolase promoter control. *Neuron* **5,** 187–197.

38. Gloster, A., Wu, W., Speelman, A., et al. (1994) The T alpha 1 alpha-tubulin promoter specifies gene expression as a function of neuronal growth and regeneration in transgenic mice. *J. Neurosci.* **14,** 7319–7330.

39. Mayford, M., Baranes, D., Podsypanina, K., and Kandel, E. R. (1996) The 3'-untranslated region of CaMKII alpha is a cis-acting signal for the localization and translation of mRNA in dendrites. *Proc. Natl. Acad. Sci. USA* **93,** 13,250–13,255.

40. Brenner, M., Kisseberth, W. C., Su, Y., Besnard, F., and Messing, A. (1994) GFAP promoter directs astrocyte-specific expression in transgenic mice. *J. Neurosci.* **14,** 1030–1037.

4

Measuring Blood Pressure in Small Laboratory Animals

Klaas Kramer and René Remie

Summary

The most common techniques currently employed for monitoring blood pressure (BP) in conscious rats and mice are the tail cuff and the exteriorized catheter that feeds a pressure transducer located outside the cage. There are, however, considerable drawbacks associated with these methods, which in many respects make each of these techniques undesirable as an accurate means of obtaining pressure measurements.

Recent studies have shown that measurements of physiological variables, such as electrocardiogram (ECG), heart rate (HR), and body temperature (BT), from freely moving rats and mice by using implantable radiotelemetry were more efficient, reliable and less labour intensive when compared to measurement techniques described in the literature so far. Nowadays, measurement of BP by radiotelemetry has been described and validated for many laboratory animal species, including rats and mice. The implantable radiotelemetry technique can circumvent many of the problems associated with conventional methods (tail cuff; exteriorized catheters) of BP monitoring in mice and rats. This chapter describes the surgical aspects of the radiotelemetry techniques currently used to monitor and measure blood pressure in awake animals.

Key Words: Blood pressure; tail cuff; indwelling catheters; radiotelemetry; small laboratory animals; rat, mouse; surgical techniques.

1. Introduction

Blood pressure (BP) measurement is one of the basic techniques in biomedical research. The majority of physiological and pharmacological knowledge on blood pressure, its regulation, and the influence of drugs on the cardiovascular system has been derived from experiments with acutely prepared, anesthetized or immobilized laboratory animals. The most commonly used sites of measurement are the carotid artery or the femoral artery.

Although it is valuable, this information is obscured by direct effects of anesthesia and surgical intervention. General anesthesia, for example, has a considerable impact on baseline blood flow and myocardial function (pres-

From: *Methods in Molecular Medicine, Vol. 108: Hypertension: Methods and Protocols*
Edited by: J. P. Fennell and A. H. Baker © Humana Press Inc., Totowa, NJ

sure). Surgery can, amongst other things, introduce local vasomotion, thus disturbing the normal hemodynamic parameters. Therefore it is sometimes impossible to use these techniques to measure delicate effects on blood pressure and heart rate, and the need for refined methods becomes apparent.

The two most commonly used techniques for measuring BP in small laboratory animals such as mice and rats are the indirect tail cuff method and direct measurement by exteriorized catheters connected to pressure transducers. Brockway and Hasler *(1)* and Kramer and Kinter *(2)* described the disadvantages of these methods. In the case of the tail cuff method, the fundamental nature of this technique is such that measurements can be unreliable or inaccurate if:

1. The animal moves
2. The animal is subjected to loud noises or other stressors
3. Vasoconstriction occurs

In the case of the exteriorized catheters, the most prominent factor limiting the useful life of this technique is patency (ability to infuse liquids and to take blood samples) of vascular catheters, especially those used for blood withdrawal or pressure measurement. There is also a risk of infection involving exteriorized vascular catheters or lead wires when using this method *(3)*. Bazil et al. *(4)* reported that BP and heart rate (HR) remained increased after implanting arterial catheters and showed in their study with conscious spontaneously hypertensive rats the benefits of using the radiotelemetry system compared with the two other systems described above.

Radiotelemetry with an implantable transmitter, which minimizes exposure to stress, provides a way to obtain accurate and reliable measurements from awake and freely moving animals *(5)* and can be a valuable tool for the pharmacological screening of new compounds *(6)*. BP measurements via radiotelemetry have been described for small laboratory animals from rabbits to mice *(5)*.

Recently, Mills et al. *(7)* published a validation study of BP measurements in mice in which it appeared to be possible to implant a BP transmitter to monitor systolic, diastolic, and mean BP as well as HR and locomotor activity by radiotelemetry in freely moving mice. The most important advantage is the possibility for the direct and accurate measurement of the effects of cardiovascular drugs, and the freedom from artefacts caused by the added stress seen when using conventional techniques. From an animal welfare point of view, telemetry has another advantage: the possibility of group housing the animals. This is very difficult in animals having an exteriorized catheter, as cage mates will gnaw on the stoppers closing the catheters, leading to the untimely death of the animal. This chapter describes the surgical aspects of the radiotelemetry techniques currently used to monitor and measure blood pressure in awake animals.

1.1. Tail Cuff

A common technique currently employed for monitoring BP in conscious rats and mice is the tail cuff device (8–12). The tail cuff method has the advantage of being noninvasive. The technique is dependent on maintaining a minimum amount of blood flow in the tail, and any physiological, pharmacological, or environmental factor that affects tail blood flow will affect the BP measurement. In addition, mice are subject to the stress of handling, heating, and restraint, to which they do not seem to adapt, even after considerable training. This was concluded by various authors in view of the significantly higher HRs found in trained mice during tail cuff BP measurements vs intraarterial measurements in the same, conscious animals (9,13). Further comparative studies into the accuracy of the tail cuff method of BP measurement in mice are needed to determine its eventual value.

Findings in rats may be extrapolated to mice because of the similarities of the tail cuff techniques in these two species. Considerable measurement errors have been found using the tail cuff technique in rats (14). Bunag et al. (15) reported that systolic arterial pressure measurements with this method in conditioned Sprague-Dawley rats may deviate from measurements obtained by simultaneous aortic cannulation by as much as 37 mmHg. Such errors result in additional variability in data. In light of the fact that only a few momentary measurements are possible in rats that are subjected to stimuli such as handling, restraint, and heating (14), this high variability may interfere with the detection of small chronic changes in pressure. Those stimuli are all inherent to the tail-cuff method.

1.2. Exteriorized Catheters

Another common technique currently employed for monitoring BP in conscious rats and mice is the use of an exteriorized catheter that refers pressure to a transducer located nearby (13,16–21). This technique involves placement of an open-lumen catheter in an artery and exteriorizing it at a site inaccessible to the animal, usually in the nape of the neck or at the crown of the head. Measurements of pulsatile arterial pressure and HR can thus be obtained. However, accurate measurements of systolic and diastolic pressure are difficult to obtain because there is often a poor dynamic response due to the small size of the catheters used for cannulation of mice arteries, significant catheter compliance, and a relatively long length of conduit from the point of cannulation to the transducer. The resulting damping renders measurements of systolic and diastolic pressure unreliable.

Probably the most significant drawback of this technique is that catheter patency is short-lived. A carefully conducted study on BP measurement in mice using exteriorized catheters showed a failure rate of 50% by the end of the fourth week after implantation *(13)*. Personal communications with several investigators using this technique in mice indicate that catheters typically remain patent for 1–2 wk.

There appear to be no documented scientific studies on whether the use of exteriorized catheters in mice results in stress artefacts. However, in rats, significantly higher levels of systolic and mean BP (both +17 mmHg) have been found when recorded by indwelling and exteriorized catheters vs implanted radiotelemetry devices *(4)*. The authors hypothesized that the differences in BP and HR were due to the stress associated with performing cardiovascular measurements through externalized catheters.

1.3. Radiotelemetry

The radiotelemetry technique can circumvent many of the problems associated with conventional methods (tail cuff, exteriorized catheters) of BP monitoring in mice and rats. The implantable devices provide accurate and reliable measurements of systolic, diastolic, and mean BP as well as HR and locomotor activity from freely moving rats and mice single-housed in their home cages *(3,4,7,22)*.

1.3.1. Telemetry and Data Acquisition System

The commercially available radiotelemetry system for rats and mice (Data Sciences International [DSI], St. Paul, MN) used in all studies mentioned below measures systolic, diastolic, and mean BP as well as HR and locomotor activity *(3,4,7,8,21–31)*. Components of the radiotelemetry system used in these studies have been described in more detail before *(3,7)*. In brief, the implantable rat (DSI) or mouse (DSI) BP transmitter provides a direct measure of arterial pressure. The transmitter signals are coded in a pulse position modulated serial bit stream, which is received and monitored by the receiver (DSI) placed underneath the animal's cage.

The signals from the receiver are consolidated by the multiplexer (DSI) and are stored and analyzed by an IBM-compatible personal computer with analyzing software (DSI). In order to compensate for changes in atmospheric pressure, ambient barometric pressure is also measured and subtracted from the telemetered pressure by the data collection system.

Systolic, diastolic, and mean BP as well as HR and locomotor activity are monitored and stored every 5 min for 10 s. Systolic, diastolic, and mean BP as well as HR data are extracted from the BP waveform. Locomotor activity is obtained by the system by monitoring changes in the received signal strength that occur upon movement of the animal. Changes in signal strength of more than a predetermined threshold generate a digital pulse, which is counted by the acquisition system. It is important to note that for detection of activity the transmitter has to move. Therefore, with the transmitter implanted intraperitoneally, slight head movements during grooming or eating are not registered as activity.

1.3.2. Blood Pressure Transmitters

For blood pressure measurements the fluid-filled catheter is placed into the appropriate blood vessel (usually the abdominal aorta, thoracic aorta, femoral artery, pulmonary artery, or carotid artery) *(7,22)*. The transmitters consist of a hermetically sealed thermoplastic cylinder housing (for rats, length 30 mm and diameter 14 mm; and for mice, length 24 mm and diameter 10 mm), coated with silicone elastomer to provide the necessary biocompatibility. Total weight of the rat implant is 9.0 g and of the mouse implant is 3.4 g; volume displacement is 4.5 mL and 1.9 mL, respectively.

A transmitter contains an amplifier, a battery, radiofrequency electronics, a low-viscosity fluid-filled catheter (for rats, diameter 0.7 mm, length 8 cm; and for mice, diameter 0.4 mm, length 5 cm) attached to the sensor located in the body of the transmitter and a magnetically activated switch that allows the device to be turned on and off in vivo. The lumen of the catheter is filled with a low-viscosity fluid, while the distal 2 mm of the thin-walled tip is filled with a blood-compatible gel that prevents blood from entering the catheter lumen. An antithrombogenic film is applied to the distal 1 cm of the catheter. A suture tab moulded into the housing provides three sites for securing the device during implantation.

As described above, blood pressure catheters in these species are usually inserted into the abdominal aorta just caudal to the left renal artery, while the body of the transmitter is positioned in the peritoneal cavity. Because the device was developed for abdominal aorta implantation, its use has not been feasible in studies where peritoneal volume is critical, i.e., in pregnant mice. Butz and Davisson *(22)* developed an alternative approach for measuring BP in mice, whereby thoracic aorta implantation of the pressure-sensing catheter is combined with subcutaneous placement of the transmitter body along the right flank. For this study they used female C57BL/6 or BPH/5 mice, a strain derived from the cross of inbred hypertensive and hypotensive mouse strains. The carotid artery was used to insert the catheter, which was advanced until the tip was located in the aortic arch. The results of their study showed that the abovementioned approach is a reliable method to measure, under stress-free conditions, mean arterial pressure and HR recordings for 50–60 d in mice weighing 22 g on average but as small as 17 g, even before, during, and after pregnancy.

Although placing the BP catheter in the carotid rather than in the abdominal aorta of the mouse can permit a less invasive operation procedure and does not interfere with peritoneal volume, one must be aware of the fact that the circle of Willis (circulus arteriosus cerebri) is not completely developed, or shows large variation in some strains of mice and thus the carotid approach is not advised for these strains *(32,33)*.

The pressure transmitters have been calibrated by the manufacturer and have a continuous-use battery life up to 6 mo for rat BP implants and up to 2 mo for mouse BP implants. However, since the battery power can be switched off using a magnet, battery life of the implant can be considerably extended.

2. Materials

2.1. Animals

Animals should be allowed to acclimatize to their new environment for a period of 7–14 d. This is to make sure that metabolic and hormonal changes as a result of a stressful transport are eliminated. It is a good habit to keep a record of body weight, food, and water consumption. A severe loss of body weight and a reduced intake of food and water is a strong indication that the animal is in pain, and adequate measures should be taken. Given the fact that small rodents do not vomit during induction of anesthesia, it is not necessary to deprive them of food prior to the operation.

2.2. Anesthetic

Inhalation anesthesia is preferred to injectable anesthesia, as it allows for a better control of the anesthetic depth. We routinely use Isoflurane in combination with oxygen and nitrous oxide or air (50%–50%). The concentration of Isoflurane depends strongly on the strain and the concomitant use of nitrous oxide. Following induction, it is most convenient to maintain anesthesia using a face mask. Ensure that waste and excess anesthetic gases are removed using a validated gas-scavenging system, in order to protect the technician from unknown side effects. Since anesthetics block the thermoregulating centre in the brain, animals should be kept at normal body temperature. Hypothermia can easily cause the untimely death of an animal.

2.3. Suture Materials

1. Sutures: As a rule of thumb, always use absorbable suture materials unless something requires fixation. In the operations described in this chapter, nonabsorbable sutures are used only for fixation of the transmitter body. In rats, the maximum suture size is 4-0 for closure of the abdominal cavity; in mice a 5-0 or 6-0 suture will do. Inside the animal, only 6-0 and 7-0 sutures should be used. Avoid excessively tight sutures, as this allows bacteria to be protected in tissues made

ischemic by pressure. Also avoid too many sutures making large ischemic portions, which can result in infection.

2. Surgical microscope: Do not use a binocular dissection microscope, as it has a very small depth of focus.
3. Surgical cannulation forceps: This is a special forceps to fix the catheter during introduction, without the risk of damaging the catheter (S&T surgical tools).
4. 25-Gauge hypodermic injection needle.
5. Surgical tools:
   a. Scalpel.
   b. Anatomical forceps (straight and 90° angled).
   c. Jewellers forceps (Dumont no. 4 and 5).
   d. Irridectomy scissors.
   e. Cotton wool sticks.
   f. Sterile gauze.
6. Tissue adhesive (Vet-Seal, B|Braun Surgical GmbH, Melsungen Germany).

2.4. Solutions

1. Saline (0.9 g NaCl in 100 mL water).
2. Iodine solution (0.1 % in water).
3. Chlorhexidine in alcohol (0.5% in 70% alcohol).
4. Lidocaine solution (2% in water).

All solutions used should be sterile and used at body temperature.

2.5. Radiotelemetry System

1. Transmitter: Implantable rat (TA11PA-C40, Data Sciences International, St. Paul, MN) or mouse (TA11PA-C20, DSI) BP transmitters.
2. Receiver (RPC-1, DSI).
3. Multiplexer (Data Exchange Matrix, DSI).
4. Ambient pressure barometer (APR-1, DSI).
5. IBM-compatible personal computer with data collection and analyzing software (Dataquest, A.R.T., DSI).

3. Methods

3.1. Transmitter Implantation

3.1.1. Preoperative Procedures

The small telemetric transmitters are implanted under anesthesia (injected or inhaled), either subcutaneously or in the peritoneal cavity of the animals through a midline laparotomy (*see* **Note 1**). All animals are prepared for surgery in a room separate from the operating theater.

1. Clip the abdominal area (*see* **Note 2**).
2. Disinfect the animal (iodine or chlorhexidine in alcohol).

3. Place on a sterile silicon plate, cover with a sterile drape, and place under a binocular operation microscope on a thermostatically controlled heating pad that maintains body temperature at 36–37°C during the operation.

3.1.2. Surgery (Abdominal Aorta)

1. Make a 2–3-cm-long midline incision immediately caudal to the xiphisternum.
2. Open the straight abdominal muscle (over the white line) and gently retract the intestines with warm saline-soaked sterile gauze, permitting access to the abdominal aorta from the left renal artery to the iliac bifurcation.
3. Using the operation microscope, carefully isolate the lower abdominal aorta and separate it from the vena cava.
4. For additional vasodilatation, irrigate the exposed part of the aorta with 2% lidocaine solution.
5. Place an occlusion ligature around the abdominal aorta just caudal to the left renal artery (*see* **Note 3**).
6. Once the occlusion suture is in place, apply some tension in the cranial direction to temporarily occlude the blood flow in the aorta.
7. Immediately after closing the aorta, puncture a small hole about 2 mm cranial to the iliac bifurcation using a 25-gage hypodermic injection needle bent at a 90° angle. Using the hollow side of the needle as a guide, insert the catheter of the transmitter upstream into the aorta over a length of 5–6 mm with the aid of a vessel cannulation forceps (*see* **Note 4**). The tip should now be located about 2 mm caudal to the left renal artery.
8. Clean the area with a cotton wool stick and seal the catheter insertion site with a minimal application of tissue adhesive (15–20 µL) (*see* **Note 5**).
9. Slowly release the tension on the occlusion suture and observe the catheter entry site for leakage.
10. Irrigate the cannulated aorta again with 2% lidocaine to prevent vessel spasm.
11. Cover the insertion site with a 3 × 5 mm cellulose fiber patch. Secure the patch to the surrounding tissues with tissue adhesive (Vet-Seal, B|Braun Surgical GmbH, Melsungen Germany); this serves to both anchor the catheter and foster connective tissue growth.
12. When the catheter is fixed in place, remove the gauze and flood the peritoneal cavity with warm sterile saline before gently massaging the intestines back into place.
13. Position the transmitter body in the peritoneal cavity, and incorporate the suture rib on the transmitter housing into the abdominal wall closure with an absorbable suture (*see* **Note 6**).
14. To complete the operation, close the skin incision again using absorbable suture material (4-0 for rats and 5-0 for mice).

3.1.3. Surgery (Carotid Artery)

1. Anesthetise the animals and shave and disinfect the neck.
2. Place the animals on their back on a heated surgical surface and secure the forelimbs using adhesive tape.

3. Make a ventral midline neck incision from the lower part of the mandible to the sternum (2–3 cm), and gently separate the submandibular glands by sharp dissection.

4. Isolate and retract the left common carotid artery (located just lateral to the sternohyoid muscle) using fine forceps (*see* **Note 7**).

5. Subsequently make a tiny incision using the same technique as described for the aorta.

6. Carefully insert the pressure-sensing catheter into the left carotid artery using a vessel cannulation forceps. Advance it over a distance of 10 mm so that the tip just enters the aortic arch.

7. Secure the catheter with ligatures, and tunnel the transmitter body subcutaneously to a small pouch along the right ventral flank.

8. Close the neck incision and keep the animals warm until they have fully recovered from anesthesia.

9. Another method, placing the transmitter body on the back at the midscapular region of the mouse, is described by Carlson and Wyss *(31)*. In short, the upper back is shaved and a horizontal incision is made. The transmitter is placed in the opening and sutured to both the muscle and the skin (with the suture loop around the probe) via the suture rib on the transmitter body. A separate ventral neck incision is then made, the catheter is tunneled subcutaneously to the neck, and the catheterization procedure is carried out.

3.2. Postoperative Care

1. After surgery, place the animals in an incubator (32°C) for 1 h. Return them together with their nonimplanted cage mates to a clean home cage that is partially placed on a heating pad for at least 24 h after surgery.

2. To prevent harassment of the implanted animals by their cage mates, gently rub the abdomen of each nonimplanted animal with gauze moistened with 70% ethanol, thus ensuring that all animals carry a novel, strange odor for a short period of time.

3. Besides normal food and water, provide Solid Drink (Triple-A Trading, Otterloo, the Netherlands), moistened food pellets, and food "porridge" made with 3% glucose solution for 4 d.

4. After implantation, provide adequate analgesia. Administer the NSAID Rimadyl (carprofen, Pfizer Animal Health) for 2 d after surgery. The dose for carprofen in rodents is 5–10 mg/kg po or parenterally. A single dose after surgery, or a dose every 3 h during a period of 12 h, has a beneficial effect on postsurgical recovery. Administration may be by gavage or in Jell-O.

4. Notes

1. Before implanting the transmitter body in the peritoneal cavity, make sure that the transmitter is at least at room temperature or, even better, at body temperature. Open the sterile transmitter package, remove the implant device with sterile forceps, and immerse the device in warm sterile saline. Soak the implant for at least 15 min before implantation. The reason for this is the fact that the catheter is

very hydrophilic and, if not hydrated, will absorb water from the bloodstream. This can cause the gel to recede slightly due to catheter expansion, leaving a dead space at the tip of the catheter, which could increase the risk of blood clot formation.

2. Do not use cream to remove the hair from the abdominal area of the anesthetized animals, because creams contain toxic components.

3. Occlusion of the aorta and the carotid artery can be carried out in different ways.
   a. The vessel can be dissected free from surrounding tissue and a ligature put in place. Lifting the ligature will obstruct the blood flow, allowing for easy cannulation. If you use braided suture materials, take care not to damage the vessel (and the surrounding nerves) because of the saw-blade effect of the ligature.
   b. Without further dissection, the vessels can be clamped with suitable microvascular clips (Biemer, Acland, etc.). This saves time and causes less trauma to the tissue. Remove adventitia only at the site of cannulation.

4. Cannulation with the aid of a bent needle is a reliable technique for the insertion of rigid catheters. When introducing soft catheters such as silicon, it is advantageous to use Vannas scissors to cut a small hole in the blood vessel. If the use of tissue glue is contraindicated, one could use a purse-string suture with the appropriate diameter (this, however, requires advanced microsurgical skills).

5. One should fill two (one extra for emergencies) small pipet tips with the required volume.

6. When closing the abdominal muscular layer, take care not to place the suture rib between the two muscular layers, as this will result in a hernia. Make sure that the muscles are properly approximated without putting too much tension on the suture and the knots.

7. During preparation of the carotid artery, take care not to touch or damage the vagus nerve that runs next to the artery, as this could lead to the untimely death of the animal.

References

1. Brockway, B. P. and Hassler, C. R. (1991) Application of radio telemetry to cardiovascular measurement and recording of blood pressure, heart rate, and activity in rat via radiotelemetry. *Clin. Exp. Hyper.* **3(5),** 885–895.

2. Kramer, K. and Kinter, L. B. (2003) Evaluation and applications of radio-telemetry in small laboratory animals. *Physiol. Genom.* **13(3),** 197–205.

3. Brockway, B. P., Mills, P. A., and Azar, S. H. (1991) A new method for continuous chronic measurement and recording of blood pressure, heart rate and activity in the rat via radio-telemetry. *Clin. Exp. Hyper.—Theory Practice* **A13(5),** 885–895.

4. Bazil, M. K., Krulan, C., and Webb, R. L. (1993) Telemetric monitoring of cardiovascular parameters in conscious spontaneously hypertensive rats. *J. Cardiovasc. Pharmacol.* **22(6),** 897–905.

5. Kramer, K. (2000) Applications and evaluation of radio-telemetry in small laboratory animals. Thesis, University of Utrecht, The Netherlands.

6. Van Acker, S. A. B. E., Kramer, K., Grimbergen, J. A., Van den Berg, D. J., Van der Vijgh, W. J. F., and Bast, A. (1995) Monohydroxyethylrutoside as protector against chronic doxorubicin-induced cardiotoxicity. *Br. J. Pharmacol.* **115,** 1260–1263.

7. Mills, P. A., Huetteman, D. A., Brockway, B. P., et al. (2000) A new method for measurement of blood pressure, heart rate, and activity in the mouse by radiotelemetry. *J. Appl. Physiol.* **88(5),** 1537–1544.

8. Abernathy, F. W., Flemming, C. D., and Sonntag, W. B. (1995) Measurement of cardiovascular response in male Sprague-Dawley rats using radiotelemetric implants and tail-cuff sphygmomonometry: A comparative study. *Toxicol. Meth.* **5(2),** 89–98.

9. Krege, J. H., Hodgin, J. B., Hagaman, J. R., and Smithies, O. A. (1995) A noninvasive computerized tail-cuff system for measuring blood pressure in mice. *Hypertension* **25,** 1111–1115.

10. Esther, C. R., Howard, T. E., Marino, E. M., Goddard, J. M., Capecchi, M. R., and Bernstein, K. E. (1996) Mice lacking angiotensin-converting enzyme have low blood pressure, renal pathology, and reduced male fertility. *Lab. Invest.* **74(5),** 953–965.

11. Gross, V., Lippoldt, A., and Luft, F. C. (1997) Pressure diuresis and natriuresis in DOCA-salt mice. *Kidney Int.* **25(5),** 1364–1368.

12. Schlager, G. and Sides, J. (1997) Characterization of hypertensive and hypotensive inbred strains of mice. *Lab. Anim. Sci.* **47(3),** 288–292.

13. Mattson, D. L. (1998) Long-term measurement of arterial blood pressure in conscious mice. *Am. J. Physiol.* **271(2 Pt 2),** R564–R570.

14. Bunag, R. D. (1983) Facts and fallacies about measuring blood pressure in rats. *Clin. Exper. Hyper.—Theory Practice* **A5(10),** 1959–1681.

15. Bunag, R. D., McCubbin, J. W., and Page, I. H. (1971) Lack of correlation between direct and indirect measurements of arterial pressure in un-anaesthetized rats. *Cardiovasc. Res.* **5,** 24–31.

16. Remie, R., Van Dongen, J. J., and Rensema, J. W. (1990) Permanent cannulation of the iliolumbar artery. In *Manual of Microsurgery on the Laboratory Rat. (1990)* van Dongen, J. J., Remie, R., Rensema, J. W., and van Wunnik, G. H. J., eds. Elsevier, Amsterdam, pp. 231–243.

17. Chen, X. M., Li, W. G., Yoshida, H., et al. (1997) Targeting deletion of angiotensin type 1B receptor gene in the mouse. *Am. J. Physiol.* **41(3),** F299–F304.

18. Desai, K. H., Sato, R., Schauble, E., Barsh, G. S., Kobilka, B. K., and Bernstein, D. (1997) Cardiovascular indexes in the mouse at rest and with exercise—new tool to study models of cardiac disease. *Am. J. Physiol.* **41(2),** H1053–H1061.

19. Oliverio, M. L., Best, C. F., Kim, H. S., Arendhorst, W. J., Smithies, O., and Coffman, T. M. (1997) Angiotensin II responses in AT(1A) receptor-deficient mice—A role for AT(1B) receptors in blood pressure regulation. *Am. J. Physiol.* **41(4),** F515–F520.

20. Wiesel, P., Mazzolai, L., Nussberger, J., and Pedrazzini, T. (1997) Two-kidney, one clip and one-kidney, one clip hypertension in mice. *Hypertension* **29(4)**, 1025–1030.

21. Balakrishnan, S., Tatchum-Talom, R., and McNeill, J. R. (1998) Radiotelemetric versus externalized catheter monitoring of blood pressure: effect of vasopressin in spontaneous hypertension. *J. Pharmacol. Toxicol. Meth.* **40(2)**, 87–93.

22. Butz, G. M. and Davisson, R. L. (2001) Long-term telemetric measurement of cardiovascular parameters in awake mice: a physiological genomics tool. *Physiol. Genom.* **5**, 89–97.

23. Guiol, C., Ledoussal, C., and Surge, J.-M. (1992) A radio-telemetry system for chronic measurement of blood pressure and heart rate in the unrestrained rat. Validation of the method. *J. Pharmacol. Toxicol. Meth.* **38**, 99–105.

24. Lemmer, B., Witte, K., Minors, D., and Waterhouse, J. (1995) Circadian rhythms of heart rate and blood pressure in four strains of rat: differences due to, and separate from, locomotor activity. *Biol. Rhythm Res.* **26(5)**, 493–504.

25. Van Vliet, B. N., Hu, L., Scott, T., Chafe, L., and Montani, J. -P. (1996) Cardiac hypertrophy and telemetered blood pressure 6 wk after baroreceptor denervation in normotensive rats. *Am. J. Physiol.* **271**, R1759–R1769.

26. Vleeming, W., Van de Kuil, A., Te Biesebeek, J. D., Meulenbelt, J., and Boink, A. B. T. J. (1997) Effect of nitrite on blood pressure in anaesthetized and free-moving rats. *Food Chem. Toxicol.* **35**, 615–619.

27. Irvine, R. J., White, J., and Chan, R. (1997) The influence of restraint on blood pressure in the rat. *J. Pharmacol. Toxicol. Meth.* **38**, 157–162.

28. Anderson, N. H., Devlin, A. M., Graham, D., et al. (1999) Telemetry for cardiovascular monitoring in a pharmacological study. New approaches to data analysis. *Hypertension* **33(part II)**, 248–255.

29. Kramer, K., Voss, H. -P., Grimbergen, J. A., et al. (2000) Telemetric monitoring of blood pressure in freely moving mice: A preliminary study. *Lab. Anim.* **34**, 272–280.

30. Davisson, R. L., Hoffmann, D. S., Butz, G. M., et al. (2002) Discovery of a spontaneous genetic mouse model of preeclampsia. *Hypertension* **39(2)**, 337–342.

31. Carlson, S. H. and Wyss, M. J. (2000) Long-term telemetric recording of arterial pressure and heart rate in mice fed basal and high NaCl diets. *Hypertension* **35**, e1–e5.

32. Barone, F. C., Knudsen, D. J., Nelson, A. H., Feuerstein, G. Z., and Willette, R. N. (1993) Mouse strain differences in susceptibility to cerebral ischemia are related to cerebral vascular anatomy. *J. Cereb. Blood Flow Metab.* **13(4)**, 683–692.

33. Ward, H.B., Baker, T. G., and McLaren, A. (1988) A histological study of the gonads of T16H/XSxr hermaphrodite mice. *J. Anat.* **158**, 65–75.

II

ASSESSMENT OF FREE RADICALS IN ENDOTHELIAL DYSFUNCTION

5

Analysis of Superoxide Anion Production in Tissue

Michela Zanetti, Livius V. d'Uscio, Timothy E. Peterson, Zvonimir S. Katusic, and Timothy O'Brien

Summary

Endothelial production of oxygen free radicals, especially superoxide anion (O_2^-), is an important mechanism of vascular dysfunction in hypertension. Overproduction of oxygen free radicals, mainly O_2^- occurs in human hypertension and in a wide variety of animal models. Thus, analysis of O_2^- generation represents a useful tool for identifying oxidative stress in hypertension. Among the methods used for O_2^- detection, the chemiluminescent probe lucigenin has been widely shown to be a useful method for detecting and quantifying the O_2^- formation. On the other hand, staining by the oxidative fluorescent probe dihydroethidine, which is freely permeable to cell membranes, is suitable to monitor *in situ* production of O_2^- and to provide a reliable marker of its intracellular presence. Dihydroethidine is oxidized in the presence of O_2^- to a fluorescent marker product, which is rapidly intercalated into DNA. Thus, nuclei are the primary fluorescent structures labeled. By simply incubating experimental samples in the presence of dihydroethidine followed by analysis of fluorescence, this method allows rapid and specific detection of intracellular oxidative stress due to superoxide anion generation.

Key Words: Superoxide anion; dihydroethidine; oxygen free radicals; oxidative stress.

1. Introduction

Reactive oxygen species (ROS) play a crucial role in the pathogenesis of vascular endothelial dysfunction. Among them, superoxide anion (O_2^-) is an important and powerful cellular oxidant that can induce vascular injury as well as mediate the production of other ROS such as hydrogen peroxide and peroxynitrite. Although many approaches to measuring O_2^- in chemical systems have been described *(1)*, its detection in intact tissues is difficult and prone to experimental artifacts. In fact, O_2^- is scarcely permeable to cell membranes and is confined within the cellular compartment where it is generated *(2)*. The objective of this chapter is to describe the procedure for the analysis of O_2^- production in tissues and cultured cells of hypertensive and atherosclerotic models, with emphasis on the technical aspects of each assay.

From: *Methods in Molecular Medicine, Vol. 108: Hypertension: Methods and Protocols*
Edited by: J. P. Fennell and A. H. Baker © Humana Press Inc., Totowa, NJ

The detection of O_2^- can be performed using a variety of assays. Unfortunately, the most sensitive and specific technique, electron spin resonance (ESR), is not readily available to many laboratories and requires labor-intensive methodologies *(3,4)*. Other assays such as the use of aconitase and cytochrome-*c* reduction may not be suitable for the detection of O_2^- in intact vessels and may also react with other ROS such that the specificity of these assays for O_2^- production may be questioned *(5,6)*. Recently, two assays have survived intense scrutiny in the literature and have emerged as the assays of choice for the general laboratory to measure O_2^- production in intact vessels. These include the lucigenin chemiluminescence assay (*see* Chapter 6) and the dihydroethidium fluorescence assay *(1)*.

The oxidative fluorescent probe dihydroethidium (also called hydroethidine, DHE) allows the detection of the cellular compartments of O_2^- generation in intact tissues. DHE is the sodium borohydride-reduced derivative of ethidium bromide *(7,8)*. This compound is a lipophilic cell-permeable dye that can be rapidly oxidized to ethidium bromide or a fluorescent marker product by O_2^- produced within the cell *(7,9,10)*. In the cytosol, DHE exhibits blue fluorescence (excitation$_{max}$ 365 nm, emission$_{max}$ 420 nm); however once this probe is oxidized to ethidium bromide by O_2^-, it binds to DNA and stains the cell nucleus red *(7,11)*. It has recently been demonstrated that DHE is oxidized to an unknown fluorescent molecule that is different from ethidium. This new product bound to DNA is fluorescent (emission$_{max}$ 567 nm) with 488-nm excitation *(10)*.

Previous work has been conducted to investigate the specificity of DHE for superoxide *(12–15)*. Dose–response studies have demonstrated that DHE does not undergo oxidation by singlet oxygen, hydroxyl radical, hydrogen peroxide, nitric oxide, and peroxynitrite. However, DHE oxidation by O_2^- will decrease rapidly in the presence of hydroxyl radical *(16)*. DHE and ethidium bromide are generally photostable under normal light *(12)*. However, photoconversion of DHE to ethidium bromide has been described following exposure to short-wavelength illumination and long exposures to full-spectrum UV light *(17)*. Thus, avoiding long exposures to normal illumination while handling is recommended. Exposure to high concentrations (>100 μM) of ethidium bromide results in acute cell toxicity, by interfering with mithochondrial respiration *(18)*. Nonetheless, the standard imaging conditions used for DHE staining to detect O_2^- production allow detection of ethidium bromide in the range between 10 nM and 30 μM, way below the range of ethidium toxicity *(12)*.

DHE is used for the detection and imaging of the cellular site of O_2^- generation in cultured cells and tissue samples. The assay basically includes DHE staining of biological samples and analysis of fluorescence (outlined under **Subheading 3.1.**) by confocal or fluorescence microscopy. Ethidium bromide or a fluorescent marker product derived from oxidation of DHE is stable for 1 h, which can be fixed into tissues *(7)* and used for end-point analyses *(12)*. The method is suitable to evaluate intracellular O_2^- production; extracellular generation of ethidium will be excluded provided that cell membranes remain intact, in accord with the use of ethidium in cell viability assays. Fluorescence intensity due to DHE oxidation is an indicator of the amount of O_2^- generated within the cell and a 1:1 molar ratio for the interaction of DHE with O_2^- has been reported *(19)*. However, this assay does not represent the method of choice to quantify O_2^- production *(20)* but is ideally used to demonstrate the cellular location of vascular O_2^- generation. So far, use of DHE for O_2^- detection has been described in flow cytometry *(9,11,21–25)*, in spectrofluorimetry *(5,26)*, and in digital imaging microphotography *(12–14,27–29)*.

The objective of this chapter is to describe procedure for O_2^- production in tissues of different animal models, and can easily be adapted to assay O_2^- production in cultured cells. The advances of DHE for detecting of O_2^-· production are (1) sensitivity and selectivity for O_2^-, and (2) cellular localization of O_2^- production, while lucigenin-enhanced chemiluminescence is useful for quantification of O_2^- production. The use of two independent methods for determining O_2^- production minimizes potential errors of assay interpretation.

2. Materials

1. Dihydroethidium. Store at –20°C. Air sensitive, use under a nitrogen or argon atmosphere. Although this compound is generally photostable compared with other fluorescent dyes, protection from light is recommended, especially when in solution. Under this form the compound is susceptible to oxidation. Prepare a fresh working stock for each new experiment. It is toxic, therefore use gloves when handling.
2. Dimethyl sulfoxide (DMSO).
3. Acetone.
4. Ethidium bromide. It is a mutagen, avoid contact and manipulate under hood.
5. Deionized water.
6. Fluorescence detection equipment—fluorescence microscope, camera, and image analysis software.
7. Phosphate-buffered saline (PBS).
8. Modified Krebs-Ringer bicarbonate solution: 118.3 mM NaCl, 4.7 mM KCl, 2.5 mM CaCl$_2$, 1.2 mM MgSO$_4$, 1.2 mM KH$_2$PO$_4$, 25.0 mM NaHCO$_3$, 0.026 mM calcium sodium EDTA, and 11.1 mM glucose, at pH 7.4.
9. 4% paraformaldehyde. Store at 4°C.
10. 1X Trypsin-EDTA. Store at 4°C.

3. Methods

3.1. Dihydroethidium Staining

3.1.1. Dihydroethidium Staining of Unfixed Frozen Tissue Sections

This section describes DHE staining of unfixed frozen tissue sections. Several modifications to this method can be performed to adapt DHE staining to different biological samples. Staining of fresh tissue (*see* **Subheading 3.1.2.**) and cultured cells (*see* **Subheading 3.1.3.**) are described below.

1. Prepare dihydroethidium as a fresh 1 M stock solution in DMSO, then dilute further to 2×10^{-6} M in acetone. Dilute pure DMSO in the same way (without dihydroethidium) in acetone; use this solution for the unlabeled sections.
2. Cut unfixed frozen tissue into 30-μm-thick sections and place them on glass slides. One extra section in each experimental group should be cut and exposed to the DHE-free solution (unlabeled samples) (*see* **Note 1**).
3. Apply topically dihydroethidium or DHE-free solutions on each section, covering the entire surface with fluid. Incubate sections in a light-protected humidified chamber at 37°C for 30 min (*see* **Note 2**).

3.1.2. Dihydroethidine Staining of Fresh Tissue

1. After harvesting, remove the surrounding connective tissue in ice-cold gassed (94% O_2 and 6% CO_2) modified Krebs-Ringer bicarbonate solution.
2. Cut into segments and place in warm (37°C) modified Krebs-Ringer bicarbonate solution for 30 min in plastic culture dishes (*see* **Note 1**).
3. After this period, remove Krebs solution and incubate samples with DHE diluted in Krebs (2×10^{-6} mol/L, stock solution prepared in DMSO) or DHE-free solution for 30 min at 37°C followed by a 15-min wash in DHE-free Krebs.
4. Split segments longitudinally and place them on a Krebs-moistened cover slip.

3.1.3. Dihydroethidine Staining of Adherent Cells

1. For adherent cells, DHE stock solution is prepared in DMSO, then further diluted in PBS to reach a final concentration of 2×10^{-6} M.
2. Remove medium, rinse twice with PBS, then incubate cells in PBS containing DHE at 37°C for 30 min.
3. Cells can then be rinsed and resuspended in PBS and the imaging protocol follows as described below.

3.2. Detection of Fluorescence

The next step in this process involves detection of fluorescence generated by DHE oxidation by O_2^-. This can be accomplished by the use of a fluorescent microscope equipped with an appropriate camera coupled with imaging software for data acquisition and eventually for calculation of emission fluorescence intensity of the samples. Details for analysis using flow cytometry or spectrofluorimetry are outlined in **Note 3**.

3.2.1. Preliminary Preparations

Turn on instrument and perform function checks according to manual.

3.2.2. Parameters

1. Consult manufacturer for optimal settings. These may vary according to instrument. Set instrument according to ethidium bromide optics parameters (excitation 488–510 nm; emission 590–620 nm) or fluorescent marker product (emission$_{max}$ 567 nm) (*10,12–14,29*).
2. After incubation, eliminate extra staining solution, cover slip, and place sections under the microscope. Depending on sections and type of tissue, a 10X–40X objective can be used. Analysis of unlabeled sections first for background autofluorescence image record is necessary (*see* **Note 4**).
3. Identical photomultiplier settings are used for image acquisition of all samples. Once developed, fluorescence due to DHE oxidation by O_2^- lasts for approx 60 min (*11*) (*see* **Note 5**).

4. Notes

1. The amount of vascular O_2^- production may be regulated by the intracellular and extracellular superoxide dismutase activity and in addition, there may be heterogeneity of superoxide dismutase activity in different vessels (*30*). Thus, a CuZn superoxide dismutase inhibitor sodium diethyldithiocarbamate (10 m*M*) can be added for a 30-min equilibration period.
2. In this protocol, a 37°C light-protected humidified chamber has been used for sample incubation. Since this piece of equipment may not always be available, an oven set at 37°C can be used; in this case, glass slides can be incubated on a covered tray. Remember to put a wet towel at the bottom of the tray, so that sections do not dry out.
3. Multiple analytical techniques can be utilized to detect changes in fluorescence following DHE staining in kinetic and end-point analyses. To this aim, methods such as flow cytometry (*9,11,21–25*) and spectrofluorimetry (*8,26*) have all proven to be very effective. For both flow cytometry and spectrofluorimetry, instrument settings are set as follows: excitation 488 nm with a 5-nm slit and emission 610 nm with a 20-nm slit. For flow cytometry, cells need to be in suspension. Adherent cells that physiologically do not grow in suspension can be stained as outlined under **Subheading 3.1.3.**, rinsed in PBS, trypsinized, and centrifuged at 150*g*, 4°C, for 5 min. After aspiration of trypsin, gently disrupt pellet by flicking tube on bottom of metal rack and resuspend cell pellet in PBS. Use 0.5 ml for small pellets, increasing to a maximum of 1 mL for larger pellets. Analysis of adherent cells in flow cytometry may be biased by disruption of cell

membrane due to manipulation for technical preparation. To avoid this problem simultaneous staining of an extra sample to assess cell viability (i.e., 10-μg/mL propidium iodide diluted in deionized water) in flow cytometry is strongly recommended.

4. Fluorescence detection sensitivity is severely compromised by background signals, which may originate from endogenous sample constituents (auto-fluorescence) or from nonspecifically bound probe. Selecting appropriate optical filters can minimize this problem.

5. When exposed to excitation light, the fluorescent dye fades within 60 min. In order to prevent this photobleach, ProLong antifade reagent (Molecular Probes) provides an excellent fluorescence stabilization and lasts for 24 h (unpublished observations).

Acknowledgments

Supported by National Heart, Lung, and Blood Institute grants HL-53524, HL-58080, HL-66958, and the Mayo Foundation. The authors thank Dr. E. Roder for helpful assistance during preparation of the manuscript.

References

1. Münzel, T., Afanas'ev I. B., Kleschyov, A. L., and Harrison D. G. (2002) Detection of superoxide in vascular tissue. *Arterioscler. Thromb. Vasc. Biol.* **22,** 1761–1768.

2. Lynch, R. E. and Fridovich I. (1978) Permeation of the erythrocyte stroma by superoxide radical. *J. Biol. Chem.* **253,** 4697–4699.

3. Xia Y. and Zweier J. L. (1997) Superoxide and peroxynitrite generation from inducible nitric oxide synthase in macrophages. *Proc. Natl. Acad. Sci. USA* **94,** 6954–6958.

4. Xia Y., Tsai A. L., Berka V., and Zweier J. L. (1998) Superoxide generation from endothelial nitric-oxide synthase. A Ca^{2+}/calmodulin-dependent and tetrahydrobiopterin regulatory process. *J. Biol. Chem.* **273,** 25804–25808.

5. Barbacanne, M. A., Souchard, J. P., Darblade, B., et al. (2000) Detection of superoxide anion released extracellularly using cytochrome c reduction, ESR, fluorescence and lucigenin-enhanced chemiluminescence techniques. *Free Radic. Biol. Med.* **29,** 388–396.

6. Gardner, P. R., Rainieri, I., Epstein, L. B., and White, C. W. (1995) Superoxide radical and iron modulate aconitase activity in mammalian cells. *J. Biol. Chem.* **270,** 13399–13405.

7. Bucana, C., Saiki, I., and Nayar, R. (1986) Uptake and accumulation of the vital dye hydroethidine in neoplastic cells. *J. Histochem. Cytochem.* **34,** 1109–1115.

8. Gallop, P. M., Paz, M. A., Henson, E., and Latt, S. A. (1984) Dynamic approaches to the delivery of reporter reagents into living cells. *Bio. Techniques* **2,** 32–36.

9. Rothe G. and Valet G. (1990) Flow cytometric analysis of respiratory burst activity in phagocytes with hydroethidine and 2',7'-dichlorofluorescin. *J. Leukoc. Biol.* **47,** 440–448.

10. Zhao, H., Kalivendi, S., Zhang, H., et al. (2003) Superoxide reacts with hydroethidine but forms a fluorescent product that is distinctly different from ethidium: potential implications in intracellular fluorescence detection of superoxide. *Free Radic. Biol. Med.* **34,** 1359–1368.

11. Carter, W. O., Narayanan, P. K., and Robinson, J. P. (1994) Intracellular hydrogen peroxide and superoxide anion detection in endothelial cells. *J. Leuk. Biol.* **55,** 253–258.

12. Bindokas, V. P., Jordan, J., Lee, C. C., and Miller, R. J. (1996) Superoxide production in rat hippocampal neurons: selective imaging with hydroethidine. *J. Neurosci.* **16,** 1324–1336.

13. Miller, F. J., Jr., Gutterman, D. D., Rios, C. D., Heistad D. D., and Davidson, B. L. (1998) Superoxide production in vascular smooth muscle contributes to oxidative stress and impaired relaxation in atherosclerosis. *Circ. Res.* **82,** 1298–1305.

14. Suzuki, H., Swei, A., Zweifach, B. W., and Schmid-Schonbein, G. W. (1995) In vivo evidence for microvascular oxidative stress in spontaneously hypertensive rats. Hydorethidine microfluorography. *Hypertension* **25,** 1083–1089.

15. Vanden Hoek, T. L., Li, C., Shao, Z., Schumacker, P. T., and Becker, L. B. (1997) Significant levels of oxidants are generated by isolated cardiomyocytes during ischemia prior to reperfusion. *J. Mol. Cell Cardiol.* **29,** 2571–2583.

16. Prutz W. A. (1984) Inhibition of DNA-ethidium bromide intercalation due to free radical attack upon DNA. *Radiat. Environ. Biophys.* **23,** 1–18.

17. Swannell, R. P. J., Caplin, R., Nedwell, D. B., and Williamson, F. A. (1992) An investigation of hydroethidine as a flurescent vital stain for prokaryotes. *FEMS Microbiol Lett.* **101,** 173–182.

18. Miko, M. and Chance, B. (1975) Ethidium bromide as an uncoupler of oxidative phosphorylation. *FEBS Lett.* **54,** 347–352.

19. Biziukin, A. V. and Korkina, L. G. (1994) Use of the fluorescent indicator hydroethidine to study the oxidative metabolism of phagocytes. *Klin. Lab. Diagn.* **1,** 41–42.

20. Benov, L., Sztejnberg, L., and Fridovich, I. (1998) Critical evaluation of the use of hydroethidine as a measure of superoxide anion radical. *Free Radic. Biol. Med.* **25,** 826–831.

21. Edwards, B. S., Kuckuck, F., and Sklar L. A. (1999) Plug flow cytometry: An automated coupling device for rapid sequential flow cytometric sample analysis. *Cytometry* **37,** 156–159.

22. Filatov, M. V., Varfolomeeva, E. Y., Ivanovm, and E. I. (1995) Flow cytofluorometric detection of inflammatory processes by measuring respiratory burst reaction of peripheral blood neutrophils. *Biochem. Mol. Med.* **55,** 116–121.

23. Olive, P. L. (1989) Hydroethidine: a fluorescent redox probe for locating hypoxic cells in spheroids and murine tumours. *Br. J. Cancer* **60,** 332–338.

24. Perticarari, S., Presani, G., Mangiarotti, M. A., and Banfi E. (1991) Simultaneous flow cytometric method to measure phagocytosis and oxidative products by neutrophils. *Cytometry* **12,** 687–693.

25. Shi T., Eaton A. M., and Ring D. B. (1991) Selection of hybrid hybridomas by flow cytometry using a new combination of fluorescent vital stains. *J. Immunol. Methods* **141,** 165–175.

26. Saiki I., Bucana C. D., Tsao J. Y., and Fidler I. J. (1986) Quantitative fluorescent microassay for identification of antiproliferative compounds. *J. Natl. Cancer Inst.* **77,** 1235–1240.
27. Becker, L. B., Vanden Hoek, T. L., Shao, Z. H., Li, C. Q., and Schumacker, P. T. (1999) Generation of superoxide in cardiomyocytes during ischemia before reperfusion. *Am. J. Physiol.* **277,** H2240–H2246.
28. Frisbee J. C. and Stepp D. W. (2001) Impaired NO-dependent dilation of skeletal muscle arterioles in hypertensive diabetic obese Zucker rats. *Am. J. Physiol.* **281,** H1304–H1311.
29. Zanetti, M., d'Uscio, L. V., Kovesdi, I., Katusic Z. S., and O'Brien T. (2003) In vivo gene transfer of inducible nitric oxide synthase to carotid arteries from hypercholesterolemic rabbits. *Stroke* **34,** 1293–1298.
30. Brandes, R. P., Barton, M., Philippens, K. M., Schweitzer, G., and Mügge, A. (1997) Endothelial-derived superoxide anions in pig coronary arteries: evidence from lucigenin chemiluminescence and histochemical techniques. *J. Physiol.* **500,** 331–342.

6

Measurement of Vascular Reactive Oxygen Species Production by Chemiluminescence

Tomasz J. Guzik and Keith M. Channon

Summary

Reactive oxygen species (ROS) play important roles in the pathogenesis of vascular disease states. In particular, superoxide anion participates in endothelial dysfunction mainly owing to its rapid interaction with NO, but also as it causes direct biological effects and serves as a progenitor for many other ROS. Detection of ROS in intact tissues and cells is much more difficult than in chemical systems. We describe advantages and potential pitfalls of chemiluminescent methods of vascular ROS detection. Lucigenin and luminol-enhanced chemiluminescent methods are described in the detection of vascular superoxide and peroxynitrite production and NAD(P)H oxidase activity. We also describe the use of new chemiluminescent probes, including cypridina luciferin analogs (coelenterazine; CLA and MCLA) and pholasin. The validity of some of these chemiluminescent methods (in particular lucigenin-enhanced chemiluminescence) recently has been questioned. It has been suggested that lucigenin itself, especially at high concentrations (>50 µmol/L), may produce superoxide via redox cycling. Using intact human vascular rings and vascular homogenates, we show that lucigenin, particularly at lower concentrations (5 µmol/L), provides an accurate assessment of the rate of superoxide production as assessed by close correlations with the SOD inhibitable ferricytochrome c reduction assay. Chemiluminescent techniques provide a useful approach for vascular ROS measurements, but should be always interpreted in the context of measurements obtained using other complementary techniques.

Key Words: Reactive oxygen intermediates; superoxide; peroxynitrite; chemiluminescence; lucigenin; NADPH oxidase; endothelial dysfunction; vessel; human; luminol; nitric oxide; homogenate; vascular ring; endothelium; method.

1. Introduction

Reactive oxygen species (ROS) produced by vascular cells, including endothelial cells, vascular smooth muscle cells, and adventitial fibroblasts, play important roles in the physiology and pathology of vascular wall (*1*). Superoxide production is increased in vascular pathologies including hypertension,

From: *Methods in Molecular Medicine, Vol. 108: Hypertension: Methods and Protocols*
Edited by: J. P. Fennell and A. H. Baker © Humana Press Inc., Totowa, NJ

hypercholesterolemia, and diabetes. Reliable measurements of superoxide production in vascular tissues are therefore critical for understanding the mechanisms of vascular dysfunction in various pathologies.

Increasing interest in the roles of reactive oxygen species in the regulation of vascular and endothelial function requires measurement of reactive oxygen species production in a specific, sensitive, and practically convenient manner *(2)*. Several approaches to measure reactive oxygen species, including electron paramagnetic resonance (EPR) or ferricytochrome-*c* reduction assay can be successfully applied in immune cells in which reactive oxygen species production occurs at very high levels, as an oxidative burst, following appropriate stimulations. In blood vessels (and to a lesser extent in cultured vascular cells), in which reactive oxygen species production occurs constitutively at much lower levels, many of these methods are limited by insufficient sensitivity and other practical considerations

1.1. Chemiluminescent Probes

Chemiluminescent probes are small molecules that can cross plasma membranes and detect intracellular reactive oxygen species, providing sensitive and convenient alternatives to the nonchemiluminescent methods. Chemiluminescent detection of reactive oxygen species is based on the interaction between selected reactive oxygen species and a chemiluminescent probe with the emission of photons that can be detected by luminometer or a scintillation counter. The exact stoichiometry of these reactions is not uniform, so it is not advised to use chemiluminescent methods for absolute quantitation of reactive oxygen species production. However, chemiluminescent methods do provide very powerful techniques for accurate quantitative comparisons of reactive oxygen species production in vascular tissues and cells. Chemiluminescent methods also allow accurate determination of basal, unstimulated vascular superoxide production in intact vascular segments, which makes them suited to reactive oxygen species measurements that are closer to physiological conditions—for example, with intact nitric oxide production from the endothelium. Measurement of "real-time" superoxide production also allows investigation of the effects of different agents such as oxidase inhibitors or substrates in a convenient manner. However, chemiluminescent techniques should be used as one approach to vascular reactive oxygen species determination that is complemented and validated by other techniques such as ferricytochrome-*c* reduction assays or dihydroethidium fluorescence in frozen sections *(2)* (*see* Chapter 5). Several chemiluminescent probes have been used for detection of reactive oxygen species; the most commonly used are lucigenin and luminol (*see* **Table 1**). Lucigenin is relatively specific for detection of superoxide, although reduc-

Table 1
Detection of Reactive Oxygen Species by Chemiluminescence

Chemiluminescent probe	Reactive oxygen species detected
Lucigenin	Superoxide
Luminol	Peroxynitrite, superoxide, hydrogen peroxide*
Coelenterazine	Peroxynitrite, superoxide*
CLA, MCLA	Superoxide, peroxynitrite*
Pholasin	Superoxide, peroxynitrite, ? hydrogen peroxide*

*Appropriate control experiments with suitable inhibitors need to be performed to determine which of the radicals are being detected under specific experimental conditions (**Table 3**).

tants such as dithionite may cause lucigenin to emit light without superoxide. Luminol has been used for detection of superoxide anion, peroxynitrite as well as hydrogen peroxide. Other newer probes include the cypridina luciferin analogs coelenterazine, CLA, and MCLA, which are less commonly used but are considered relatively specific for superoxide anion. Pholasin has been used introduced recently, but its specificity for reactive oxygen species in vascular applications is not fully determined.

1.2. Luminometer Type and Setup

Either single-tube or multichannel luminometers or scintillation counters can be used for chemiluminescent detection of vascular reactive oxygen species. Most currently available luminometers are provided with a computerized system for online monitoring of luminescence in response to addition of various substrates or stimulants (**Fig. 1**). We recommend that single-tube luminometers are used for basal measurements from intact cells or vessels. Although these assays are more laborious (one measurement usually takes around 30 min), they provide the higher sensitivity that is required for basal reactive oxygen species production from vascular tissues. Multichannel luminometers offer greatly increased throughput, but compromise sensitivity (*see* **Note 1**).

1.3. Lucigenin-Enhanced Chemiluminescence

Lucigenin (*bis-N*-methylacridinium) has been employed extensively to study superoxide generation from vascular tissues *(3)*, spermatozoa, chondrocytes, macrophages, and hepatocytes *(4)*. Lucigenin-enhanced chemiluminescence has been used to assess xanthine oxidase *(5)*, NADPH oxidase in phagocytic and vascular cells *(6,7)*, and to monitor mitochondrial superoxide production in intact cells *(8)*.

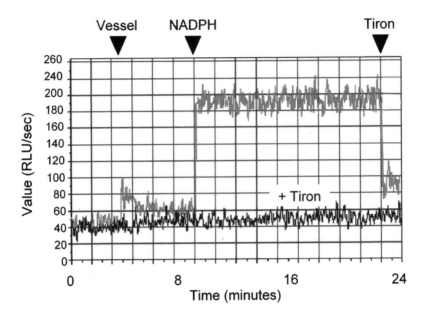

Fig. 1. Example recording of lucigenin-enhanced chemiluminescence. Segments of human saphenous vein were trimmed from excess of adventitia and equilibrated in oxygenated Krebs-HEPES buffer at 37°C. After recording background reading, the vessel was added to the vial containing Krebs-HEPES with lucigenin (5 μ*M*) in a 30-mL scintillation vial in a Berthold FB12 single-tube luminometer. Chemiluminescence was recorded using dedicated software. Then NADPH (100 μ*M*; as a substrate) was administered, resulting in increased chemiluminescence, following which recording was paused and Tiron (1 m*M*) added to the vial. The lower line shows chemiluminescence from a similar vessel preincubated with Tiron prior to measurement and stimulation with NADPH.

To detect superoxide, lucigenin is first reduced to produce the lucigenin cation radical (*see* **Fig. 2**). Superoxide is then capable of reducing lucigenin cation to dioxetane, which decomposes, producing two molecules of N-methylacridone, one of which is in the excited state and emits photon upon relaxation to ground state. Measurement of the photon emission from this reaction allows for very sensitive determination of superoxide generation.

Use of lucigenin-enhanced chemiluminescence for the detection of superoxide has several advantages over other available methods, but it may also suffer from certain pitfalls as discussed later (*see* **Table 2**). One of the major advantages is high specificity for superoxide anion. Unlike other chemiluminescent probes, lucigenin does not produce light in response to peroxynitrite, hydrogen peroxide, or hydroxide anions.

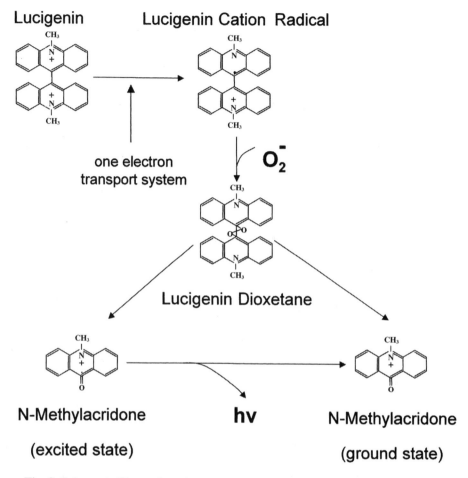

Fig. 2. Schematic illustration of the reaction pathway leading to lucigenin-enhanced chemiluminescence. Lucigenin is first reduced, usually by the same biological system that produces superoxide. Superoxide anion (O_2^-) reacts with reduced lucigenin to generate a photon (*h*ν).

The potential limitations of lucigenin have been highlighted by several authors, with the caution that lucigenin may undergo redox cycling, resulting in artificial generation of superoxide anion, especially in conditions of high biological oxidoreductase activity (reviewed in **ref. 2**). The true importance of redox cycling has been controversial, but most investigators believe that at low concentrations of lucigenin (less than 20 μ*M*), redox cycling does not invalidate measurements.

2. Materials

1. Krebs-HEPES buffer: 99 mM NaCl, 4.7 mM KCl, 1.2 mM MgSO$_4$, 1 mM KH$_2$PO$_4$, 1.9 mM CaCl$_2$, 25 mM NaHCO$_3$, 11.1 mM glucose, and 20 mM HEPES, pH 7.44 (stable at 4 °C for 7 d).

2. Krebs-Henseleit buffer: 120 mM NaCl, 4.7 mM KCl, 1.2 mM MgSO$_4$, 1.2 mM KH$_2$PO$_4$, 2.5 mM CaCl$_2$, 25 mM NaHCO$_3$, and 5.5 mM glucose.

3. Chemiluminescent probes: lucigenin (Sigma); luminol (Sigma); CLA; coelenterazine (Molecular Probes); pholasin (Knight Scientific, UK). These probes are light sensitive; 100X stock solutions of lucigenin and luminol should be prepared in Krebs HEPES buffer fresh for each experiment (heat to 37°C to dissolve well). Stock solutions (1000X) of CLA, coelenterazine, or pholasin should be made up and aliquots should immediately be stored at –20°C. Do not refreeze.

4. Oxidase substrates (NADH; NADPH; xanthine; arachidonic acid). NADH and NADPH stock solutions should be made in Krebs-HEPES buffer as required; store at 4°C. Xanthine is difficult to dissolve—it should be prepared as 10 mM stock in Krebs-Hepes buffer. Add NaOH to dissolve, heat to 37°C, and then titrate back to pH 7.4.

5. Oxidase inhibitors (diphenyliodonium chloride [DPI]; apocynin; allopurinol; rotenone; Sigma). 1000X stock solutions should be prepared in dimethyl sulfoxide DMSO by vigorous shaking; stable at 4°C for up to 2 mo. L-NAME, L-NMMA (Calbiochem)-Prepare in double-distilled water; store at 4°C and –20°C, respectively.

6. Superoxide scavengers: Superoxide dismutase (SOD); PEG-SOD; Tiron; Mn(III)tetrakis (4-benzoic acid) porphyrin chloride (MnTBAP) (Sigma).

7. Protease inhibitors (e.g., Complete; Roche, or similar).

8. Phenylmethylsulfonyl fluoride (PMSF; Sigma).

9. Homogenization buffer: 20 mM HEPES buffer containing 10 mM EDTA, containing protease inhibitors and PMSF (1 mM).

10. Luminometer: either single-tube (e.g.- Berthold FB12) or multichannel.

11. Plastic 30-mL scintillation vials (Beckmann).

3. Methods

3.1. Chemiluminescence Measurements From Blood Vessels and Cells

Vascular reactive oxygen species can be determined by chemiluminescence from intact blood vessels or intact cells or from vascular homogenates.

3.1.1. Intact Blood Vessels

1. Harvest blood vessels carefully and store in Krebs-HEPES buffer on ice until directly prior to measurement. Flush the vessel lumen delicately immediately after harvest, to remove blood, and dissect away excess adipose tissue from the adventitia, using micro instruments. Cut into equal rings of appropriate size (*see* **Note 2**).

2. Following storage on ice, gently cut open individual vessel rings longitudinally to expose the endothelial surface and equilibrate in Krebs-HEPES buffer at 37°C for 30 min immediately before measuring. We prefer to use oxygenated buffer (bubbled with 95% O_2, 5% CO_2) during equilibration, and keep the vessel and buffer in semidark conditions inside a closed water bath.

3. Place 2 mL prewarmed Krebs-HEPES buffer into the luminometer vial, then add an appropriate volume of stock solution of lucigenin to achieve the desired final concentration (*see* **Subheadings 1.3.** and **3.1.4.**). Allow dark adaptation by recording background luminescence for 5 min; levels should fall to virtually undetectable levels within 1–2 min. Working in a semidark environment, and in particular avoiding direct illumination of the work area by fluorescent lighting, minimizes the need for prolonged adaptation of solutions when placed in the luminometer.

4. Pause recording and add the vessel ring to the vial. After a 20-s delay to allow decay of light-stimulated chemiluminescence, recommence recording for 10 min. During this time the "basal" chemiluminescence should rise to a plateau within a few minutes.

5. In order to measure maximal NADPH oxidase activity, pause the recording, and add small volumes of stock solutions of either NADH (100 μM), NADPH (100 μM), or other oxidase substrates directly to the luminometer vial, mix very gently, then record for an additional 10 or 15 min, after a 20-s delay.

6. At the end of the recording period, specificity for superoxide can be checked by the addition of SOD (450 U/mL final concentration) or the superoxide scavenger Tiron (10 mM) into the vial. This approach typically results in only partial (70 to 80%) inhibition of the signal, due to limited tissue penetration. Separate experiments where a superoxide scavenger is preincubated with the vessel ring, and is present in the assay vial, are preferred if quantitative comparisons are required.

7. After measurements, retrieve vessel samples from the luminometer vials, place in open Eppendorf tubes, and dry overnight in a 60°C oven or heating block. Weigh the dried tissue specimens.

8. Obtain mean chemiluminescent readings during the plateau phase of each recording period, subtract the background reading and express the integrated values (relative light units [RLU]/s) of chemiluminescence and per milligram of dry weight. This method of expressing readings from chemiluminescence is widely used in the literature (*9,10*) and is generally more reproducible than wet (fresh) vessel weight (*see* **Note 2**).

3.1.2. Intact Cells

1. To achieve uniform experimental conditions, culture cells without fetal calf serum (FCS) for at least 24 h prior to measurements, as FCS may contain substances that may either stimulate (such as angiotensin II) or inhibit (such as steroid hormones) cellular reactive oxygen species production. Note that phenol red may possess some estrogen-like properties. Similarly, growth phase and the degree of confluence may substantially affect reactive oxygen species generation, and should be determined in preliminary experiments for each cell type.

2. In experiments involving inhibitors such as PEG-SOD, add to the cultures at least 6 h prior to the measurements to achieve complete intracellular penetration of this compound.

3. For reactive oxygen species determinations from cell suspensions, wash monolayers in Krebs-HEPES buffer, briefly trypsinize cells (0.1% trypsin in PBS) to release from the dish, pipet to disperse well, wash in Krebs-HEPES, and remove residual medium and trypsin by centrifugation and resuspension in Krebs-HEPES. For uniformity, allow cells to incubate for at least 30 min at 4°C prior to measurements. Count cell number in the suspension, and aliquot an equal number of cells for use in each of the parallel experiments. The optimal number of cells to be used needs to be individually determined for each cell type, as described for vessel weight in **Note 2**. Add the aliquot of cells into the prepared luminometer vial, and proceed with reactive oxygen species recording as described under **Subheading 3.1.1.**

4. For determinations of basal reactive oxygen species production in cells grown in monolayers, cells should be passaged into 6- or 12-well plates containing a round glass cover slip, and allowed to grow to appropriate confluence as described above. Prior to reactive oxygen species determination, wash cell monolayers gently in cold Krebs-HEPES, and maintain the plate at 4°C. Carefully pick up cover slips from the wells using a needle with a bent tip, then transfer the cover slips, cell side up, using fine forceps, into the prepared luminometer vial, and proceed with reactive oxygen species recording as described under **Subheading 3.1.1.**

5. For cells stimulated with appropriate substrates (e.g., PMA, NADPH) *(11)*, chemiluminescent signals may be sufficient to use cells grown directly in a mulitplate format, or cell suspensions aliquoted into multiple wells, in a multi-channel luminometer (*see* **Subheading 1.2.**).

3.1.3. Vascular/Cell Homogenates

Measurements of reactive oxygen species (in particular superoxide anion) may be performed using protein homogenates prepared from vascular tissue or cells. This approach is especially valuable for the determination of maximal oxidase activity following stimulations with oxidase substrates. The method is not limited by penetration of substrates or inhibitors into intact tissue or cells, and multiple parallel experiments may be performed from homogenates prepared from a single pool of tissue or cells.

1. Snap-freeze vessel tissue sample or pelleted cells in liquid nitrogen immediately after harvest and washing to remove residual blood or medium, and store at –80°C. On the day of measurement, homogenize on ice in 20 mM HEPES buffer containing 1 mM EDTA, protease inhibitors (complete; Roche), and PMSF (1 mM). Pellet tissue debris at 800g for 10 min, and retain the supernatant for further analysis.

2. Determine protein concentrations to allow equalization for protein content. Homogenates should be diluted with buffer to equalize protein concentrations in

each of the samples to be compared. Homogenates may be stored for up to 8 h at 4°C. These should not be freeze-thawed, as this leads to significant loss of oxidase activity.

3. After recording background readings from 2 mL Krebs-HEPES buffer containing an appropriate concentration of lucigenin, add a portion of the protein homogenate and measure chemiluminescence as described under **Subheading 3.1.1.** Substrates for various oxidases (NADPH, 100 μM; NADH-100 μM; xanthine 1 μM; succinate, 3 μM) may be added after recording basal reactive oxygen species generation, and the resulting chemiluminescence recorded for an additional 10 min. For protein homogenates, stimulated with appropriate substrates (e.g., NADPH), chemiluminescent signals may be sufficient to use a multiplate format in a multichannel luminometer (*see* **Subheading 1.2.** and **Note 1**).

4. The quantity of tissue or cell protein homogenate used in each assay needs to be determined in preliminary experiments to ensure that the response is quantitative and linear across the range of protein quantity used, in both basal and stimulated conditions. Activity in a specific fraction of the total homogenate (e.g., total, membrane-associated, cytosolic) may be measured by subcellular fractionation of protein homogenates by centrifugation.

3.1.4. Concentrations of Lucigenin for Reactive Oxygen Species Detection Assays

Early studies of superoxide production by lucigenin-enhanced chemiluminescence typically used either 250 μM or 500 μM final lucigenin concentration. As a result of suggestions that at these high concentrations lucigenin undergoes redox cycling resulting in artificial self-generation of superoxide in the presence tissues, lower concentrations of lucigenin (5–20 μM) are recommended for vascular superoxide determinations *(6,7)*. Using 5 μM lucigenin decreases sensitivity, but avoids significant redox cycling. In order to increase sensitivity higher concentrations of lucigenin such as 20 or even 50 μM may be used (*see* **Fig. 3**). We measured superoxide production in parallel using 5, 20, 50, and 250 μM lucigenin in both protein homogenates and intact vessel segments of human saphenous vein obtained from patients undergoing coronary artery bypass surgery, showing a close correlation despite the difference in lucigenin concentration (**Figs. 4** and **5**). Thus, lucigenin appears to provide a valid approach to measuring the relative magnitude of superoxide production, in a linear and quantitative fashion, in any one experimental system. However, the quantitative nature of this relationship may vary greatly under different conditions in different systems *(2)* (*see also* **Note 2**). Nevertheless, the potential problem of redox cycling of lucigenin should always be critically addressed, and findings should ideally be validated using independent methods such as SOD inhibitable ferricytochrome-*c* reduction measurements and/ or EPR or dihydroethidium staining.

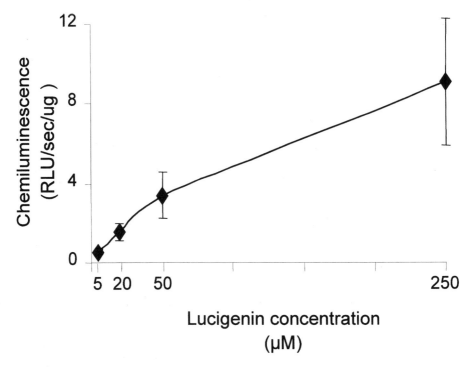

Fig. 3. Effect of lucigenin concentrations on chemiluminescence recorded from vascular homogenates. Lucigenin-enhanced chemiluminescence was measured from serial aliquots of vascular protein homogenate (50 µg) stimulated with NADH (100 µM), using concentrations of lucigenin ranging from 5 to 250 µM) (horizontal axis) dissolved in Krebs-HEPES buffer (n = 6 experiments). Chemiluminescence was recorded for 10 min, averaged, and, after subtracting background, expressed as RLU/s/µg of protein.

3.2. Measurement of Vascular Reactive Oxygen Species Using Other Chemiluminescent Probes

Several other chemiluminescent probes may be used for determination of reactive oxygen species production from tissues, cells, or homogenates, in exactly the same way as described for lucigenin under **Subheadings 3.1.1.– 3.1.3.** These probes can be used to measure different reactive oxygen species species, with varying specificity, under different conditions (**Table 2**).

3.2.1. Luminol-Enhanced Chemiluminescence

While lucigenin-enhanced chemiluminescence appears to be specific for superoxide, luminol has been shown to interact with numerous reactive oxygen species produced in vascular tissues or cells (including peroxynitrite,

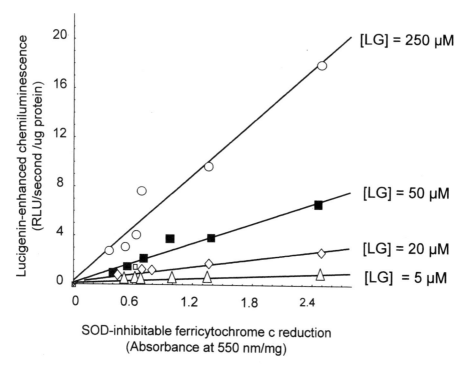

Fig. 4. Relationship between lucigenin-enhanced chemiluminescence and ferricytochrome-*c* reduction assays (protein homogenates). Superoxide generation from saphenous vein homogenates stimulated with NADH were compared using lucigenin-enhanced chemiluminescence (in concentrations of 5, 20, 50, or 250 μ*M*) with measurements conducted using SOD-inhibitable ferricytochrome-*c* reduction assay (80 μ*M* ferricytochrome-*c*; 400 U/mL SOD). Increasing lucigenin concentration progressively increased the chemiluminescence signal, but the relationship with ferricytochrome-*c* reduction remained linear across the range of lucigenin concentrations tested.

superoxide, hydrogen peroxide, and hydroxyl radical). Luminol reacts with reactive oxygen species to yield an unstable luminol endoperoxide that generates light. Predominant reactive oxygen species species detected by luminol may vary in relation to experimental conditions. Therefore it is vital to characterize luminol-enhanced chemiluminescence using a panel of specific inhibitors and stimulants before using it in experimental comparisons (**Table 3**).

3.2.1.1. LUMINOL-ENHANCED CHEMILUMINESCENCE IN VASCULAR TISSUES

Luminol-enhanced chemiluminescence can be performed using fresh vascular segments in a manner similar to those described for lucigenin-enhanced chemiluminescence *(12–14)* (**Subheading 3.4.1.**), except using 500 μ*M*

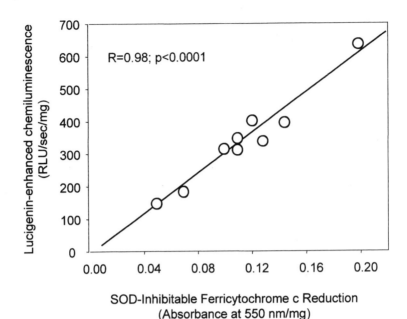

Fig. 5. Relationship between lucigenin-enhanced chemiluminescence and ferricytochrome-*c* reduction assays (intact vessels). Correlation of measurements of NADH-stimulated superoxide generation measured from intact blood vessels using lucigenin (5 μ*M*) enhanced chemiluminescence with SOD-inhibitable ferricyto-chrome-*c* reduction assay. Experiments were performed on consecutive segments of saphenous vein obtained from nine patients undergoing coronary artery bypass surgery *(3)*.

Table 2
Advantages and Disadvantages of Lucigenin-Enhanced Chemiluminescence for Detection of Vascular Superoxide Production

Advantages	Disadvantages
Access to intracellular sites of superoxide production	Requirement for initial one-electron reduction by biological system (Luc to Luc^{+2})
Specificity for superoxide	
Sensitivity higher than other methods	Possibility of auto-oxidation of Luc^+
Minimal cellular toxicity	at high concentrations
Convenient, simple and rapid assay	
Possibility of online measurement of changes in superoxide production	

Table 3
Methods That May Be Used in Discrimination of The Most Common Sources of Luminol-Enhanced Chemiluminescence in Vascular Tissues

Reactive oxygen species detected	Characterization of luminol-enhanced chemiluminescence
Superoxide	Inhibition by SOD or SOD mimetic
	Often increased in response to NOS inhibitors
	(may be inhibition in conditions of NOS dysfunction)
	Inhibition by NO donors
	No inhibition by catalase
Peroxynitrite	Scavenging by uric acid and ebselen
	Inhibition by SODor SOD mimetic
	Inhibition by NOS inhibitors
	Increase by NO donors* (often concomitant stimulation of
	superoxide release by NADPH or PMA is required)
	No inhibition by catalase
Hydrogen peroxide	Inhibition by catalase
	Often inhibition by SOD and SOD mimetics

*A large NO excess can inhibit peroxynitrite-dependent luminol-enhanced chemiluminescence.

luminol in 2 mL of Krebs-Henseleit buffer. To validate specificity of luminol-enhanced chemiluminescence for peroxynitrite, control measurements in the presence of the peroxynitrite scavenger ebselen (50 μM), the superoxide scavenger Tiron (10 mM), or catalase (1000 U/mL) to remove hydrogen peroxide should be included in the protocol (**Table 3**).

3.2.1.2. Peroxynitrite Measurements Using Luminol-Enhanced Chemiluminescence

In human blood vessels, luminol-enhanced chemiluminescence is significantly inhibited by NOS inhibitors (100 µM L-NAME and 100 µM L-NMMA), as well as by superoxide scavengers (400 U/mL SOD; 10 mM Tiron). It was also almost completely abolished by ebselen (50 µM) or urate (250 µM) (15). These data suggest that luminol-enhanced chemiluminescence largely reflects peroxynitrite formation in human vessels. Recently, similar observations were described for mouse aorta (16), indicating again that luminol-enhanced chemiluminescence mainly reflects peroxynitrite formation.

3.2.2 Cypridina Luciferin Analogs

3.2.2.1. COELENTERAZINE (2-(4-HYDROXYBENZYL)-6-(4-HYDROXYPHENYL)-8-BENZYL-3,7-DIHYDROIMIDAZO [1,2-A]PYRAZIN-3-ONE)

Coelenterazine is a very sensitive chemiluminescent probe that has been recommended by Tarpey and colleagues to detect superoxide anion *(17)*. Coelenterazine is highly sensitive and appears less susceptible than lucigenin to artificially-enhanced luminescence, but it may not be specific and can interact with peroxynitrite. Coelenterazine was used in concentrations of 5–50 μ*M* in PBS buffer to measure chemiluminescence from intact vascular rings and cells in culture *(17)*. We found that coelenterazine is characterized by 100–1000-fold higher background chemiluminescence than lucigenin (even at high concentrations). This background can be reduced 10-fold by addition of EDTA (100 μ*M*) and desferroxamine (100 μ*M*) and in some experiments DETC (100 μ*M*) in the PBS buffer. Coelenterazine (10 μ*M*) gives very high sensitivity; basal chemiluminescence from vascular rings is 100-fold higher than with lucigenin. These signals are significantly inhibited by Tiron (10 m*M*; by 40%) but in contrast to lucigenin-enhanced chemiluminescence are not consistently inhibited by preincubation with PEG-SOD. It may be necessary to preincubate the tissues in PBS containing EDTA and desferroxamine (100 μ*M*) to improve the characteristics of vascular coelenterazine chemiluminescence. A recent study indicates that there is a very strong correlation between superoxide production measured using either coelenterazine or lucigenin-enhanced chemiluminescence *(18)*.

3.2.2.2. CLA (2-METHYL-6-PHENYL-3,7-DIHYDROIMIDAZO [1,2-A]PYRAZIN-3-ONE) AND MCLA (2-METHYL-6-(4-METHOXYPHENYL)-3,7-DIHYDROIMIDAZO [1,2-A]PYRAZIN-3-ONE)

CLA and MCLA have similar properties as coelenterazine, and similar experimental conditions should be applied *(19)*. They are difficult to use because of very high background chemiluminescence, but were successfully applied in measurements of superoxide anion at concentrations of 1 μ*M* by several authors *(19,20)*.

3.2.3. Pholasin

Pholasin is a glycoprotein derived from *Pholas dactylus*, described in 1986, which has been recently used successfully to measure reactive oxygen species production from inflammatory cells *(21)*. Pholasin can react with a variety of reactive oxygen species (specificity not yet determined) to form oxypholasin and light as a by-product; the protein reacts only once with reactive oxygen species and the luminescent product then degrades rapidly, leading to a greater accuracy when establishing real-time kinetics of superoxide release. In studies of reactive oxygen species release by activated neutrophils, Pholasin was found to have a 50- to 100-fold greater sensitivity than luminol in detecting superoxide release. Pholasin was used at final concentration of 5 μg/μL and chemiluminescence was measured in PBS.

4. Notes

1. The choice of luminometer or scintillation counter has a substantial impact on the exact practical details of the assay setup. The assay conditions should be optimized and validated for an individual machine and assay conditions, and cannot necessarily be extrapolated from one machine to another. Scintillation counters should be used in out-of-coincidence mode to measure light photons, and provide high sensitivity. However, scintillation counters that have been used extensively for high-activity radioactivity measurements suffer from photomultiplier bleaching that reduces sensitivity and increases background, making them unsuitable for detecting low-level chemiluminescence. Luminometers are popular, as they are cheaper and more convenient for dedicated use. Single-tube luminometers are sensitive, and usually accept vials suitable for chemiluminescent measurement from intact vessels. Because of the kinetics of enzymatic reactions, the optimal temperature for enzymatic generation of superoxide anions should be 37°C. Although reactive oxygen species-generating reactions proceed at room temperature, it is preferable that the internal chamber of the luminometer be maintained at a constant temperature of 37°C. More important than *absolute temperature* is to ensure *constant temperature*. Temperature drift as the machine warms up, or as the sample vial and contents equilibrate to machine temperature, causes significant "drift" in the luminescent signal that may invalidate quantitative comparisons. Integral temperature control is common in multichannel luminometers, which use a multiwell plate format and allow for measurement of large numbers of samples in parallel. Compared with single-tube luminometers, sensitivity is compromised, truly continuous online monitoring of luminescence in all channels may not be possible, and addition of cell or tissue samples, or reagents to the reactions may be difficult to synchronize. Nevertheless, multichannel luminometers are particularly suited for reactive oxygen species determination in vascular homogenates or cells aliquoted into multiwell plates, and when maximal oxidase activities (e.g., stimulated by NADPH) are to be determined. Both single-tube and multichannel luminometers may have automatic injectors for direct dispensing of reagents into the vial or wells, without opening the machine and exposing the system to light.

2. The optimal size of vessel rings should be determined in preliminary experiments, to ensure that (1) the size of tissue used is sufficient to generate a consistently measurable signal; and (2) the response of the assay system remains linear and quantitative across a range of tissue mass. For studies in human blood vessels, using 30-mL Beckmann vials in a Berthold FB12 luminometer, we use 2–3 mg

dry weight segments. As far as possible, the same mass and size of tissue should be used in each experiment, to reduce variability due to factors that cannot be systematically controlled for. In animal studies (e.g., rabbit or rat aorta), the uniform shape and size of vessel rings makes this easier to achieve, whereas human vessels from different patients usually vary in shape and size. In order to achieve sufficient signals, there may be a need to pool segments of aorta from more than one of identical animals for the experiment.

As most studies express reactive oxygen species production per dry weight of tissue (high degree of correlation with protein content), the size and weight of vessels segments used in parallel experiments should be similar.

References

1. Griendling, K. K., Sorescu, D., and Ushio-Fukai, M. (2000) NAD(P)H oxidase: role in cardiovascular biology and disease. *Circ. Res.* **86,** 494–501.
2. Munzel, T., Afanas'ev, I. B., Kleschyov, A. L., and Harrison, D. G. (2002) Detection of superoxide in vascular tissue. *Arterioscler. Thromb. Vasc. Biol.* **22,** 1761–1768.
3. Guzik, T. J., West, N. E. J., Black, E., et al. (2000) Vascular superoxide production by NAD(P)H oxidase: association with endothelial dysfunction and clinical risk factors. *Circ. Res.* **86,** e85–e90.
4. Gyllenhammar, H. (1989) Effects of extracellular pH on neutrophil superoxide anion production, and chemiluminescence augmented with luminol, lucigenin or DMNH. *J. Clin. Lab. Immunol.* **28,** 97–102.
5. White, C. R., Darley-Usmar, V., Berrington, W. R., et al. (1996) Circulating plasma xanthine oxidase contributes to vascular dysfunction in hypercholesterolemic rabbits. *Proc. Natl. Acad. Sci. USA* **93,** 8745-8749.
6. Li, Y., Zhu, H., Kuppusamy, P., Roubaud, V., Zweier, J. L., and Trush, M. A. (1998) Validation of lucigenin (bis-N-methylacridinium) as a chemilumigenic probe for detecting superoxide anion radical production by enzymatic and cellular systems. *J. Biol. Chem.* **273,** 2015–2023.
7. Skatchkov, M. P., Sperling, D., Hink, U., et al. (1999) Validation of lucigenin as a chemiluminescent probe to monitor vascular superoxide as well as basal vascular nitric oxide production. *Biochem. Biophys. Res. Commun.* **254,** 319–324.
8. Li, Y., Zhu, H., and Trush, M. A. (1999) Detection of mitochondria-derived reactive oxygen species production by the chemilumigenic probes lucigenin and luminol. *Biochim. Biophys. Acta* **1428,** 1–12.
9. Bauersachs, J., Bouloumi, A., Fraccarollo, D., Hu, K., Busse, R., and Ertl, G. (1999) Endothelial dysfunction in chronic myocardial infarction despite increased vascular endothelial nitric oxide synthase and soluble guanylate cyclase expression: role of enhanced vascular superoxide production. *Circulation* **100,** 292–298.
10. Huraux, C., Makita, T., Kurz, S., et al. (1999) Superoxide production, risk factors, and endothelium-dependent relaxations in human internal mammary arteries. *Circulation* **99,** 53–59.

11. Li, J. M., Mullen, A. M., Yun, S., et al. (2002) Essential role of the NADPH oxidase subunit p47(phox) in endothelial cell superoxide production in response to phorbol ester and tumor necrosis factor-alpha. *Circ. Res.* **90**, 143–150.
12. Radi, R., Cosgrove, T. P., Beckman, J. S., and Freeman, B. A. (1993) Peroxynitrite-induced luminol chemiluminescence. *Biochem J.* **290**, 51–57.
13. Iesaki, T., Gupte, S. A., Kaminski, P. M., and Wolin, M. S. (1999) Inhibition of guanylate cyclase stimulation by NO and bovine arterial relaxation to peroxynitrite and H_2O_2. *Am. J. Physiol.* **277**, H978–985.
14. Wang, P. and Zweier, J. L. (1996) Measurement of nitric oxide and peroxynitrite generation in the postischemic heart. Evidence for peroxynitrite-mediated reperfusion injury. *J. Biol. Chem.* **271**, 29223–29230.
15. Guzik, T. J., West, N., Pillai, R., Taggart, D., and Channon, K. M. (2002) Nitric oxide modulates superoxide release and peroxynitrite formation in human blood vessels. *Hypertension* **39**, 1088–1094.
16. Laursen, J. B., Somers, M., Kurz, S., et al. (2001) Endothelial regulation of vasomotion in apoE-deficient mice: implications for interactions between peroxynitrite and tetrahydrobiopterin. *Circulation* **103**, 1282–1288.
17. Tarpey, M. M., White, C. R., Suarez, E., Richardson, G., Radi, R., and Freeman, B. A. (1999) Chemiluminescent detection of oxidants in vascular tissue. Lucigenin but not coelenterazine enhances superoxide formation. *Circ. Res.* **84**, 1203–1211.
18. Ng, D. S., Maguire, G. F., Wylie, J., et al. (2002) Oxidative stress is markedly elevated in lecithin:cholesterol acyltransferase-deficient mice and is paradoxically reversed in the apolipoprotein E knockout background in association with a reduction in atherosclerosis. *J. Biol. Chem.* **277**, 11715–11720.
19. Skatchkov, M. P., Sperling, D., Hink, U., Angggard, E., and Munzel, T. (1998) Quantification of superoxide radical formation in intact vascular tissue using a cypridina luciferin analog as an alternative to lucigenin. *Biochem. Biophys. Res. Commun.* **248**, 382–386.
20. Teranishi, K. and Shimomura, O. (1997) Coelenterazine analogs as chemiluminescent probe for superoxide anion. *Anal. Biochem.* **249**, 37–43.
21. Swindle, E. J., Hunt, J. A., and Coleman, J. W. (2002) A comparison of reactive oxygen species generation by rat peritoneal macrophages and mast cells using the highly sensitive real-time chemiluminescent probe pholasin: inhibition of antigen-induced mast cell degranulation by macrophage-derived hydrogen peroxide. *J. Immunol.* **169**, 5866–5873.

7

A Guide to Wire Myography

Angela Spiers and Neal Padmanabhan

Summary
Wire myography is an in vitro technique that allows us to examine functional responses and vascular reactivity of isolated small resistance arteries. Vessels from various species, including transgenic models, and vascular beds can be examined in a variety of pathological disease states. Vessels are dissected, cleaned, and then mounted onto a four-channel myograph under isometric techniques. Each vessel is then normalized to determine maximum active tension development. This allows the standardization of initial experimental conditions, an important consideration when examining pharmacological differences between vessels.

Key Words: Wire myography; small resistance arteries; normalization; isometric.

1. Introduction

There is a wide range of techniques available to study the function of vascular smooth muscle, ranging from isolated single cells to whole-body methods. This chapter will concentrate on a popular in vitro technique that examines the functional and mechanical properties of isolated small arterial segments.

Mulvany and Aalkjaer *(1)* suggested that small arteries with internal diameters of less than 500 µm, which contribute substantially to the peripheral resistance, be considered as resistance arteries. The importance of these vessels lies in their ability to regulate the distribution of blood to peripheral organs, through variation of their diameter and hence resistance to flow. Wire myography is a technique developed by Mulvany and Halpern *(2)* for the investigation of both active and passive properties of small arteries under isometric conditions in vitro (**Fig. 1**).

This technique is applicable to the study of isolated vessels, with internal diameters between 100–400 µm, independent of homeostatic mechanisms, such as blood flow or autonomic nervous system control *(3)*. The technique has been adapted to the study of blood vessels from a variety of animal species

From: *Methods in Molecular Medicine, Vol. 108: Hypertension: Methods and Protocols*
Edited by: J. P. Fennell and A. H. Baker © Humana Press Inc., Totowa, NJ

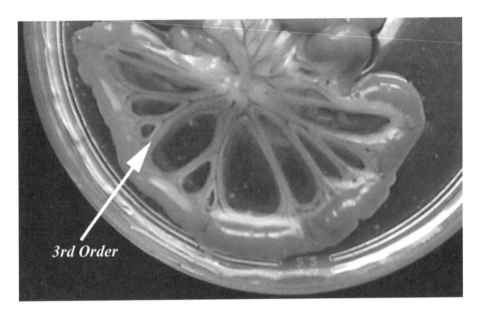

Fig. 1. Rat mesenteric arcade. Arrow shows the third-order vessel to be dissected.

(including transgenic models) and vascular beds in various pathological states, including diabetes, hypertension or cardiac failure *(4–7)*.

The four-channel myograph is most commonly used, because it allows the simultaneous study of four vessels in individual organ baths. Other models (such as two-channel myographs), to which the techniques described in this chapter are equally applicable, are also available. Myography starts with the careful dissection of small arteries, with a diameter of 200–400 µm, from an appropriate species and vascular bed. They are then mounted on a four-channel wire myograph and "normalized"—a procedure to determine maximum active tension development and standardize experimental conditions *(8)*. Quantitative structural and functional comparisons can then be made *(9)*. This chapter will consider these steps in turn.

2. Materials

1. Myograph: Four channel multimyograph, e.g., model 610M available from Danish MyoTechnologies (DMT) A/S.
2. Data recording: Linseis four-channel chart recorder or Powerlab system supplied by DMT.
3. Dissecting instruments: Fine watchmakers' spring scissors and fine forceps (e.g., from InterFocus Fine Science Tools, cat. no. 12).
4. Krebs salt solution: Physiological salt solution (PSS) had the following composition: 118.4 mM NaCl, 4.7 mM KCl, 1.2 mM MgSO$_4$, 1.2 mM KH$_2$PO$_4$, 24.9 mM

NaHCO$_3$, 2.5 mM CaCl$_2$, 11.1 mM glucose, 0.023 mM EDTA. pH will be 7.4 when solution gassed with 95% O$_2$ and 5% CO$_2$ mixture.

5. Potassium salt solution: Potassium physiological salt solution (KPSS) had the following composition: 125 mM KCl, 1.2 mM MgSO$_4$, 1.2 mM KH$_2$PO$_4$, 24.9 mM NaHCO$_3$, 2.5 mM CaCl$_2$, 11.1 mM glucose. pH will be 7.4 when solution gassed with 95% O$_2$ and 5% CO$_2$ mixture.

3. Methods

The methods outlined here describe (1) the preparation of resistance arteries, (2) mounting of the vessels, (3) the normalization procedure, (4) assessment of tissue viability, and (5) construction of a cumulative concentration response curve (CCRC).

3.1. Preparation of Resistance Arteries

3.1.1. Source of Arteries

Small vessel myography was historically devised with rat mesenteric resistance vessels in mind; however, the technique can be applied to other small vessels. Examples include human subcutaneous resistance vessels, myometrium and omental resistance arteries, and human small coronary arteries *(10)*. Mouse vessels commonly used are the caudal, mesenteric, carotid, and aorta *(11)*. For the purpose of this chapter, we will concentrate on rat mesenteric arteries and human subcutaneous arteries.

3.1.2. Dissection of Arteries

3.1.2.1. Rat Mesenteric Resistance Arteries

1. Sacrifice rats by CO$_2$ inhalation.
2. Approximately 10 cm from the pylorus, remove intestine including the superior mesenteric artery.
3. Place mesenteric arcade into a Petri dish with a thick layer of clear silicone gel in base. Cover with cold PSS.
4. Pin out arcade in an anticlockwise direction, taking care to avoid stretch. Veins should now be on top of arteries (*see* **Note 1**).
5. Identify third order branches of the arterial tree (**Fig. 1**).
6. Using fine spring scissors, carefully dissect and clean of connective tissue under a dissecting microscope (*see* **Note 2**). To prevent trauma, avoid contact with artery.
7. Divide dissected artery into four segments, each approx 2 mm in length (*see* **Note 3**).

3.1.2.2. Human Subcutaneous Resistance Arteries

1. A subcutaneous gluteal fat biopsy approx 1.5 cm × 0.5 cm × 1.5 cm, is excised under local anesthesia with 1% lignocaine *(9)* (*see* **Note 4**).

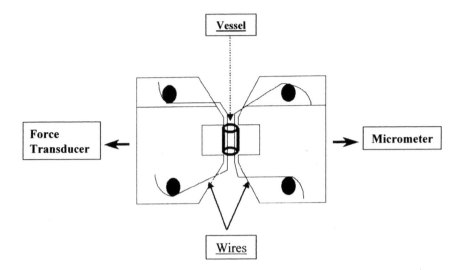

Fig. 2. Mulvany–Halpern myograph (not to scale). The force transducer is connected to a specially designed myo-interface and thus to a chart recorder, allowing the force across the vessel wall to be recorded. The preparation is bathed in Krebs solution that could be extracted using a suction device. The myograph is kept at 37°C during the experiments by a built-in heater.

2. Place into ice-cold PSS and transfer to the laboratory immediately (*see* **Note 5**).
3. The fat biopsy is placed into a dissecting Petri dish and vessels are carefully removed under a dissecting microscope. Vessels of the correct size may be difficult to locate, and dissection may take from 30 min to 2 h to complete.
4. PSS in the Petri dish should be replaced regularly during the procedure. The biopsy may be secured gently with entomology pins; this may assist the operator when looking for vessels lying within the fat. When handling the vessel, care should be taken to avoid direct contact.
5. The dissected vessel should then be divided into four segments each approx 2 mm in length (*see* **Note 3**).

3.2. Mounting of Vessels (Fig. 2)

1. Wash baths four times with distilled water.
2. Wash baths four times with cold PSS.
3. Add 5 mL of Krebs solution to each bath, turn on heat and gas. Put covers on.
4. Carefully clean up vessel if required. Excess connective tissue and fat adherent to the vessel should be removed carefully, taking care not to handle the vessel directly.
5. Cannulate vessel with first wire in Petri dish or directly onto wire previously fixed to left myograph head. In our experience it is easier and less traumatic to the vessel to cannulate it with the first wire while still in the Petri dish.

6. If the vessel was cannulated in the Petri dish, transfer wire and vessel to left myograph head. (For diagrams consult myograph manual.)

7. Mount second wire. Ensure that wire is straight and not too long (*see* **Note 6**). Insert into lumen by holding wire with forceps and sliding along the top of the first wire. This can be done from either the near or far end but may be easier from the near end. Wire should be inserted in one fluid motion to avoid trauma to vessel.

8. Close jaws gently, ensuring second wire slides underneath first wire. This will prevent wires from crossing over.

9. Secure wire underneath screws. Ensure wires are taut. Vessel length should not exceed 2 mm (*see* **Note 3**).

10. Open jaws slightly and adjust the wires until they are on the same plane.

11. Close jaws gently until wires are "just touching."

12. Measure vessel length using previously calibrated eyepiece in dissecting microscope. Position hairline of eyepiece over the far end of the segment and take measurement (for normalization purposes this measurement is known as a_1; units are ocular divisions). Next, position hairline over near end of segment and take measurement (denoted a_2). Both of these measurements are recorded onto the normalization experiment sheet. (**Fig. 3**).

13. Read myograph micrometers with wires "just touching" (this measurement is known as X_0, units micrometers, and is needed for normalization procedure.) Again note measurement onto normalization experiment sheet (**Fig. 3**).

14. Return baths to base unit.

3.3. Normalization for Passive Force

Once vessels have been mounted, they are washed with PSS and left to equilibrate for 30 min before being normalized. All baths are maintained at 37°C and gassed with a mixture of 95% O_2 and 5% CO_2 throughout the experimental procedure.

The aim of normalization is to set vessels to standard initial conditions. Some studies have indicated that the initial passive conditions (resting tension) under which vessels are placed may have an impact on any pharmacological differences observed (*12*). It is therefore important to standardize initial conditions to ensure that the physiological responses of the vessels are assessed in a reliable manner. It should be noted that although attempts are made to standardize conditions, it is impossible to mimic in vivo parameters. By removing the vessel from the tethering of the connective tissue, the pressure–length and pressure–diameter relationships are unavoidably altered (*13*). The axial length and tension in wire-mounted preparations will therefore differ from in vivo conditions.

Mulvany and Halpern (*2*) addressed the issue of setting initial conditions and developed the technique of normalization. This determines the internal circumference a vessel would have if relaxed and under a transmural pressure

DATE:

EXPERIMENTER:
MYOGRAPH No:

Tissue type:	1		
alpha 0·1635	2 delta 0·7825		
a1 0	beta		
a2 4·93	Xo 7163		
yo 2	Lo		
2 x vessel length 3·8516			

Tissue type:	2		
alpha	2 delta		
a1	beta		
a2	Xo		
yo	Lo		
2 x vessel length			

Tissue type:	3		
alpha	2 delta		
a1	beta		
a2	Xo		
yo	Lo		
2 x vessel length			

Tissue type:	4		
alpha	2 delta		
a1	beta		
a2	Xo		
yo	Lo		
2 x vessel length			

NORMALISATION

	force (y)	micro (x)	kPa
1	7	7422	1·84
2	18	7512	4·72
3	31	7553	7·84
4	46	7581	11·26
5	60	7601	14·30

	force (y)	micro (x)	kPa
1			
2			
3			
4			
5			

NORMALISATION

	force (y)	micro (x)	kPa
1			
2			
3			
4			
5			

	force (y)	micro (x)	kPa
1			
2			
3			
4			
5			

l100 (IC100)	341
l1 (IC1)	
l2	0·99
X1	7542
y1	
kPa	
mmHg	
mmHg	
(from length/tension curve)	

l100	
l1	
l2	
X1	
y1	
kPa	
mmHg	
mmHg	
(from length/tension curve)	

l100	
l1	
l2	
X1	
y1	
kPa	
mmHg	
mmHg	
(from length/tension curve)	

Fig. 3. Normalization experiment sheet.

of 100 mmHg (IC_{100}). Once the IC_{100} of a vessel is ascertained, it is set to 0.9 of this value, as maximum active tension development is optimal at this point (IC_1). The point of maximum active tension development can be calculated from the passive internal circumference/tension relationship of the vessel.

The artery is incrementally stretched using the micrometer and the passive force measured (F) using the chart recorder. Wall tension (T) is calculated by dividing the force by twice the segment length (previously measured using the micrometer eyepiece). The internal circumference can be calculated from the micrometer readings and the knowledge that the diameter of each wire is 40 μm. The equivalent increase in pressure can be determined by applying the Laplace equation:

$$P_1 = \frac{\text{wall tension}}{\text{internal circumference}/2\pi}$$

Note that the Laplace equation assumes that the wall of the artery is thin and that pressure is unaffected by the curvature caused by the wires. In practice, this technique involves taking micrometer readings and chart recording readings and entering them into a computer or hand-held programmable calculator. Details of the normalization computer program are included with the user's manual included with the myograph (*see* **Note 7**).

1. An initial micrometer reading is noted with wires just touching (X_0).
2. Myograph heads are then opened very slightly—this equates to zero wall force— and the corresponding chart recorder reading (known as Y_0) is noted on the normalization experiment sheet (**Fig. 3**).
3. Wires are then moved apart at 1-min intervals and the corresponding wall force, Y (chart reading) and new micrometer reading, X, are taken (**Fig. 3**).
4. Values Y and X are noted and entered into the computer or hand-held calculator.
5. The procedure is repeated approx 5 times or until the effective pressure exceeds 100 mmHg (13.3 kPa). At that point the computer fits an exponential curve to the internal circumference–pressure data and the intersection of the 100 mmHg isobar is calculated. This gives the IC_{100}.
6. The computer then displays the micrometer reading necessary to set the vessel to 0.9 of IC_{100}, i.e., IC_1. The micrometer should be adjusted to this reading. As described previously, this is the point at which optimal maximum active tension is expected.
7. Following normalization, vessels are washed with fresh PSS and allowed to equilibrate.

3.4. Viability of Tissue

To obtain optimum data from tissues, it is important to ensure that the technique of isolating and mounting tissue has had no adverse effects on functional response (3).

Our practice is to test contractile ability using the response to high-potassium depolarization and a standard vasoconstrictor (norepinephrine, NE) and endothelium-dependent vasodilation using acteylcholine (ACh). Both the contractile and vasodilator responses may vary from tissue to tissue and between species. Preliminary experiments may have to be carried out in order to determine what is acceptable in any specific preparation.

Following a rest period of 40 min after normalization, vessels are subjected to a series of three depolarisations with 125 mM KPSS.

1. Add 5mls of KPSS to each bath.
2. Once contraction has reached plateau, wash with PSS and allow to relax to baseline.
3. Repeat three times.
4. Add NE to the bath to a final concentration of 10^{-5} M. When contraction has peaked, test vasodilator response by the addition of ACh to a final concentration of 3×10^{-6} M.
5. If vessels fail to contract to either KPSS or NE, or do not relax to ACh; they should be excluded from further study.

3.5. Concentration Response Curves

Most of the results obtained from wire myography are from looking at the response of the vessel to agonists or antagonists that have been added to the bath. This is usually done in the form of a CCRC, also known as a dose–response curve. In order to achieve receptor saturation, large ranges of concentrations are required, so CCRC are usually logarithmic. This typically produces a curve of sigmoidal shape, with the segment between 20 and 80% of the maximal response being approximately linear.

When performing a vasoconstrictor CCRC, a suitable time interval should be left between each dose until contraction begins, at which point each subsequent dose should be added when contraction has peaked. Once the higher concentrations are reached, desensitization, or tachyphylaxis, may occur. This is a reduced response to the agonist when the agonist is continually present at the receptor (14) (see **Note 8**).

In vasodilator curves, each vessel is first contracted to 80% of its maximum using a suitable agonist, e.g., NE. Once the vessel starts to relax, subsequent doses of agonist should be added when the response has leveled off. In vasodilator curves a common problem is spontaneous relaxation, where the vessel will fail to maintain contraction and relax to baseline either before or during the CCRC. If this happens, the vessel should be washed with fresh PSS and allowed to rest before a further attempt is made.

When designing an experimental protocol for wire myography, care should be taken with the order in which agonists are used. Certain agonists are irreversible and so cannot be washed out; these should always be used last.

It may be helpful to denude the endothelium of blood vessels when looking at endothelium-dependent vascular responses. This can be done in either a mechanical manner using a hair and rubbing it along the endothelium, or by infusing the vessel with antibody and complement *(15)*. If removing the endothelium by mechanical means, care should be taken to avoid damaging the vascular smooth muscle cells.

3.6. Data Analysis

Contractile responses can be expressed as an increase in active effective pressure (P, mmHg), calculated as an increase in isometric tension (T) above resting tension divided by the normalized internal radius. Responses of the vessels to agonists can be expressed as the percent of the response to a standard vasoconstrictor such as NE or KPSS.

Myography results are often expressed in terms of the EC_{50} values, this being the concentration required to produce 50% of the maximum response. The EC_{50} can be derived from fits of each separate curve (calculated directly by interpolation in Microsoft Excel spreadsheets, using the "Forecast" function). To facilitate analysis, values may be expressed as the PD_2—which is the negative logarithm of the corresponding EC_{50} and is a whole number. For example, an EC_{50} of 1.5×10^{-6} would give a corresponding PD_2 value of 5.820. The advantage of using PD_2 as opposed to EC_{50} is that whole numbers are more suitable for use in statistical analysis. Maximum responses can be taken directly from the CCRCs. Since some responses will not achieve a clear maximum even at the highest concentration of agonist, EC_{50} values can not be calculated; in this instance, area under the curve (AUC) may be used.

4. Notes

1. Identification of arteries: It is possible to identify small resistance arteries by their helical shape and distinct wall. In contrast, veins are more flaccid structures, and it may be difficult to clearly identify their walls. Veins also have a larger lumen than arteries. When dissecting rat mesentery, if excised arcade is correctly pinned in an anticlockwise direction, veins should lie directly on top of arteries. Human subcutaneous vessels are more difficult to locate and the dissection process may be protracted.
2. Instruments: Fine forceps and watchmakers' spring scissors should be used in dissection and cleaning of small arteries. For human tissue it may be useful to use spring scissors with a cutting blade of approx 6 mm. This will facilitate access to vessels lying deep within the fat of the biopsy.
3. Length of segments: Vessel length should not exceed 2 mm. If length is longer than this it may interfere with the normalization process. If length exceeds 2 mm, the top of the vessel should be carefully cut where it protrudes from the jaws, to prevent this area being stretched during normalization. When gaining experience in the mounting technique it may be advantageous to photocopy a ruler marked

in millimeters and place it underneath the dissecting Petri dish just before cutting your segments.

4. Gluteal biopsy: Biopsies are usually taken from the upper outer quadrant of the buttock under local anesthetic. A minor operations set with scalpel, blunt-nosed forceps, and two artery forceps is required. After sterilization of the appropriate area, the skin is anesthetised with approx 5 mL of 1% lignocaine (without epinephrine). An oval incision approx 1.5 × 0.5 cm is made and fat adherent to the skin is excised to a depth of approx 1.5 cm. It is usually possible to excise a cone of fat (with the skin at the apex) 2–3 cm in diameter without causing excessive bleeding. It may be necessary to place a deep absorbable suture to achieve hemostasis. The skin is closed with interrupted or subcuticular sutures. Alternative sources of tissue include the edge of an abdominal incision being performed for some other reason, and omental fat. In these cases it is important to avoid diathermy.

5. Storage of dissected vessels: As the dissection process may exceed 2 h, it can be helpful to store vessels in PSS and use them the following day. McIntyre *(16)* demonstrated that functional responses are unaffected by overnight storage at 4°C.

6. Wires: Stainless steel wire of 40 μm should be straight and of the correct length (approx 2 cm) to ease the mounting procedure. If the wire is curved, it may damage the endothelium when it is passed through the lumen. If the vessels to be used are very small, 20-μm wire is available.

7. Normalization program: The Basic program Normalization is available from DMT. The user manual is being updated to include details of the theory behind normalization and comprehensive explanations of terms and equations used. In the past this could be programmed into a Hewlett Packard hand-held computer. These are now unavailable, but the program can be compiled onto an EXCEL spreadsheet. Alternatively, there is now a normalization plug-in available for the Powerlab data acquisition software. The Basic Normalisation program is:

```
    PRINT "Enter value for normalisation e.g. 0.9" : INPUT RATIO
    Ok_
    LIST 10-100
    10 PRINT "Enter value for normalisation e.g. 0.9" : INPUT RATIO
    20 PRINT "Enter microscope calibration"; : INPUT DELTA
    22 DELTA2 = DELTA*2
    30 PRINT "Enter micrometer reading - wires touching"; : INPUT X0
    40 PRINT "Enter internal circumference of wires"; : INPUT L0
    45 PRINT : PRINT
    48 '
    49 ' Second set of parameters
    50 PRINT "Enter transducer calibration"; : INPUT ALPHA
    60 PRINT "Enter vessel length - start"; : INPUT A1
    70 PRINT "Enter vessel length - finish"; : INPUT A2
    80 PRINT "Enter baseline trace reading - zero force"; : INPUT Y0
```

```
88 '
89 ' Calculate twice segment length
90 AA=ABS(A1-A2)*DELTA2 : PRINT : PRINT "twice vessel length = ";
AA
96 PRINT
98 '
99 ' Enter points on resting tension - i.c. determination
100 I=0
110 I=I+1
120 PRINT : PRINT
122 PRINT "If calculation is required before effective pressure is greater "
123 PRINT "than 13.3 kPa then input 999 as next micrometer reading."
125 PRINT "Enter micrometer reading (";I;")"; : INPUT X(I)
126 IF X(I) = 999 THEN GOTO 192
130 PRINT "Enter trace reading (";I;")"; : INPUT Y(I)
150 T(I)=(Y(I)-Y0)*(ALPHA/(AA)) ' Wall tension (N/m)
160 L(I)=((X(I)-X0)*2+L0) ' Internal circumference (um)
170 P(I)=T(I)/(L(I)/(2000*PI)) ' Effective pressure (kPa)
180 PRINT "effective pressure (";I;")"" = ";P(I)
190 IF P(I)<13.3 THEN GOTO 110 ELSE N=I
191 GOTO 199
192 IF P(I) > 10 THEN GOTO 199
193 PRINT "Effective pressure is less than 10 kPa therefore not useful "
194 PRINT "information can be gained from calculation at this stage. "
195 PRINT "Either continue normalization or redo. To continue type"
196 PRINT "'continue' to redo input any letter"
197 INPUT B$ : IF B$ = "continue" THEN GOTO 125
198 GOTO 10
199 ' Regression of points to T=A exp(B L)
200 XSUM=0 : X2SUM=0 : YSUM=0 : Y2SUM=0 : XYSUM=0
210 FOR I=1 TO N
220 XSUM=XSUM+L(I)
230 X2SUM=X2SUM+L(I)*L(I)
240 YSUM=YSUM+LOG(T(I))
250 Y2SUM=Y2SUM+LOG(T(I))*LOG(T(I))
260 XYSUM=XYSUM+L(I)*LOG(T(I))
270 NEXT I
280 X=X2SUM-(1/N)*(XSUM*XSUM)
290 Y=Y2SUM-(1/N)*(YSUM*YSUM)
300 Z=XYSUM-(1/N)*(XSUM*YSUM)
Ok_
310 R2=Z*Z/(X*Y)
320 B=Z/X
330 A=EXP(YSUM/N-B*XSUM/N)
```

```
340 PRINT : PRINT
350 PRINT "a="; A
360 PRINT "b="; B
370 PRINT "r = "; R2 ' coefficient of determination
380 PRINT
390 '
499 ' Iteration to solve L100 = (2 pi A exp(B L100))/p100
500 LEST=L(N) ' seed estimate of L100
510 FL=2000*PI*A*EXP(B*LEST)/P100 ' Value of L with this estimate
530 LEST=LEST+(LEST-FL)/20 ' new estimate of L100
540 'PRINT LEST optional control for convergence
550 IF ABS(FL-LEST)>.1 THEN GOTO 510 ' reiterate until equation
560 ' approx solved
599 ' Final calculations
600 L100=LEST
600 L100=LEST
610 L1=RATIO*L100
620 PRINT "Diameter at L(100) = "; L100/PI ' Normalized lumen
621 PRINT
622 LRATIO = (L100/PI)*RATIO
625 PRINT "Diameter at L"; RATIO ; " = " ; LRATIO
630 X1=X0+(L1-L0)/2
640 PRINT "micrometer setting = "; X1 ' setting for i.c. = 0.9 L100
700 PRINT "Enter final trace reading at " ; RATIO ; :INPUT TRACE : PRINT
TRACE
700 PRINT "Enter final trace reading at " ; RATIO ; :INPUT TRACE : PRINT
TRACE
710 T = (TRACE - Y0) * (ALPHA/(AA)) 'final tension (N/m)
720 P = T/(L1/(2000*PI)) 'final pressure (kPa)
730 PRINT "Effective pressure at "; RATIO ; " = " ; P ; " kPa"
740 PRINT " Equivalent to " ; 7.51 * P ; "mmHg"
741 PRESS = (A*EXP(B*L1))/(L1/(2000*PI))
742 PRESS = PRESS*7.518796992#
747 PRINT "Pressure reiterated from length/tension curve = "; PRESS
750 PRINT "Do you wish to calculate parameters for new ratio? y or n" :
INPUT Q$
: PRINT Q$
760 IF Q$ = "n" THEN GOTO 800
770 PRINT "Calculate for new diameter ratio eg 0.8"
775 PRINT "Enter value for new ratio" : INPUT RATIO : PRINT RATIO
780 GOTO 610
800 END
```

8. Vasomotion: Quite often in small isolated arteries, vasomotion may be observed. This phenomenon has long been noted and its exact cause is still unclear. It is periodic, rhythmic oscillation of vascular tone *(17)* and may be an important mechanism in the regulation of local blood flow.

In practical terms for wire myography, vasomotion can make interpretation of CCRCs very difficult. It may begin during the normalization period or upon stimulation of the vessels with agonists and is unpredictable *(18)*. If a vessel exhibits severe vasomotion, it will most probably have to be excluded from study, as overcoming vasomotion during the course of an experiment is extremely difficult, if not impossible.

References

1. Mulvany, M. J. and Aalkjaer, C. (1990) Structure and function of small arteries. *Physiol. Rev.* **70,** 921–961.
2. Mulvany, M.J. and Halpern, W. (1977) Contractile properties of small arterial resistance vessels in spontaneously hypertensive and normotensive rats. *Circ. Res.* **41,** 19–26.
3. Angus, J. A. and Wright, C. E. (2000) Techniques to study the pharmacodynamics of isolated large and small blood vessels. *J. Pharmacol. Toxicol. Meth.* **44,** 395–407.
4. Heagerty, A. M., Aalkjaer, C., Bund, S. J., Korsgaard, N. and Mulvany, M. J. (1993) Small artery structure in hypertension: dual processes of growth and remodeling. *Hypertension* **21,** 391–397.
5. Angus, J. A., Ferrier, C. P., Kirshnankutty, S., Kaye, D. M., and Jennings, G. L. (1993) Impaired contraction and relaxation in skin resistance arteries from patients with congestive heart failure *Circ. Res.* **27,** 204–210.
6. Kelly, C. J. G., Spiers, A., Gould, G. W., Petrie, J. R., Lyall, H., and Connell, J. M. C. (2002) Altered vascular function in young women with polycystic ovary syndrome. *J. Clin. Endocrinol. Metab.* **2,** 742–746.
7. Rizzoni, D., Portei, E., Guelfi, D., et al. (2001) Structural alterations in subcutaneous small arteries of normotensive and hypertensive patients with non-insulin dependent diabetes mellitus. *Circulation* **103,**1238–1244.
8. Lew, M. J. and McPherson, G. A. (1996) Isolated tissue techniques. In *The Pharmacology of Vascular Smooth Muscle* (Garland, C. J. and Angus, J. A., eds.), Oxford University Press, Oxford, pp. 25–41.
9. Aalkjaer, C., Pedersen, E. B., Danielsen, H., et al. (1986) Morphological and functional characteristics of resistance vessels in advanced uraemia. *Clin. Sci.* **71,** 657–663.
10. Ashworth, J. R., Warren, A. Y., Baker, P. N., and Johnson, I. R. (1996) A comparison of endothelium-dependent relaxation in omental and myomental resistance arteries in pregnant and non-pregnant woman. *Am. J. Obstet. Gynecol.* **175,** 1307–1312.

11. Daly, C. J., Deighan, C., McGee, A., et al. (2002) A knockout approach indicates a minor vasoconstrictor role for vascular α_{1b}-adrenoceptor in mouse. *Phys. Genom.* **9,** 85–91.

12. McPherson, G. A. (1992) Assesing vascular reactivity of arteries in the small vessel myograph. *Clin. Exp. Pharm. Phys.* **19,** 815–825.

13. Lew, M. J. and Angus, J. A. (1992) Wall thickness to lumen diameter ratios of arteries from SHR and WKY: comparison of pressurised and wire-mounted preparations. *J. Vasc. Res.* **29,** 435–442

14. Rang, H.P and Dale, M.M (eds.) (1991) *Pharmacology*. Churchill Livingstone, Edinburgh.

15. Juncos, L. A., Ito, S., Carretero, O. A., and Garvin, J. L. (1994) Removal of endothelium-dependent relaxation by antibody and complement in afferent arterioles. *Hypertension* **23** (suppl. I), I54–I59.

16. McIntyre, C. A., Williams, B. C., Lindsay, R. M., McKinght, J. A., and Hadoke, P. W. F. (1998) Preservation of vascular function in rat mesenteric resistance arteries following cold storage, studied by small vessel myography. *Br. J. Pharm.* **123,** 1555–1560.

17. Nilsson, H. and Aalkjaer, C. (2003) Vasomotion mechanisms and physiological importance. *Mol. Interventions* **3,** 79–89.

18. Angus, J. A. and Cocks, T. M. (1996) Pharmacology of human isolated large and small coronary arteries. In *The Pharmacology of Vascular Smooth Muscle* (Garland, C. J. and Angus, J. A., eds.), Oxford University Press, Oxford, pp. 276–305.

III

Nucleic Acid Techniques

8

Selection of Candidate Genes in Hypertension

Charles A. Mein, Mark J. Caulfield, and Patricia B. Munroe

Summary

Essential hypertension is a common disease with multifactorial etiology affecting up to 10 million individuals in the United Kingdom alone. Current knowledge of the genetic contribution to this trait is restricted to a number of rare variants that produce hypertensive phenotypes in a Mendelian fashion and to genes highlighted by work on blood pressure regulation in rodent models. Recent advances in comparative genomics, genome-wide scans for linkage, transcriptomics, proteomics, and metabolomics allow a systematic approach to the prioritization of candidate genes for hypertension and other complex traits. We review the current state of play in these fields related to hypertension and show, with a particular example, how these data may help target genetic studies in the future.

Key Words: Hypertension; blood pressure; genetic linkage; genome wide scan; candidate gene; proteomics; transcriptomics; metabolomics.

1. Introduction

Essential hypertension affects up to 10 million people in the United Kingdom and is a major risk factor for stroke, renal failure and coronary artery disease (www.who.int/en/index.html). It is now clear from epidemiological and family studies that genetic and environmental factors contribute to the phenotype, but thus far the identity of genes causing the condition remain to be elucidated *(1)*. During the past decade two main approaches have been utilized for determining the genes causing complex diseases such as hypertension: candidate gene studies and genome-wide screening. In the candidate gene approach a gene of known function is tested for association with the disease; in the genome-wide screening approach polymorphic markers at known location in the genome are analyzed and candidate genes mapping to the linked interval are subsequently tested for disease association. In this chapter we give a historical perspective on the selection of candidate genes in hypertension and then discuss a strategy to follow using genome-wide screen results.

From: *Methods in Molecular Medicine, Vol. 108: Hypertension: Methods and Protocols*
Edited by: J. P. Fennell and A. H. Baker © Humana Press Inc., Totowa, NJ

In hypertension research, the selection of candidate genes has traditionally been based on their established effects on the cardiovascular system and blood pressure (BP) control. There are three main sources from which candidates have been derived: (1) from information available on the physiology and pharmacology of BP regulation, (2) from analysis of rare Mendelian disorders that have extreme BP levels as part of the phenotype, and (3) from studies of experimental models.

1.1. Physiology and Pharmacology of Blood Pressure Control

The regulation of BP is complex and is dependent on the integrated action of the cardiovascular, endocrine, neural, and renal systems. Hypertension results when one or more of these systems stops working optimally. One well-recognized regulatory system is the renin–angiotensin system (RAS), a key modulator of vascular tone, salt-water homeostasis, and BP levels. Some of the most successful therapeutic drugs for lowering BP levels (angiotensin-converting enzyme inhibitors and angiotensin type II receptor antagonists) are inhibitors of this system (2,3).

In recent years all of the primary components of the RAS (angiotensinogen, angiotensin-converting enzyme, angiotensin type II receptor, and aldosterone) have been studied as candidate genes for hypertension. One of the most intensively studied has been angiotensinogen. Early genetic studies implicated this gene to have a primary role in the etiology of hypertension (4,5). However, subsequent analyses suggested that genetic variants have only a minor influence on BP levels, but functional variants and mechanisms have yet to be determined (6,7).

Many other genes from different physiological pathways have also been assessed, primarily using association studies with human volunteers. Data from analysis of a few, namely the β2 adrenergic receptor and guanine nucleotide-binding protein (G protein), β polypeptide 3 (GNB3), have found positive association with hypertension, but there are also negative studies reported for each (8–11). Lack of reproducibility of association is a recurrent theme in genetic studies of complex traits and hypertension is no exception, but it is probably fair to say that many of the studies were statistically underpowered to demonstrate association. Therefore, it is prudent to reassess some candidate genes in larger cohorts to really discover if they contribute to essential hypertension.

1.2. Mendelian Disorders

There are four monogenic disorders that have hypertension as part of the phenotype: glucocorticoid remediable hyperaldosteronism (GRA), Liddle's syndrome, apparent mineralocorticoid excess (AME), and Gordon's syndrome.

The genes responsible for each condition have now been discovered and, interestingly, the majority are involved in the same physiological pathway—that of sodium reabsorption in the distal nephron of the kidney *(12–15)*. Researchers initiated these studies not only to discover the causative genes for these rare disorders but also to potentially identify new candidate genes for essential hypertension, with the assumption that more subtle susceptibility variants within the same gene are disease-predisposing.

A chimeric gene resulting from an unequal crossover between 11-βhydroxylase promoter and aldosterone synthase was found to be the cause of GRA *(12)*. Studies have subsequently been performed on aldosterone synthase as a candidate gene for essential hypertension and there is suggestive evidence for association *(16–18)*. Mutations in 11-βhydroxy steroid dehydrogenase cause AME *(14)*. There are some data suggesting that this gene plays a role in essential hypertension in association with salt sensitivity *(19,20)*. Liddle's syndrome is caused by mutations in the epithelial sodium channel *(13)*. Studies of the three subunits of the channel in hypertensive patients from different ethnic groups provide conflicting data on its role, with positive association reported in black and Japanese cohorts *(21–23)*, but no consistent evidence of association in Caucasians *(24,25)*.

Mutations in the WNK1 and WNK4 kinases (members of a novel serine threonine kinase family of proteins) cause Gordon's syndrome *(15)*. Recent data support WNK1 and WNK4 as being inhibitors of the thiazide-sensitive NaCl cotransporter (NCCT). In Gordon's syndrome there is loss of inhibition of the NCCT, which in turn leads to increased sodium reabsorption and hypertension in affected individuals *(26)*. Only one study has been performed so far assessing the role of the WNK kinases in essential hypertension. Erlich and colleagues reported a single variant in the WNK4 gene and found association of this intronic variant with essential hypertension *(27)*. There are no studies in the literature as yet on the WNK1 gene. By assessing the monogenic forms of hypertension, a previously unrecognized pathway regulating sodium homeostasis and several new candidate genes for essential hypertension were found. This research has therefore proved extremely valuable, and time will tell if any of the genes are a cause of essential hypertension: further work is first required.

1.3. Experimental Models

There are numerous inbred rat strains that have hypertension or a related phenotype. These have now been studied for over a decade to try and determine the loci influencing BP levels. It is hoped that the discovery of a BP gene in an experimental model will not only provide important information on the physiological systems regulating BP levels but will also provide a source of good candidate genes for the human condition. Genome-wide screening using polymorphic markers has now been performed for many hypertensive inbred strains, and numerous chromosomal regions have been found to harbor BP loci *(28–31)*. Congenic mapping has subsequently been used to try and confirm the presence of a quantitative trait locus (QTL) and to reduce the size of the chromosomal region in which it resides *(32–35)*.

Two BP QTLs were mapped to chromosome 10 in the stroke-prone spontaneously hypertensive rat (SHRSP) strain in the early 1990s *(28,29)*. Subsequently analysis of the Dahl salt-sensitive hypertensive strain also revealed two BP loci on chromosome 10 *(36,37)*. Congenic mapping has now been performed in the Dahl strain confirming two loci and excluding inducible nitric oxide synthase and angiotensin-converting enzyme as the causative genes *(38)*. In the SHRSP congenic mapping also confirms BP loci and excludes the WNK4 gene as a QTL *(39)*.

A segment on the long arm of human chromosome 17 is syntenic to BP region on rat chromosome 10. Some studies have found linkage between chromosome 17 and essential hypertension *(40–43)*, although other larger studies with additional microsatellite markers have not confirmed this observation *(44,45)*. At this time the role of human chromosome 17 is not clear. However, with mapping studies in the rat being so consistent and with the net closing in on the causative genes, studies of the syntenic genes in humans will answer the question of whether the gene also plays a role in the human condition. Translation of other rat QTLs to human loci is ongoing; only time will tell if comparative mapping will prove to be a fruitful resource of candidate genes. It may be that BP QTLs differ between species.

The approach whereby candidate genes are selected based on their role in a monogenic form of the trait or from a known physiological pathway have led to important increases in our understanding of hypertension. However, an alternative approach is to use the burgeoning global tools available to study the genome, transcriptome, proteome, and metabolome in a systematic way that is less dependent on our imperfect understanding of disease etiology (*see* **Fig. 1**). The challenge is to weave these disparate threads of evidence together to gain a more complete appreciation of the cause of the disease. It is possible to start an investigation using any one of these technologies and draw corroborating evidence from other fields in support of a candidate gene. In the methods section we will discuss the genome-wide screen approach to studying complex disease tying in the study of RNA, proteins, and metabolites to prioritize candidate gene selection. As an illustration, a genomic region on chromosome 2 that shows suggestive evidence of linkage has been chosen. This region was selected because it demonstrates the concepts rather than for the strength of evidence for linkage to hypertension.

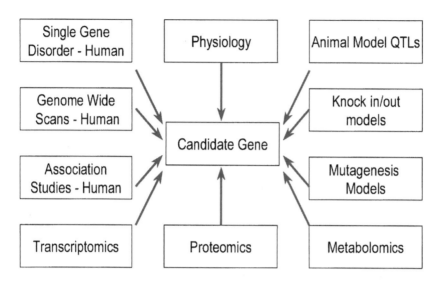

Fig. 1. Schematic of strategy used to prioritize candidate genes for complex disease.

2. Methods

2.1. Genome-Wide Screens for Hypertension

Genome-wide scans for linkage to Mendelian traits have been successful for the monogenic syndromes with a hypertensive component as described above. A similar strategy may be applied to complex traits, such as essential hypertension, but the approach is modified to utilize smaller pedigree sizes and nonparametric statistical methods *(46–48)*.

A genome-wide screen for linkage to a complex trait typically yields several regions of a large size, anything up to 20 or even 40 million base pairs, for which there is some statistical support. An example is the recent Medical Research Council funded British Genetics of Hypertension (BRIGHT) study of Caulfield et al. *(44)*. This is the largest study to date in a single ethnic group (1599 sib pairs), and four loci with genome-wide significance were found ($p < 0.05$). Given an estimated 35,000 genes in the genome, each of these regions could contain up to 500 genes. The challenge is to identify which of these loci represent a true positive result (given the weak statistical evidence from a single study, any one locus may be a false positive) and which gene(s) within a particular locus is contributing to the linkage signal.

Once a region of linkage is found, the next step is to compare linkage results from other populations with a similar phenotype to identify common regions between studies. There is currently no database in which these data are deposited for hypertension; therefore a search of original journal articles must be made in PubMed (www.ncbi.nlm.nih.gov/Entrez). At the time of writing there are 24 published genome screens for hypertension or related phenotypes (systolic/diastolic BP, etc., see Samani or Garcia for reviews *[49,50]*). Taken together, nine loci have met Lander and Kruglyak's criteria for significance (LOD > 3.6 or genome-wide $p < 0.05$) and 36 fall into their suggestive category (3.6 > LOD > 2.2) *(51)*. First impressions might suggest that this is an ample resource for gene mappers. However, it is disappointing to report that, in common with other complex traits, there is limited overlap between regions indicated in each genome screen. Potential reasons for this include differences between ethnicities of patient cohorts, diagnostic criteria, imprecision of estimated positions in linkage, marker map identities, and so forth *(52–54)*. However, the main factor is probably the size of studies to date, which lack power to detect genes of modest, but important effect *(47,55)*.

2.2. Chromosome 2q22-2q33

A recent publication highlighted a region on chromosome 2q as a susceptibility locus for hypertension *(44)*. This region had a LOD score of 1.76 at marker D2S142 and the LOD −1 interval is 25 cM between markers D2S151 and D2S355 and spans approx 60 Mb of genomic DNA *(44)*. This region is large but may be considered typical of first-generation genome screen results.

Using the human genome reference sequence (www.ensembl.org, www.ucsc.org, www.ncbi.nlm.nih.gov) as a scaffold rather than more traditional genetic maps, it is possible to locate accurately markers used between studies and thereby compare linkage results. There are five other genome screens for hypertension or BP phenotypes that report linkage to this region and overlap with the BRIGHT study (**Fig. 2**). The patient cohorts in these studies are drawn from a variety of ethnic groups—Caucasian *(56)*, Amish *(57)*, Mexican American *(58)*, Chinese *(59)*, and Finnish *(60)* and differ in size from a modest number of 47 sib pairs *(60)*, to the largest screen to date, 1599 sib pairs *(44)*. In addition there is overlap with regions identified in two genomewide screens for preeclampsia in Icelandic *(61)* and in Australian and New

---

Fig. 2. (*opposite page*) Genome screens for hypertensive traits at a locus on 2q. 1, Caulfield et al., 2003; 2, Hsueh et al., 1999; 3) Atwood et al., 2000; 4, Perola et al., 2000; 5, Zhu et al., 2001; 6, Krushkal et al., 1999; 7, Arnigrimson et al., 1999; 8, Moses et al., 2000; 9, Syntenic regions in rat: horizontal shading, four regions on rat chromosome 3; diagonal shading, rat chromosome 11; vertical shading, rat chromosome 6; checkered shading, rat chromosome 9. The candidate gene bone morphogenic receptor 2 is indicated with a white diamond. Horizontal bars indicate the position of microsatellite markers along the chromosome.

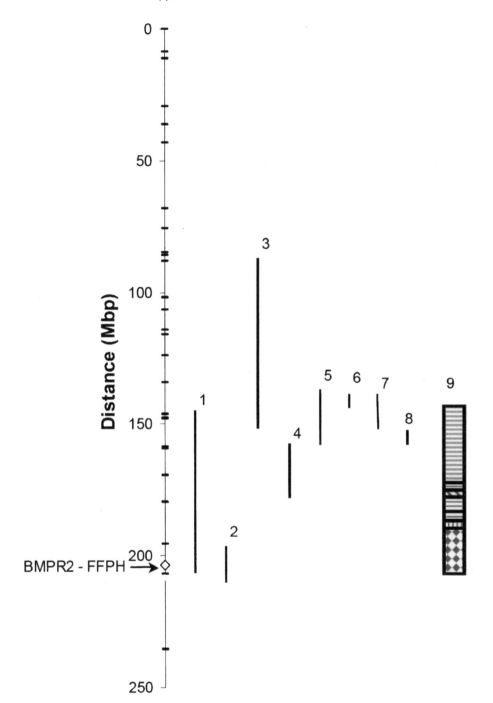

Zealand cohorts *(62)*. Given the poor positional information inherent in genome screens for complex traits *(52)* and despite the different study designs, it is possible that these linkages represent signals from the same locus, or possibly loci *(52)*. Interestingly, the gene responsible for primary pulmonary hypertension (PPH1), the bone morphogenic protein receptor 2 (BMPR2), maps within this region and so represents a good positional candidate (**Fig. 2**) *(63,64)*.

2.3. Potential Candidate Genes

The 60-Mb interval on chromosome 2q22-q33 contains 272 RefSeq genes, 1922 mRNAs, and 67,411 ESTs. A perusal of the 272 RefSeq genes highlights a few potential candidate genes, one of which is the gene encoding BMPR2 (as mentioned previously). Primary pulmonary hypertension is a rare autosomal dominant disorder that is characterized by intimal fibrosis and plexiform lesions of the precapillary pulmonary arteries and raised pulmonary artery pressure *(65)*. The pathogenesis of the disorder is not fully understood; however, it is feasible that different mutations in BMPR2 lead to essential hypertension. PPH1 is a heterogeneous condition, and a recent study has found a second locus mapping to chromosome 2q31 *(66)*. This region is also within the BRIGHT study chromosome 2 (LOD–1) interval, and the causative gene will possibly represent another candidate.

A nitric oxide synthase trafficker (NOSTRIN) also maps to the region. This protein was recently discovered using the yeast two-hybrid system, and is highly expressed in vascular endothelial cells *(67)*. It has been postulated that NOSTRIN is involved in the trafficking and targeting of endothelial nitric oxide synthase and therefore could represent an excellent candidate gene. There are several other promising candidates; these include a family of voltage-gated sodium channels, several subunits of voltage-gated calcium channels, and a serine–threonine kinase. In addition there are 12 genes in the region that are expressed three times above average levels in the kidney; these could all represent candidates too, as the kidney demonstrates disease pathology. There are probably many other potential candidate genes in the 60-Mb region on chromosome 2q31-q33. However, it is difficult, based on the information that is available from PubMed alone, to prioritize genes. Reducing the size of the region and bringing in information from other sources is a vital process before embarking on expensive individual candidate gene analysis.

2.4. Animal Models of Hypertension

Parallels between the genetic analysis of rodent models of disease and linkage results in human studies may be drawn upon to lend support to individual loci or genes as candidates. Many genome-wide screens have now been performed using the hypertensive rodent models available and, consistent with the picture emerging in human linkage studies, linkage is seen on each of the rat chromosomes with exception of rats 6, 11, and 15 *(68)*.

There is currently no database of rodent hypertensive loci, therefore the researcher, as with human studies, is dependent on published reviews and papers to ascertain overlapping regions *(68)*. However, with the recent completion of the human genome sequence and the ever-improving rat and mouse sequencing projects, syntenic regions can now be easily identified *(31)*. These aligned genomes are available online at a number of general genome annotation web sites such as UCSC server, Ensembl, or NCBI, along with a variety of specific sites (*see* **Notes 1** and **2**).

As linkage data provide limited positional information, each BP-related region in the rodent model is large, as in human studies. To improve resolution, congenic mapping approaches may be used *(32)*. Interestingly, a single linkage peak may break down using a congenic approach but will reveal several tightly linked disease genes *(69–71)*, and this appears to be the case for a hypertension locus in the distal region of rat chromosome 2 *(72,73)*. This observation should be borne in mind when results of initial linkage screens in disparate species are compared. To date none of the genes underlying rodent linkage peaks or congenic effects has been cloned.

2.5. Human Chromosome 2q22-2q33 and Rat Syntenic Regions

Human chromosome 2q22-2q33 shows synteny with seven different regions of the rat genome: four separate regions on rat chromosome 3 (36 Mb), one on chromosome 6 (0.817 Mb), one on chromosome 11 (2.155 Mb), and one on chromosome 9 (16.72 Mb) (www.ensembl.org, www.ncbi.nlm.nih.gov, www.genome.ucsc.edu, and **Fig. 2**). Rat chromosome 6 and rat chromosome 11 have not previously been linked to hypertensive traits *(68)*. Therefore genes syntenic to rat chromosomes 6 and 11 although not completely excluded, may take a lower priority. Rat chromosome 9 was linked to hypertension in a cross between spontaneously hypertensive rat (SHR) and Wistar-Kyoto rats *(74)*, and a congenic mapping strategy confirmed this region *(75)*. Further congenic mapping narrowed this to a 2.4-cM region, the syntenic region of which lies 15 Mb distal to the locus on human chromosome 2 *(76)*. It therefore unlikely that the linkage signals on rat chromosome 9 and human 2 are derived from variants of the same gene.

The majority of the linked human chromosome 2 region is syntenic to several regions of rat chromosome 3 (**Fig. 2**). There are two distinct regions of rat chromosome 3 linked to hypertensive-related traits *(68)*. In addition, Matsumoto and colleagues and Clarke et al. have both detected BP loci mapping to a large area of rat chromosome 3 *(77,78)* (**Fig. 3**). There is a considerable difference between the marker order used in these analyses and that of

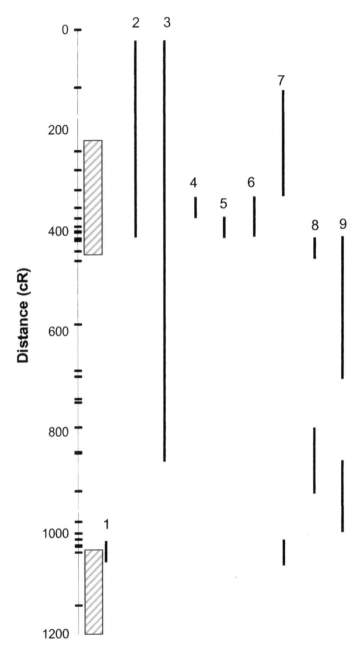

Fig. 3. Genome screen results for hypertension-related traits on rat chromosome 3. The diagonal shaded boxes show regions syntenic with hypertension loci on human chromosome 2q22-2q33. Regions linked to hypertensive-related traits in rat crosses. 1, Cicila et al., 1994; blood pressure and cardiac mass; 2, Clarke et al., 1996; hypertersion; 3, Matsumoto et al., 1996; salt-induced hypertension; 4, Hamet et al.,

previous maps *(68)* and sequence data from the genome sequencing projects (www.ensembl.org, www.ncbi.org, and www.genome.ucsc.edu). Therefore the precise location of these loci is unclear, however completion of the rat sequence should prompt a reevaluation of the data and resolve these queries.

Several other studies have shown consistent linkage to the proximal *(79,80)* or distal ends of rat chromosome 3 *(79,81,82)* with hypertensive phenotypes (**Fig. 3**). In addition, linkage to heart rate *(83)*, kidney mass *(84)*, and cardiac mass *(85)* have been reported to the proximal region of chromosome 3, although these are unlikely to be to the same gene (**Fig. 3**). In summary it is probable that rat chromosome 3 has at least two hypertension-related loci, and both of these regions share synteny with the human chromosome 2 locus (**Fig. 3**). Congenic mapping of these regions has yet to be undertaken.

2.6. Knock-In, Knockout, and Transgenic Animal Models

Alternative genetic models in the rodent that may help prioritize candidate genes for hypertension are knockout, knockin, transgenic models, and ethylnitrosurea (ENU) mutagenesis models. Knockout, knock-in, and transgenic models have been used to test the role of genes within a hypothesis-driven approach. A search of the mouse mutation database (http://research.bmn.com/mkmd/) for the term BP reveals 114 loci. There is currently no program to knock out each mouse gene across the genome to assay their function systematically. A systematic approach has been used to target genes randomly using ENU mutagenesis and to link those to phenotype. Several national programs are using this technology (e.g., MRC Harwell Mutagenesis program, NIH Mouse Mutagenesis for Developmental Defects and European Mouse Mutant Archive (EMMA), *see* **Note 2**), but currently none has reported a BP phenotype.

2.7. Transcriptomics

Clearly, for a gene to represent a good candidate it must be expressed in the relevant tissue. For chronic diseases with multiple tissue involvement this is not a simple issue, as both spatial and temporal expression patterns are important. There are several online databases of tissue expression patterns, and these provide a first clue about the expression pattern of a gene. Expressed sequence tags are sequences cloned from RNA libraries from a variety of tissues, organisms, and developmental stages, and two useful databases of these are dbEST

Fig. 3. (*continued*) 1998; kidney mass; 5, Garrett et al., 1998; blood pressure; 6, Cicila et al., 1999; blood pressure and cardiac mass; 7, Kreutz et al., 1999; heart rate; 8, Sebkhi et al., 1999; cardiac mass; 9, Kato et al., 1999; blood pressure. Horizontal bars indicate the position of microsatellite markers along the chromosome.

and Unigene (*see* **Note 3**). These databases, while useful, do have drawbacks in that they favor genes that are expressed at high copy number and it is often unclear from which tissue and at which time point.

The technology now exists to assay the entire transcriptome of a tissue in a single experiment using DNA or RNA microarrays or chips, or serial analysis of gene expression (SAGE) *(86)*. Several online databases store genome-wide expression profiles from a variety of tissues and species using microarrays, including Gene Expression Atlas *(87)*, TissueInfo *(88)*, and SAGEmap *(89)*, and each shows a good level of concordance *(90)* (*see* **Note 3**). These are all important resources giving background expression in many tissues; of particular interest in hypertension studies are the kidney profiles. It is possible to compare a list of expressed genes from these experiments with a list of genes within linked regions to help prioritize candidate gene selection. For a complex disease it would be advantageous to have expression data from specific tissues at particular time points in development.

To date there are no published reports of expression patterns from essential hypertensive patients, because of the ethical and practical difficulties of obtaining the appropriate tissue. Geraci et al. have circumvented this issue in primary pulmonary hypertension (PPH) by using cadaverous material. Geraci et al. identified 307 genes from a total of 6800 that showed differential expression between six PPH samples and six control tissues *(91)*. As has been done for a variety of tumor types, they were able to define a set of genes whose expression patterns define the disease phenotype. Although this is an intriguing look at end-stage disease, it would be useful to examine expression patterns over an expanded time course to investigate disease progression. This is obviously possible only in animal models of hypertension.

To date there are only a handful of experiments looking at expression levels in rodent models of disease. Okuda et al. examined differences in gene expression patterns using the Affymetrix gene chip system to look for differences between SHR strains and control rats *(92,93)*. Surprisingly, only a small number of genes were consistently changed between sources *(92,93)*. The gene expression patterns in other rat models have also been examined, for example, in smooth muscle in SHR *(94)*, progression to heart failure *(95)*, and two congenic strains *(72,96)*. Currently these data are available from published papers or directly from the authors. It would be a valuable resource if a database conforming to the Minimum Information About a Microarray Experiment (MIAME) *(97)* standards were set up to store this data.

2.8. Human Chromosome 2q22-2q33 Expression Patterns

As discussed, expression patterns from online databases in basic tissue types may help to prioritize genes as candidates. A cross-comparison of the 272 refseq genes within the linked region on 2q22-2q33 to the Gene Expression

Atlas shows 12 genes that are expressed in human kidney to a level three times over background. Moreover, of this set of 12 genes there are nine annotated with a mouse equivalent and five of these show expression in the murine kidney sample in the Gene Expression Atlas. Six of these genes lie in the upper syntenic region of rat chromosome 3 and therefore in the current schema represent good candidate genes. However, none of these genes overlaps with those cited in targeted expression profiling in the hypertensive models outlined above *(91,93–95)*.

2.9. Proteomics

The study of the protein component of a tissue or fluid, the proteome, may give insight into the likelihood that a gene is a good candidate. RNA expression levels show a limited correlation with the level of protein within a cell and cannot tell us of the posttranslational modifications important to a cell's function. It is now possible to interrogate the entire protein component of two systems to identify differences. In conventional proteome analysis, proteins are separated by charge and mass using two-dimensional gel electrophoresis (2GE) to identify those that differ between samples *(98–101)*. Additional methods such as affinity chromatography, ion exchange, size exclusion, and high-performance liquid chromatograpy (HPLC) may be used to improve the sensitivity of this method *(98–101)*. Proteins of different abundance may then be identified by peptide mass mapping, whereby the protein is degraded to smaller peptides using proteases such as trypsin or chemical reagents such as cyanogen bromide (CNBr) and the mass of these is determined by mass spectroscopy *(98–101)*. As each peptide will give a unique mass, these can be compared to a database of known peptide masses to identify the protein. It is now possible to analyze the proteome of any tissue or bodily fluid. Perhaps even more so than with expression studies it is essential that the precise tissue, timing, and experimental conditions are controlled in proteome studies.

There are several online databases of 2GE experiments listed at WORLD-2DPAGE (*see* **Note 4**), which focus mainly on particular disease states and for which only a minority of protein spots have been identified *(102)*. Current projects to identify global protein component in large numbers of tissues are limited to the industrial sector (Celera, OxfordGlycoSciences, GeneProt) (*see* **Note 4**) *(102)*. There is, however, a growing literature of proteomic studies that may inform hypertension research. Targeted proteomics investigates a subset of the proteome, focusing on proteins that have a potential involvement in a system of interest. Brooks et al. studied sodium transporter abundance in knockout mice for either Na^+H^+ exchanger type 3 (NHE3) or the Na^+Cl^- cotransporter (NCC) *(103)*. They measured levels of six other sodium transporters in whole kidney preparations and found increases in protein level of the sodium phosphate cotransporter and the γ-subunit of the epithelial sodium channel in NHE3 knockouts and the upregulation γ-subunit of the epithelial sodium channel in NCC knockout mice, thereby demonstrating a compensatory mechanism *(103)*.

A more global approach was taken by Thongboonkerd et al., who used a rat model of hypoxia-induced hypertension *(104)*. Kidney capsules from animals subjected to either sustained or episodic hypoxia were compared using two-dimensional electrophoresis. A total of 248 different protein spots were identified on each gel, and 25 spots showed a significantly different level of expression, which resolved to 14 different proteins *(104)*. A similar strategy was taken by Taurin et al. who examined vascular remodeling of the aorta produced by ouabain inhibition of the $Na^+K^+ATPase$. A total of 158 protein spots were induced and 104 suppressed. Peptide mass fingerprinting was then used to identify 24 of these proteins *(105)*. These data are only available in journal format, and in the future these should be made available in a standard electronic format to allow querying. None of these resources identifies any genes in 2q22-2q33 and therefore do not aid in candidate gene prioritization.

2.10. Future Approaches to Candidate Gene Prioritization

2.10.1. Genome-Wide Screens for Linkage Disequilibrium

Linkage screens for complex traits are widely recognized to have low power and limited positional accuracy *(106–109)*. It is anticipated that the next generation of genetic study design, the genome-wide screen for linkage disequilibrium (LD), and the non-random association of tightly linked variants, will overcome these hurdles *(106–109)*. It is likely that a panel of tens if not hundreds of thousand of markers will be necessary (compared to the hundreds in linkage analysis) *(110)*. Before these can be realized, however, concerns surrounding the underlying LD structure, statistical methods, and technical costs need to be addressed *(110–113)*. Despite these reservations some preliminary genome-wide screens for LD have been conducted. Notably, Ozaki et al. screened the genome with 65,671 single-nucleotide polymorphic markers in a cohort of 94 Japanese patients with myocardial infarction and identified, among others, polymorphisms in the lymphotoxin-α gene associated with the trait *(114)*. In the next few years, projects of this type will lead to novel candidate genes for hypertension.

2.10.2. Metabolomics

The study of metabolites, metabolomics, may help to yield new subphenotypes that coexist with a complex trait and therefore provide a stronger correlation between genotype and phenotype. In principle, the metabolite component of any fluid may be analyzed using a combination of nuclear magnetic resonance spectroscopy, chromatography, and mass spectroscopy. This has yet to be used to examine either a model of hypertension or samples from hypertensive individuals. However, proof of principle has been seen in single-celled organisms *(115)* and in nutrition and toxicology studies *(116–118)*.

3. Concluding Remarks

In summary, lots of data are available to help in prioritizing candidate genes. The challenge, however, is to integrate the data and to make the most efficient use of it. In our view, natural-language parsing methods need to be implemented to make the best use of published data. Bioinformatic approaches need to be developed to collate and rank genes using researcher-tailored queries so that experimental protocols are optimally designed. It is hoped that this type of analysis will lead to an increased understanding of human essential hypertension.

4. Notes

1. Genomics databases: Ensembl, www.ensembl.org; University of California at Santa Cruz Genome Browser http://genome.ucsc.edu; National Centre for Biotechnology Information, www.ncbi.nlm.nih.gov/entrez.
2. Rat and mouse genome mapping resources: Rat Genome Database, http://rgd.mcw.edu/maps, http://ratmap.hgc.jp/menu/Genome.html; Otsuka GEN Research Institute, http://ratest.uiowa.edu; Wellcome Trust Centre for Human Genetics, www.well.ox.ac.uk/rat_mapping_resources; Rat Map, http://ratmap.gen.gu.se; Mouse Knockout and Mutation Database, http://research.bmn.com/mkmd; MRC Harwell Mutagenesis Program, www.mut.har.mrc.ac.uk; NIH Mouse Mutagenesis for Developmental Defects, www.mouse-genome.bcm.tmc.edu; European Mouse Mutant Archive (EMMA) http://www.gsf.de/ieg/index.html
3. Transcriptomics resources dbEST http://www.ncbi.nlm.nih.gov/dbEST/ UNIGENE http://www.ncbi.nlm.nih.gov/entrez/query.fcgi?db=unigene Serial Analysis of Gene Expression (SAGEmap) http://www.ncbi.nlm.nih.gov/SAGE/ Tissueinfo http://icb.mssm.edu/services/tissueinfo/query Gene Expression Atlas http://expression.gnf.org/cgi-bin/ 4. Proteomics resources WORLD-2DPAGE http://us.expasy.org/ch2d/2d-index.html Celera http://www.celera.com OxfordGlycoSciences http://www.ogs.com GeneProt http://www.geneprot.com

Acknowledgments

We are extremely grateful to the Medical Research Council, The British Heart Foundation, Joint Research Board, and The Special Trustees of St Bartholomew's Hospital for funding. We would like to thank Richard Dobson and Daniel Buchan for bioinformatics support, and Edwin Garcia and Steven Newhouse for comments on the manuscript.

References

1. Ward, R. (1990) Familial aggregation and genetic epidemiology of blood pressure. In *Hypertension: Pathophysiology, Diagnosis and Management* (eds. Laragh, J. H. and Brenner, B. M., eds.) Raven Press, New York pp. 81–100.
2. Nicholls, M. G. and Robertson, J. I. (2000) The renin-angiotensin system in the year 2000. *J. Hum. Hypertens.* **14**, 649–666.
3. Perazella, M. A. and Setaro, J. F. (2003) Renin-angiotensin-aldosterone system: fundamental aspects and clinical implications in renal and cardiovascular disorders. *J. Nucl. Cardiol.* **10**, 184–196.
4. Jeunemaitre, X., Soubrier, F., Kotelevtsev, Y., et al. (1992) Molecular basis of human hypertension: role of angiotensinogen. *Cell* **71**, 169–180.
5. Caulfield, M., Lavender, P., Farrall, M., et al. (1994) Linkage of the angiotensinogen gene to essential hypertension. *N. Engl. J. Med.* **330**, 1629–1633.
6. Lalouel, J. M., Rohrwasser, A., Terreros, D., Morgan, T., and Ward, K. (2001) Angiotensinogen in essential hypertension: from genetics to nephrology. *J. Am. Soc. Nephrol.* **12**, 606–615.
7. Sethi, A. A., Nordestgaard, B. G., and Tybjaerg-Hansen, A. (2003) Angiotensinogen gene polymorphism, plasma angiotensinogen, and risk of hypertension and ischemic heart disease: a meta-analysis. *Arterioscler. Thromb. Vasc. Biol.* **23**, 1269–1275.
8. Brand, E., Herrmann, S. M., Nicaud, V., et al. (1999) The 825C/T polymorphism of the G-protein subunit beta3 is not related to hypertension. *Hypertension* **33**, 1175–1178.
9. Tomaszewski, M., Brain, N. J., Charchar, F. J., et al. (2002) Essential hypertension and beta2-adrenergic receptor gene: linkage and association analysis. *Hypertension* **40**, 286–291.
10. Herrmann, S. M., Nicaud, V., Tiret, L., et al. (2002) Polymorphisms of the beta2 -adrenoceptor (ADRB2) gene and essential hypertension: the ECTIM and PEGASE studies. *J. Hypertens.* **20**, 229–235.
11. Siffert, W. (2003) G-protein beta3 subunit 825T allele and hypertension. *Curr. Hypertens. Rep.* **5**, 47–53.
12. Lifton, R. P., Dluhy, R. G., Powers, M., et al. (1992) A chimeric 11 beta-hydroxylase/aldosterone synthase gene causes glucocorticoid-remediable aldosteronism and human hypertension. *Nature* **355**, 262–265.
13. Shimkets, R. A., Warnock, D. G., Bositis, C. M., et al. (1994) Liddle's syndrome: heritable human hypertension caused by mutations in the b subunit of the epithelial sodium channel. *Cell* **79**, 407–414.
14. Stewart, P. M., Krozowski, Z. S., Gupta, A., et al. (1996) Hypertension in the syndrome of apparent mineralocorticoid excess due to mutation of the 11 beta-hydroxysteroid dehydrogenase type 2 gene. *Lancet* **347**, 88–91.
15. Wilson, F. H., Disse-Nicodeme, S., Choate, K. A., et al. (2001) Human hypertension caused by mutations in WNK kinases. *Science* **293**, 1107–1112.
16. Kumar, N. N., Benjafield, A. V., Lin, R. C., Wang, W. Y., Stowasser, M., and Morris, B. J. (2003) Haplotype analysis of aldosterone synthase gene (CYP11B2)

polymorphisms shows association with essential hypertension. *J. Hypertens.* **21,** 1331–1337.

17. Zhu, H., Sagnella, G. A., Dong, Y., et al. (2003) Contrasting associations between aldosterone synthase gene polymorphisms and essential hypertension in blacks and in whites. *J. Hypertens.* **21,** 87–95.

18. Lim, P. O., Macdonald, T. M., Holloway, C., et al. (2002) Variation at the aldosterone synthase (CYP11B2) locus contributes to hypertension in subjects with a raised aldosterone-to-renin ratio. *J. Clin. Endocrinol. Metab.* **87,** 4398–4402.

19. Melander, O., Orho-Melander, M., Bengtsson, K., et al. (2000) Association between a variant in the 11 beta-hydroxysteroid dehydrogenase type 2 gene and primary hypertension. *J. Hum. Hypertens.* **14,** 819–823.

20. Ferrari, P. and Krozowski, Z. (2000) Role of the 11beta-hydroxysteroid dehydrogenase type 2 in blood pressure regulation. *Kidney Int.* **57,** 1374–1381.

21. Dong, Y.B., Zhu, H.D., Baker, E.H., et al. (2001) T594M and G442V polymorphisms of the sodium channel beta subunit and hypertension in a black population. *J. Hum. Hypertens.* **15,** 425–430.

22. Iwai, N., Baba, S., Mannami, T., et al. (2001) Association of sodium channel gamma-subunit promoter variant with blood pressure. *Hypertension* **38,** 86–89.

23. Iwai, N., Baba, S., Mannami, T., Ogihara, T., and Ogata, J. (2002) Association of a sodium channel alpha subunit promoter variant with blood pressure. *J. Am. Soc. Nephrol.* **13,** 80–85.

24. Persu, A., Barbry, P., Bassilana, F., et al. (1998) Genetic analysis of the beta subunit of the epithelial Na$^+$ channel in essential hypertension. *Hypertension* **32,** 129–137.

25. Persu, A., Coscoy, S., Houot, A.M., Corvol, P., Barbry, P., and Jeunemaitre, X. (1999) Polymorphisms of the gamma subunit of the epithelial Na$^+$ channel in essential hypertension. *J. Hypertens.* **17,** 639–645.

26. Wilson, F. H., Kahle, K. T., Sabath, E., et al. (2003) Molecular pathogenesis of inherited hypertension with hyperkalemia: the Na-Cl cotransporter is inhibited by wild-type but not mutant WNK4. *Proc. Natl. Acad. Sci. USA* **100,** 680–684.

27. Erlich, P. M., Cui, J., Chazaro, I., et al. (2003) Genetic variants of WNK4 in whites and African Americans with hypertension. *Hypertension* **41,** 1191–1195.

28. Hilbert, P., Lindpaintner, K., Beckmann, J. S., et al. (1991) Chromosomal mapping of two genetic loci associated with blood-pressure regulation in hereditary hypertensive rats. *Nature* **353,** 521–529.

29. Jacob, H. J., Lindpaintner, K., Lincoln, S. E., et al. (1991) Genetic mapping of a gene causing hypertension in the stroke-prone spontaneously hypertensive rat. *Cell* **67,** 213–224.

30. Stoll, M., Kwitek-Black, A. E., Cowley, A. W., Jr., et al. (2000) New target regions for human hypertension via comparative genomics. *Genome Res.* **10,** 473–482.

31. Jacob, H. J. and Kwitek, A. E. (2002) Rat genetics: attaching physiology and pharmacology to the genome. *Nat. Rev. Genet.* **3,** 33–42.

32. Wakeland, E., Morel, L., Achey, K., Yui, M., and Longmate, J. (1997) Speed congenics: a classic technique in the fast lane (relatively speaking). *Immunol. Today* **18,** 472–477.

33. Jeffs, B., Negrin, C. D., Graham, D., et al. (2000) Applicability of a "speed" congenic strategy to dissect blood pressure quantitative trait loci on rat chromosome 2. *Hypertension* **35**, 179–187.

34. Collins, S. C., Wallis, R. H., Wallace, K., Bihoreau, M. T., and Gauguier, D. (2003) Marker-assisted congenic screening (MACS): a database tool for the efficient production and characterization of congenic lines. *Mamm. Genome* **14**, 350–356.

35. Kreutz, R. and Hubner, N. (2002) Congenic rat strains are important tools for the genetic dissection of essential hypertension. *Semin. Nephrol.* **22**, 135–147.

36. Dukhanina, O. I., Dene, H., Deng, A. Y., Choi, C. R., Hoebee, B., and Rapp, J. P. (1997) Linkage map and congenic strains to localize blood pressure QTL on rat chromosome 10. *Mamm. Genome* **8**, 229–235.

37. Sivo, Z., Malo, B., Dutil, J., and Deng, A. Y. (2002) Accelerated congenics for mapping two blood pressure quantitative trait loci on chromosome 10 of Dahl rats. *J. Hypertens.* **20**, 45–53.

38. Palijan, A., Lambert, R., Dutil, J., Sivo, Z., and Deng, A. Y. (2003) Comprehensive congenic coverage revealing multiple blood pressure quantitative trait loci on Dahl rat chromosome 10. *Hypertension* **42**, 515–522.

39. Monti, J., Zimdahl, H., Schulz, H., Plehm, R., Ganten, D., and Hubner, N. (2003) The role of Wnk4 in polygenic hypertension: a candidate gene analysis on rat chromosome 10. *Hypertension* **41**, 938–942.

40. Julier, C., Delepine, M., Keavney, B., et al. (1997) Genetic susceptibility for human familial essential hypertension in a region of homology with blood pressure linkage on rat chromosome 10. *Hum. Mol. Genet.* **6**, 2077–2285.

41. Baima, J., Nicolaou, M., Schwartz, F., et al. (1999) Evidence for linkage between essential hypertension and a putative locus on human chromosome 17. *Hypertension* **34**, 4–7.

42. Levy, D., DeStefano, A .L., Larson, M. G., et al. (2000) Evidence for a gene influencing blood pressure on chromosome 17. Genome scan linkage results for longitudinal blood pressure phenotypes in subjects from the Framingham heart study. *Hypertension* **36**, 477–483.

43. Rutherford, S., Johnson, M. P., Curtain, R.P., and Griffiths, L. R. (2001) Chromosome 17 and the inducible nitric oxide synthase gene in human essential hypertension. *Hum. Genet.* **109**, 408–415.

44. Caulfield, M., Munroe, P., Pembroke, J., et al. (2003) Genome-wide mapping of human loci for essential hypertension. *Lancet* **361**, 2118–2123.

45. Knight, J., Munroe, P. B., Pembroke, J. C., and Caulfield, M. J. (2003) Human chromosome 17 in essential hypertension. *Ann. Hum. Genet.* **67**, 193–206.

46. Risch, N. (1990) Linkage strategies for genetically complex traits. I. multilocus models. *Am. J. Hum. Genet.* **46**, 222–228.

47. Risch, N. (1990) Linkage strategies for genetically complex traits. II. The power of affected relative pairs. *Am. J. Hum. Genet.* **46**, 229–241.

48. Risch, N. (1990) Linkage strategies for genetically complex traits. III. The effect of marker polymorphism on analysis of affected relative pairs. *Am. J. Hum. Genet.* **46**, 242–253.

49. Samani, N. J. (2003) Genome scans for hypertension and blood pressure regulation. *Am. J. Hypertens.* **16**, 167–171.
50. Garcia, E. A., Newhouse, S., Caulfield, M. J., and Munroe, P. B. (2003) Genes and hypertension. *Curr. Pharm. Des.* **9**, 1679–1689.
51. Lander, E. and Kruglyak, L. (1995) Genetic dissection of complex traits: guidelines for interpreting and reporting linkage results. *Nat. Genet.* **11**, 241–247.
52. Roberts, S. B., MacLean, C. J., Neale, M. C., Eaves, L. J., and Kendler, K. S. (1999) Replication of linkage studies of complex traits: an examination of variation in location estimates. *Am. J. Hum. Genet.* **65**, 876–884.
53. Goring, H. H., Terwilliger, J. D., and Blangero, J. (2001) Large upward bias in estimation of locus-specific effects from genomewide scans. *Am. J. Hum. Genet.* **69**, 1357–1369.
54. Siegmund, D. (2002) Upward bias in estimation of genetic effects. *Am. J. Hum. Genet.* **71**, 1183–1138.
55. Suarez, B., Hampe, C., and Van Eerdewegh, P. (1994) Problems of replicating linkage claims in psychiatry. In *Genetic Approaches to Mental Disorders* (Cloninger, C., ed.) American Psychiatric Press, Washington, DC, pp. 23–46.
56. Krushkal, J., Ferrell, R., Mockrin, S., Turner, S., Sing, C. F., and Boerwinkle, E. (1999) Genome-wide linkage analysis of systolic blood pressure using highly discordant siblings. *Circulation* **99**, 1407–1410.
57. Hsueh, W. C., Mitchell, B. D., Schneider, J. L., et al. (2000) QTL influencing blood pressure maps to the region of PPH1 on chromosome 2q31-34 in Old Order Amish. *Circulation* **101**, 2810–2816.
58. Atwood, L. D., Samollow, P. B., Hixson, J. E., Stern, M. P., and MacCluer, J. W. (2001) Genome-wide linkage analysis of blood pressure in Mexican Americans. *Genet. Epidemiol.* **20**, 373–382.
59. Zhu, D. L., Wang, H. Y., Xiong, M. M., et al. (2001) Linkage of hypertension to chromosome 2q14-q23 in Chinese families. *J. Hypertens.* **19**, 55–61.
60. Perola, M., Kainulainen, K., Pajukanta, P., et al. (2000) Genome-wide scan of predisposing loci for increased diastolic blood pressure in Finnish siblings. *J. Hypertens.* **18**, 1579–1585.
61. Arngrimsson, R., Sigurard ttir, S., Frigge, M. L., et al. (1999) A genome-wide scan reveals a maternal susceptibility locus for pre-eclampsia on chromosome 2p13. *Hum. Mol. Genet.* **8**, 1799–1805.
62. Moses, E. K., Lade, J. A., Guo, G., et al. (2000) A genome scan in families from Australia and New Zealand confirms the presence of a maternal susceptibility locus for pre-eclampsia, on chromosome 2. *Am. J. Hum. Genet.* **67**, 1581–1585.
63. Deng, Z., Morse, J. H., Slager, S. L., et al. (2000) Familial primary pulmonary hypertension (gene PPH1) is caused by mutations in the bone morphogenetic protein receptor-II gene. *Am. J. Hum. Genet.* **67**, 737–744.
64. Lane, K. B., Machado, R. D., Pauciulo, M. W., et al. (2000) Heterozygous germline mutations in BMPR2, encoding a TGF-beta receptor, cause familial primary pulmonary hypertension. The International PPH Consortium. *Nat. Genet.* **26**, 81–84.

65. Runo, J. R. and Loyd, J. E. (2003) Primary pulmonary hypertension. *Lancet* **361**, 1533–1544.
66. Rindermann, M., Grunig, E., von Hippel, A., et al. (2003) Primary pulmonary hypertension may be a heterogeneous disease with a second locus on chromosome 2q31. *J. Am. Coll. Cardiol.* **41**, 2237–2244.
67. Zimmermann, K., Opitz, N., Dedio, J., Renne, C., Muller-Esterl, W., and Oess, S. (2002) NOSTRIN: a protein modulating nitric oxide release and subcellular distribution of endothelial nitric oxide synthase. *Proc. Natl. Acad. Sci. USA* **99**, 17167–17172.
68. Rapp, J. P. (2000) Genetic analysis of inherited hypertension in the rat. *Physiol. Rev.* **80**, 135–172.
69. Podolin, P. L., Denny, P., Lord, C. J., et al. (1997) Congenic mapping of the insulin-dependent diabetes (Idd) gene, Idd10, localizes two genes mediating the Idd10 effect and eliminates the candidate Fcgr1. *J. Immunol.* **159**, 1835–1843.
70. Podolin, P. L., Armitage, N., Lord, C. J., et al. (1998) Localization of two insulin-dependent diabetes (Idd) genes to the Idd10 region on mouse chromosome 3. *Mamm. Genome* **9**, 283–286.
71. Serreze, D. V., Bridgett, M., Chapman, H. D., et al. (1998) Subcongenic analysis of the Idd13 locus in NOD/Lt mice: evidence for several susceptibility genes including a possible diabetogenic role for beta 2-microglobulin. *J. Immunol.* **160**, 1472–1478.
72. McBride, M. W., Carr, F. J., Graham, D., et al. (2003) Microarray analysis of rat chromosome 2 congenic strains. *Hypertension* **41**, 847–853.
73. Dutil, J. and Deng, A. Y. (2001) Further chromosomal mapping of a blood pressure QTL in Dahl rats on chromosome 2 using congenic strains. *Physiol. Genomics* **6**, 3–9.
74. Takami, S., Higaki, J., Miki, T., et al. (1996) Analysis and comparison of new candidate loci for hypertension between genetic hypertensive rat strains. *Hypertens. Res.* **19**, 51–56.
75. Rapp, J. P., Garrett, M. R., Dene, H., Meng, H., Hoebee, B., and Lathrop, G.M. (1998) Linkage analysis and construction of a congenic strain for a blood pressure QTL on rat chromosome 9. *Genomics* **51**, 191–196.
76. Meng, H., Garrett, M. R., Dene, H., and Rapp, J.P. (2003) Localization of a blood pressure QTL to a 2.4-cM interval on rat chromosome 9 using congenic strains. *Genomics* **81**, 210–220.
77. Clark, J. S., Jeffs, B., Davidson, A. O., et al. (1996) Quantitative trait loci in genetically hypertensive rats. Possible sex specificity. *Hypertension* **28**, 898–906.
78. Matsumoto, C., Nara, Y., Ikeda, K., et al. (1996) Cosegregation of the new region on chromosome 3 with salt-induced hypertension in female F2 progeny from stroke-prone spontaneously hypertensive and Wistar-Kyoto rats. *Clin. Exp. Pharmacol. Physiol.* **23**, 1028–1034.
79. Cicila, G. T., Rapp, J. P., Bloch, K. D., et al. (1994) Cosegregation of the endothelin-3 locus with blood pressure and relative heart weight in inbred Dahl rats. *J. Hypertens.* **12**, 643–651.

80. Garrett, M. R., Dene, H., Walder, R., et al. (1998) Genome scan and congenic strains for blood pressure QTL using Dahl salt-sensitive rats. *Genome Res.* **8,** 711–723.

81. Cicila, G. T., Choi, C., Dene, H., Lee, S. J., and Rapp, J. P. (1999) Two blood pressure/cardiac mass quantitative trait loci on chromosome 3 in Dahl rats. *Mamm. Genome* **10,** 112–116.

82. Kato, N., Hyne, G., Bihoreau, M. T., Gauguier, D., Lathrop, G. M., and Rapp, J. P. (1999) Complete genome searches for quantitative trait loci controlling blood pressure and related traits in four segregating populations derived from Dahl hypertensive rats. *Mamm. Genome* **10,** 259–265.

83. Kreutz, R., Struk, B., Stock, P., Hubner, N., Ganten, D., and Lindpaintner, K. (1997) Evidence for primary genetic determination of heart rate regulation: chromosomal mapping of a genetic locus in the rat. *Circulation* **96,** 1078–1081.

84. Hamet, P., Pausova, Z., Dumas, P., et al. (1998) Newborn and adult recombinant inbred strains: a tool to search for genetic determinants of target organ damage in hypertension. *Kidney Int.* **53,** 1488–1492.

85. Sebkhi, A., Zhao, L., Lu, L., Haley, C. S., Nunez, D. J., and Wilkins, M. R. (1999) Genetic determination of cardiac mass in normotensive rats: results from an F344 × WKY cross. *Hypertension* **33,** 949–953.

86. Barczak, A., Rodriguez, M. W., Hanspers, K., et al. (2003) Spotted long oligonucleotide arrays for human gene expression analysis. *Genome Res.* **13,** 1775–1785.

87. Su, A. I., Cooke, M. P., Ching, K. A., et al. (2002) Large-scale analysis of the human and mouse transcriptomes. *Proc. Natl. Acad. Sci. USA* **99,** 4465–4470.

88. Skrabanek, L. and Campagne, F. (2001) TissueInfo: high-throughput identification of tissue expression profiles and specificity. *Nucleic Acids Res.* **29,** E102–E102.

89. Lash, A. E., Tolstoshev, C. M., Wagner, L., et al. (2000) SAGEmap: a public gene expression resource. *Genome Res.* **10,** 1051–1060.

90. Huminiecki, L., Lloyd, A. T., and Wolfe, K. H. (2003) Congruence of tissue expression profiles from Gene Expression Atlas, SAGEmap and TissueInfo databases. *BMC Genomics* **4,** 31.

91. Geraci, M. W., Moore, M., Gesell, T., et al. (2001) Gene expression patterns in the lungs of patients with primary pulmonary hypertension: a gene microarray analysis. *Circ. Res.* **88,** 555–562.

92. Okuda, T., Sumiya, T., Mizutani, K., et al. (2002) Analyses of differential gene expression in genetic hypertensive rats by microarray. *Hypertens. Res.* **25,** 249–255.

93. Okuda, T., Sumiya, T., Iwai, N. & Miyata, T. (2002) Difference of gene expression profiles in spontaneous hypertensive rats and Wistar-Kyoto rats from two sources. *Biochem. Biophys. Res. Commun.* **296,** 537–543.

94. Hu, W. Y., Fukuda, N., and Kanmatsuse, K. (2002) Growth characteristics, angiotensin II generation, and microarray-determined gene expression in vascular smooth muscle cells from young spontaneously hypertensive rats. *J. Hypertens.* **20,** 1323–1333.

95. Ueno, S., Ohki, R., Hashimoto, T., et al. (2003) DNA microarray analysis of in vivo progression mechanism of heart failure. *Biochem. Biophys. Res. Commun.* **307,** 771–777.

96. Liang, M., Yuan, B., Rute, E., et al. (2002) Renal medullary genes in salt-sensitive hypertension: a chromosomal substitution and cDNA microarray study. *Physiol. Genomics* **8,** 139–149.

97. Brazma, A., Hingamp, P., Quackenbush, J., et al. (2001) Minimum information about a microarray experiment (MIAME)-toward standards for microarray data. *Nat. Genet.* **29,** 365–371.

98. Patterson, S. D. and Aebersold, R. H. (2003) Proteomics: the first decade and beyond. *Nat. Genet.* **33** (Suppl.), 311–323.

99. Jager, D., Jungblut, P. R., and Muller-Werdan, U. (2002) Separation and identification of human heart proteins. *J. Chromatogr. B, Anal. Technol. Biomed. Life Sci.* **771,** 131–153.

100. Lee, R. T. (2001) Functional genomics and cardiovascular drug discovery. *Circulation* **104,** 1441–1446.

101. Arrell, D. K., Neverova, I., and Van Eyk, J. E. (2001) Cardiovascular proteomics: evolution and potential. *Circ. Res.* **88,** 763–773.

102. Gromov, P. S., Ostergaard, M., Gromova, I., and Celis, J. E. (2002) Human proteomic databases: a powerful resource for functional genomics in health and disease. *Prog. Biophys. Mol. Biol.* **80,** 3–22.

103. Brooks, H. L., Sorensen, A. M., Terris, J., et al. (2001) Profiling of renal tubule Na^+ transporter abundances in NHE3 and NCC null mice using targeted proteomics. *J. Physiol.* **530,** 359–366.

104. Thongboonkerd, V., Gozal, E., Sachleben, L. R., Jr., et al. (2002) Proteomic analysis reveals alterations in the renal kallikrein pathway during hypoxia-induced hypertension. *J. Biol. Chem.* **277,** 34708–34716.

105. Taurin, S., Seyrantepe, V., Orlov, S. N., et al. (2002) Proteome analysis and functional expression identify mortalin as an antiapoptotic gene induced by elevation of $[Na^+]_i/[K^+]_i$ ratio in cultured vascular smooth muscle cells. *Circ. Res.* **91,** 915–922.

106. Risch, N. and Merikangas, K. (1996) The future of genetic studies of complex human diseases. *Science* **273,** 1516–1517.

107. Teng, J. and Risch, N. (1999) The relative power of family-based and case-control designs for linkage disequilibrium studies of complex human diseases. II. Individual genotyping. *Genome Res.* **9,** 234–241.

108. Risch, N. and Teng, J. (1998) The relative power of family-based and case-control designs for linkage disequilibrium studies of complex human diseases I. DNA pooling. *Genome Res.* **8,** 1273–1288.

109. Herr, M., Dudbridge, F., Zavattari, P., et al. (2000) Evaluation of fine mapping strategies for a multifactorial disease locus: systematic linkage and association analysis of IDDM1 in the HLA region on chromosome 6p21. *Hum. Mol. Genet.* **9,** 1291–1301.

110. Kruglyak, L. (1999) Prospects for whole-genome linkage disequilibrium mapping of common disease genes. *Nat. Genet.* **22,** 139–144.
111. Couzin, J. (2002) Human genome. HapMap launched with pledges of $100 million. *Science* **298,** 941–942.
112. Terwilliger, J. D. and Weiss, K. M. (1998) Linkage disequilibrium mapping of complex disease: fantasy or reality? *Curr. Opin. Biotechnol.* **9,** 578–594.
113. Weiss, K. M. and Terwilliger, J. D. (2000) How many diseases does it take to map a gene with SNPs? *Nat. Genet.* **26,** 151–157.
114. Ozaki, K., Ohnishi, Y., Iida, A., et al. (2002) Functional SNPs in the lymphotoxin-alpha gene that are associated with susceptibility to myocardial infarction. *Nat. Genet.* **32,** 650–654.
115. Raamsdonk, L. M., Teusink, B., Broadhurst, D., et al. (2001) A functional genomics strategy that uses metabolome data to reveal the phenotype of silent mutations. *Nat. Biotechnol.* **19,** 45–50.
116. Phelps, T. J., Palumbo, A. V., and Beliaev, A. S. (2002) Metabolomics and microarrays for improved understanding of phenotypic characteristics controlled by both genomics and environmental constraints. *Curr. Opin. Biotechnol.* **13,** 20–24.
117. van Ommen, B. and Stierum, R. (2002) Nutrigenomics: exploiting systems biology in the nutrition and health arena. *Curr. Opin. Biotechnol.* **13,** 517–521.
118. Watkins, S. M. and German, J. B. (2002) Toward the implementation of metabolomic assessments of human health and nutrition. *Curr. Opin. Biotechnol.* **13,** 512–516.

9

Genome-Wide Scanning With SSLPs in the Rat

Carol Moreno, Kathleen Kennedy, Jaime Wendt Andrae,
and Howard J. Jacob

Summary

Genome-wide linkage analysis is a powerful tool for the identification of genes underlying single gene and complex genetic disorders. The most commonly used technique for performing genome wide scans for genetic studies in the rat is by analysis of simple sequence length polymorphism (SSLPs) or microsatellite markers. A sensitive and flexible method for high-throughput genotyping is described. Addition of an M13 tail to the SSLP primer eliminates the need for direct conjugation of the fluorescent dye to the primers, allowing for any combination of primer and fluorophor, and therefore for easy multiplexing of primers in the same reaction. With the use of three different dyes, it is possible to run more than five hundred genotypes in each run of the automatic sequencer. Automation in the fluorescent detection system and data tracking software for processing genotypes, contributes to the ability to genotype large number of samples rapidly and accurately.

Key Words: Genetic markers; fluorescent genotyping; linkage; SSLPs; QTL; multiplexing.

1. Introduction

Genome-wide scanning (GWS) studies are widely used to study Mendelian (single-gene) and complex, polygenic disorders without *a priori* hypotheses regarding candidate genes. For studies in experimental animals, it is typically applied to a backcross (**Fig. 1A**) or intercross (**Fig. 1B**) between affected and unaffected inbred strains. Linkage analysis for different traits allows the identification of quantitative trait loci (QTL) responsible for the regulation of complex traits *(1)*, such as arterial blood pressure. The most commonly used technique for performing genome-wide scans for genetic studies is by analysis of simple sequence length polymorphism (SSLPs), also called microsatellites, in genes.

From: *Methods in Molecular Medicine, Vol. 108: Hypertension: Methods and Protocols*
Edited by: J. P. Fennell and A. H. Baker © Humana Press Inc., Totowa, NJ

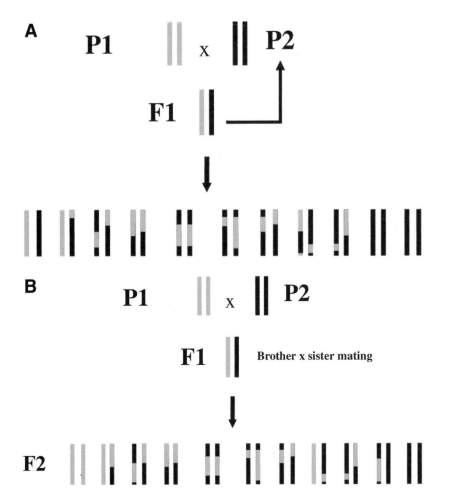

Fig. 1. **(A)** Generation of an F2 population by backcross. Two parental strains are crossed to produce F1 progeny. The F1 population is crossed with one parental strain to produce an F2 population. **(B)** Generation of an F2 population by intercross. Two parental strains are crossed to produce F1 progeny. The F1 population is brother–sister-mated to produce F2 population.

Here we describe the method for performing a genome wide scan in the laboratory rat (*Rattus novergicus*) with a fluorescent-based assay modified from Oetting et al. *(2)*, which includes the use of M13 sequencing SSLP primers and an automated DNA sequencer (Applied Biosystems 377). The addition of an M13 tail to the design of the primers eliminates the need for direct conjugation of the fluorescent dye to the primers. The ability to combine any of the three dyes to any primer allows for easy multiplexing of primers in the same reaction, reducing the number of polymerase chain reaction (PCR) reactions to perform, and therefore reducing cost and increasing flexibility. The general aim in performing a GWS is to achieve an average interval distance between loci sufficient to detect linkage to a QTL with a minimum number of genetic markers uniformly distributed across the genome. As a general rule of thumb we use a 10-cM interval as a goal, with no interval greater than 20–25 cM.

To date, more that 10,000 rat genetic markers have been published *(3,4)*. Moreover, polymorphisms of these markers across 48 species have been characterized *(5)* and are publicly available through the Rat Genome Database (RGD, www.rgd.mcw.edu). This greatly facilitates the selection of more suitable markers for the rat strains used in each cross.

1.1. Study Design Considerations

1. The selection of rat strains to study is of vital importance: Phenotypically, for a quantitative trait such as blood pressure, the difference between the control and the diseased strain should be greater than 2 SD for the trait of study. Genetically, the strains selected should be inbred and homozygous at all loci. They should also be genetically divergent, to have a high percentage of marker polymorphism.
2. Cross setup: In order to perform a genetic linkage study, the affected and unaffected inbred strains are mated to generate a first filial generation (F1). A second-generation cross is then carried either by a backcross (in which F1 animals are mated with one of the parental strains, **Fig. 1A**) or an intercross (in which F1 progeny are mated to each other, **Fig. 1B**). The second generation is then phenotyped for the trait of interest and a GWS performed.
3. Reciprocal cross design: If experiments are performed by single-cross design, in which an affected male is typically crossed with an unaffected female, they will fail to address whether the phenotypical difference between male and female animals is due to sex-linked gene(s) or to a sex-specific effect. It is recommended to use a reciprocal-cross design, in which an affected male is crossed with an unaffected female and an unaffected male is crossed with an affected female. When the F1 progeny are studied, if each sex shows the same phenotypic values independent of the direction of the cross, then the difference is sex-specific. However, if animals of a given sex from the two crosses show differences, this indicates that a sex-linked gene, a mitochondrial effect, or imprinting is affecting the phenotype.
4. Backcross vs intercross: Backcross studies are chosen when it is desired to have the maximum efficiency in detecting some of the major QTL. Intercross of F2 studies should be chosen when the purpose of the study is to detect how many QTL are segregating for that cross and to estimate their mode of inheritance.
5. How many animals to study: In dealing with polygenic diseases, you first need to have an estimate of the number of genes involved in the development of the disease. This can be calculated by the formula of Sewall Wright (*see* **Note 1**). The number of progeny that must be genotyped to map a QTL will then depend

on the difference between the strains and the number of potential loci, as calculated by Lander and Botstein *(6)*. As an example, for a trait that differs 2 SD between parental strains, and is expected to be determined by four loci, the study will need about 200 F2 animals to be studied in backcross progeny.

6. Selective genotyping of the extreme progeny: One way to increase the efficiency of QTL mapping is by selective genotyping. The individuals that provide the most linkage information are those with the most extreme phenotype, which deviate the most from the phenotypic mean. Progeny with phenotypes more than 1 SD from the mean (33% of the population) contribute 81% of the total linkage information. Progeny with phenotypes more than 2 SD from the mean (5%) contribute about 28% of the total linkage information *(6)*.

2. Materials

2.1. DNA Extraction

1. Lysis buffer (200 mL): 158 mL of sterile water, 10 mL of 2 M Tris-HCl, pH 8.5 (e.g., Sigma), 20 mL of 0.05 M EDTA (pH 8.0), 4 mL of 10% sodium dodecyl sulfate (SDS), 8 mL of 5 M NaCl, 10 µL of a 10-mg/mL stock solution of proteinase K (Sigma) for each milliliter of lysis buffer, added just before use.
2. Isopropyl alcohol and ethanol.
3. Resuspension buffer (200 mL): 199 mL of sterile water, 1 mL of 2 M Tris-HCl, pH 7.5 (e.g., Sigma), 400 µL of 0.05 M EDTA.

2.2. PCR Reaction

1. 384- or 96-well PCR plate (e.g., MJ-Research).
2. Primers (Proligo, Boulder, CO): Mixed forward and reverse primers, diluted to 0.46 µM. The forward primer of each marker set will have an M13 tail attached to the 5'-end. The sequence of the M13 tail is as follows:

    5'TGTAAAACGACGGCCAGT-XXXXXXXXXXXX3'

3. PCR mix stock solutions:
    a. dNTPs: 100 mM each of dATP, dTTP, dCTP, and dGTP, pooled in equal amounts. Dilute 10 times with water to make a final concentration of 2.5 mM for dNTP.
    b. 10X PCR buffer: 100 mM Tris-HCl (pH 8.3), 15 mM MgCl$_2$, 500 mM KCl.
    c. 5 U/µL *Taq* DNA polymerase (Promega).
    d. 1200 nM M13-primer-dye conjugate (Applied Biosystems): 5'-Fluorophore-TGTAAAACGACGGCCAGT. Fluorophores used: NED (yellow), HEX (green), and 6-FAM (blue).
4. MJ Research Tetrad Thermal Cycler.

2.3. Extraction and Gel Loading

1. 75% Isopropanol (Sigma).
2. Gel: 18 g urea (Sigma), 5 mL Long Ranger gel solution (Cambrex Bio Science), 2.5 mL 10X Tris-borate-EDTA (TBE, Fisher), 30 µL TEMED (Bio-Rad), 250 µL

10% ammonium persulfate (APS, Amresco), diluted to a final volume of 50 mL with sterile water.

3. Size standard 400-HD-Rox (Applied Biosystems): 50 μL 400HD Rox, 50 μL loading buffer; 250 μL HiDi formamide, 175 μL water.
4. Electrophoresis: TBE 1X (1:10 dilution of 10X TBE with water); eight-barrel, dual-position sample loading syringe (Kloehn).
5. Sequencer (Applied Biosystems 377-96 DNA analyzer).

2.4. Data Analysis

1. ABI Genescan and Genotyper software for gel analysis.
2. MapMaker/EXP 3.0 and MapMaker/QTL 1.1 (Whitehead Institute).

3. Methods

3.1. Primer Selection and Design

For primer selection we use Genome Scanner (http://hmgc.mcw.edu/GenScan/), a Web tool designed to assist researchers in selecting polymorphic markers for a genome scan of a cross between two strains. It uses the Allele Characterization Project dataset in combination with various genetic and Radiation Hybrid maps, which provides investigators with a means of quickly selecting informative markers in a vast number of mapping crosses, resulting in a significant savings of both time and resources.

3.2. Genotype

3.2.1. DNA Extraction

1. Add 500 μL of lysis buffer to 1 mm^3 of tissue. Place the tubes in a 55°C water bath with agitation for 2 h.
2. Add 500 μL of 100% isopropyl alcohol to each tube to precipitate the DNA.
3. Shake the tubes vigorously for 3 min.
4. Centrifuge the tubes for 15 min at 16,000g.
5. Gently pour off the liquid by decantation, being careful not to lose the DNA pellet.
6. Add 500 μL of 70% ETOH to each tube, shake the tubes, and centrifuge for 5 min at 16,000g.
7. Pour off the liquid and leave the tubes uncapped for a minimum of 1 h to allow the ETOH to evaporate.
8. Resuspend the DNA in 500 μL of resuspension buffer.
9. Shake the tubes vigorously and place in a 55°C water bath shaker for 12 h.
10. Dilute the extracted DNA to 5 ng/μL with water.

3.2.2. PCR Reaction

1. Place 30 ng of DNA (6 μL) into appropriate wells. Allow the DNA to dry overnight at room temperature. Alternately, a speed vacuum or hot block can be used.

Table 1
PCR Mix Preparation

	Stock concentration	Volume per reaction	Concentration in PCR mix	Final concentration
dNTPs	2500 μ*M*	0.48 μL	400 μ*M*	200 μ*M*
Buffer	10X	0.6 μL	2X	1X
Dye	1200 n*M*	0.75 μL	300 n*M*	150 n*M*
Taq	5 U/μL	0.144 μL	0.24 U/μL	0.12 U/μL
Water	—	1.026 μL	—	—
	Total volume	3 μL		

2. Dilute the mixed forward and reverse primers with water to 460 n*M*, and dispense 3 μL into the wells containing the dried DNA.
3. Prepare the PCR mix as shown in **Table 1** and add 3 μL of PCR mix into each well, keeping the plate on ice.
4. Seal the plate (*see* **Note 2**), centrifuge for 1 min and start PCR reaction. "Touchdown PCR" is recommended to increase specificity of the reaction and to reduce background. Cycling moves from denature to anneal with a gradual step down of the annealing temperature in between (*see* **Note 3**). Remove the plate and store at 4°C until ready to use.

3.2.3. Purifying and Loading

1. When 384 well plates have been used with different primer-conjugated dyes, pool samples into a 96-well plate (*see* **Note 4**).
2. Add 80 μL of 75% isopropyl alcohol to each well. Mix the samples a minimum of 20 times with pipet.
3. Cover plate with a rubber mat and place in a dark place at room temperature for 45 min.
4. Spin plate at 1930*g* for 1 h at 10°C.
5. Invert the plate onto a paper towel, and quick spin at 183*g*. This will pull the isopropyl alcohol out of the plate and leave the PCR product behind.
6. To prepare the gel, add Long Ranger and 10X TBE to the urea. Bring up to 50 mL with water. Bring up to solution by gentle mixing. Add TEMED and APS immediately before pouring gel. Mix and pour gel. Allow 2 h for polymerization of gel before loading the samples.
7. Electrophoresis: Add 3 μL of size standard preparation to each well containing the purified PCR product. Denature the samples by placing the plate in a heated block (95°C) for 2 min and snap-cool in ice. Insert comb in the gel for lane formation and load 1 μL of each sample with loading syringe.

3.3. Data Analysis

3.3.1. Analysis of Image

The ABI 377 sequencer will generate a digitized image of the gel. Analysis of the image and identification of the allele(s) for each individual is performed by the software provided with the sequencer (Genotyper, ABI). The software will determine the size of the bands according to the size marker. The user should assign a number to each allele according to the strain it belongs to, being 1 and 2 for rats homozygous for one allele and 3 for heterozygous. Results can then be exported to a spreadsheet for further analysis.

3.3.2. Linkage Analysis

The first step in the analysis is the construction of a genetic map. This can be done with the program MAPMAKER/EXP 3.0, publicly available from the Whitehead Institute. As a first step, a framework map is built, in which markers are grouped into 21 linkage groups assigned to one of the 21 rat chromosomes.

For QTL analysis, there are several available programs. MAPMAKER/QTL 1.1 (Whitehead Institute) uses interval mapping for detection of the genetic regions linked to a phenotype. It calculates maximum likelihood of linkage by giving a LOD score (logarithm of the odds ratio), which represents the likelihood of there being a QTL between a pair of markers vs the likelihood of not being present. A significant LOD score will indicate the presence of a QTL in a genomic area.

In calculating the threshold of significance for the LOD score, if we assume an infinite dense map, it will depend on the type of cross performed. For a backcross, a LOD of 3.2 is significant and 2.0 is suggestive. For an intercross, a LOD of 4.2 is significant and 2.8 is suggestive.

4. Notes

1. Estimation of the number of genes involved in the development of the disease by the formula of Sewall Wright:

$$n = (P - q)2$$

$$X(\sigma 2F2 - \sigma 2F1)$$

where P is the phenotype value of the healthy parental strain; q is the phenotype value for the disease parent

n is the number of segregating (heterozygous) loci expected; σ2F2 is the phenotypic variance of the F2 population (estimated from a pilot study); σ2F1 is the phenotypic variance of the F1 population (environmental variance); X is a constant that equals 8 for an intercross study and 16 for a backcross study.

2. Sealing is very important because of the small volume of the PCR reaction (3 µL). Putting adhesive foil on top of the sealer reduces the volume loss.

3. Touchdown PCR reaction:
   Denature at 95°C for 5 min
   <u>7 cycles</u>: Ramp annealing temperature down from 68 to 56°C.
   Denature: 95°C for 45 s.
   Anneal: 68°C for 45 s (down to 56°C, by decreasing 2°C each cycle).
   Extend: 72°C for 1 min.
   <u>30 cycles</u>:
   Denature: 95°C for 45 s.
   Anneal: 54°C for 45 s.
   Extend: 72°C for 1 min.
   <u>1 cycle</u>:
   Extend: 72°C for 10 min.
   Hold: 4°C.

4. The signal from genotypes run with 6-FAM dye (blue) is usually brighter than others. Dilution of the PCR product before purification can be used to normalize the signal intensity in the gel.

References

1. Lander, E. S., and Schork, N. J. (1994) Genetic dissection of complex traits. *Science* **265,** 2037–2048.
2. Oetting, W. S., Lee, H. K., Flanders, D. J., Wiesner, G. L., Sellers, T. A., and King, R. A. (1995) Linkage analysis with multiplexed short tandem repeat polymorphisms using infrared fluorescence and M13 tailed primers. *Genomics* **30,** 450–458.
3. Dracheva S. V., Remmers E. F., Chen S., et al. (2000) An integrated genetic linkage map with 1,137 markers constructed from five F2 crosses of autoimmune disease-prone and -resistant inbred rat strains. *Genomics* **63,** 202–226.
4. Watanabe, T. K., Ono, T., Okuno, S., et al. (2000) Characterization of newly developed SSLP markers for the rat. *Mamm. Genome* **11,** 300–315.
5. Jacob, H. J., Brown, D. M., Bunker, R. K., et al. (1995) A genetic linkage map of the laboratory rat, *Rattus norvegicus. Nat. Genet.* **9,** 63–69.
6. Lander, E. S. and Botstein, D. (1989) Mapping mendelian factors underlying quantitative traits using RFLP linkage maps. *Genetics* **121,** 185–199.

10

Extraction of RNA From Cells and Tissue

Ian M. Bird

Summary

Total undegraded cellular RNA, largely free of contaminating DNA, can be rapidly and easily isolated from homogenized tissue or cultured cells using acid pH guanidinium thiocyanate/phenol/chloroform extraction. Commercially available acid phenol/guanidinium thiocyanate solutions allow one-step complete solubilization of tissue or cells under conditions that inhibit RNAse activity. We describe here a detailed procedure for total RNA extraction from homogenized tissues or cultured cells using such reagents, together with additional purification steps by passage through Phase-Lock gel tubes, and recommend optional chromatographic poly(A+) RNA enrichment procedure using Mini Oligo(dT) spin columns, together with the spectrophotometric determination of RNA yield and purity.

Key Words: RNA; cells; tissue; extraction; purification.

1. Introduction

Total undegraded cellular RNA, largely free of contaminating DNA, can be rapidly and easily isolated from homogenized tissue or cultured cells using acid pH guanidinium thiocyanate/phenol/chloroform extraction *(1)*. Commercially available acid phenol/guanidinium thiocyanate solutions *(2)* such as RNAzol B (Cinna Scientific, Cleveland, OH) and TRIzol (Gibco), allow one-step complete solubilization of tissue or cells under conditions that inhibit RNAse activity. By subsequent addition of chloroform, phase separation is forced to occur and RNA is extracted into an aqueous phase, separated from the lower organic phase by an insoluble protein interphase. Guanidinium thiocyanate remains in the aqueous phase and so continues to act as an RNAse inhibitor by disrupting protein–nucleic acid interactions. However, the protein interphase is still rich in RNAse and, on accidental recovery with the aqueous phase, may result in degradation of the RNA. To eliminate this contamination, the aqueous phase can be reextracted in fresh phenol/chloroform/isoamyl alco-

From: *Methods in Molecular Medicine, Vol. 108: Hypertension: Methods and Protocols*
Edited by: J. P. Fennell and A. H. Baker © Humana Press Inc., Totowa, NJ

hol solution (*see* **Note 1**) such as PCI reagent (Eppendorf) and spun through a barrier material that separates phases of greater and lesser density. The lighter aqueous phase does not penetrate the barrier, whereas the organic phase and any residual protein interphase migrate through the barrier to become trapped underneath. Heavy-grade Phase-Lock Gel tubes (Eppendorf) are suitable for procedures using guanidinium thiocyanate, which imparts higher density to the aqueous phase *(3)*. RNA isolated by this procedure is suitable for use in Northern analysis, slot blotting, and reverse transcriptase/polymerase chain reaction (RT/PCR). Commercially available kits can be used to further isolate poly(A+) RNA-enriched fractions for use in detection or amplification of rare transcripts. We describe here a detailed procedure for total RNA extraction from homogenized tissues or cultured cells using RNAzol B, purification by passage through Phase-Lock Gel tubes, and recommend optional chromato-graphic poly(A+) RNA enrichment procedure using Mini Oligo(dT) spin columns (Qiagen), together with the spectrophotometric determination of RNA yield and purity. Ultimately, RNA quality should be further evaluated by ethidium bromide visualization following agarose/formaldehyde gel electrophoresis. Good-quality RNA is indicated not only by clear 18S and 28S subunits but also by discrete RNA bands, especially of high molecular weight, together with an absence of excess low-molecular weight (<200 bases, degraded) RNA.

2. Materials

Unless otherwise stated, all reagents are molecular biology grade.

1. Autoclave.
2. NanoPure/UltraPure (18Ω) Water.
3. Microcentrifuge, 12,000*g*.
4. Vacuum centrifuge/vacuum pump.
5. Diethyl pyrocarbonate, Sigma (cat. no. D5758).
6. Sterile, disposable 100-mm Petri dishes.
7. Chloroform.
8. Isopropanol.
9. Ethanol (200 proof).
10. RNAzol B, TelTest (cat. no. CS105).
11. Heavy-grade Phase-Lock Gel (PLG) tubes, Eppendorf.
12. Phenol/chloroform/isoamyl alcohol (PCI) reagent, InVitrogen.
13. Molecular biology-grade (MB-grade) water, Eppendorf.
14. Mussel glycogen, 1 mg/mL (MB grade), Sigma (cat no. G1767).

For extraction from tissues:

15. Sterile dissection instruments.
16. Liquid nitrogen (N*l*).
17. Polytron homogenizer with approx 0.25-in blade, Fisher (cat. no. 15338700P).

18. 2-mL Cryovials, Fisher (cat. no. 033377D).
19. 15-mL Homogenization tubes, Fisher (cat. no. 1495910B).

For cultured cells:

20. Cell scrapers, Fisher (cat. no. 087732).

For poly (A+) RNA extraction:

21. OligoTex mRNA Midi Oligo (dT) spin column kit, Qiagen (cat. no. 70042).
22. Heating block.
23. Water bath.

2.1. Solution Preparation

All glassware should be thoroughly cleaned and autoclaved before use. Wear gloves at all times and use new weighing boats with autoclaved spatulas. Weigh reagents to 1% accuracy. When using a pH meter, calibrate first for pH 4.0–7.0 range, then rinse electrode in distilled water, followed by molecular-grade water. Store magnetic stir bars in ethanol and rinse in DEPC water (*see* **step 1**) before use. Unless otherwise stated, keep solutions at room temperature. Store and handle hazardous items in accordance with safety guidelines.

1. DEPC water: Add 500 μL diethyl pyrocarbonate (DEPC) per liter to 5 L filtered deionized water in a conical flask and swirl to mix. Stand at room temperature for 4 h (to inactivate RNAses), then autoclave (liquid cycle) to deactivate DEPC/sterilize. Allow to cool overnight before making up other aqueous solutions.
2. Water, molecular biology-grade (MB grade: MB quality is essential for making solutions coming in direct contact with RNA). Store at 4°C.
3. RNAzol B: Store protected from light at 4°C.
4. CHCl$_3$: Store working stock in 100-mL bottle at 4°C.
5. Phenol/chloroform/isoamyl alcohol (PCI) solution: Store at 4°C.
6. 75% Ethanol: Dilute 75 mL of 200-proof alcohol with 25 mL MB-grade water. Store at 4°C. Replace after 1 mo.
7. Isopropanol: Store working stock in 100-mL bottle at 4°C.

Additional solutions for tissue homogenization:

8. 12% TCA: Dissolve 60 g trichloroacetic acid in DEPC water to a final volume of 500 mL. Store at 4°C.
9. Phosphate-buffered saline (PBS) pH 7.4: To 4 L DEPC water, add 6.186 g Na$_2$HPO$_4$ (MW 142), 1.633 g KH$_2$PO$_4$ (MW 137.99), and 52.60 g NaCl (MW 58.44) and adjust pH to 7.4. Adjust volume to 6 L with DEPC water. Dispense in 500-mL vol to glass bottles and autoclave on liquid cycle (lid loose!) Store at 4°C.

3. Methods

Before performing the procedure, ensure that RNAzol B, chloroform, PCI solution, isopropanol, fresh 75% ethanol, and MB-grade water are stored at 4°C. Microcentrifuge temperature should also be equilibrated to 4°C in a cold room. For optional poly(A+) RNA isolation, ensure that absolute ethanol, and appropriate reagents (mussel glycogen, 3.0 M sodium acetate, pH 5.2) are also at 4°C. Clean and store the spectrophotometer cuvette in a 50-mL tube containing DEPC water. During the procedure, keep everything on ice. Wear gloves and work over sterile napkins. Each 100-mg tissue cube processed will require four microcentrifuge rotor wells, so up to three cubes can be processed simultaneously using a 12-well rotor. Alternatively, each cell culture dish processed will require only one rotor well.

3.1. Tissue and Cell Solubilization in RNAzol B

3.1.1. Collection and Storage of Tissues

1. Place fresh weigh boats in *shallow* Styrofoam containers and add N_l into and around weigh boats. Add N_l to an additional container for transfer of processed samples to a –70°C freezer. Also place sterile Petri dishes on ice and add cold PBS.
2. Transfer freshly obtained tissues to sterile Petri dishes containing cold PBS (to rinse away blood, which contains abundant RNAse). Working *quickly* with a sterile scalpel, slice into cubes of approx 3–4 mm in size weighing approx 100 mg each. Immediately transfer cubes to weigh boats immersed in N_l, to snap-freeze the tissue.
3. Immerse appropriately labeled cryovial into Nl surrounding the weigh boat. Holding the vial with a hemostat, transfer cubes (using forceps) into the tube, cap, and transfer in Nl to –70°C freezer or Nl Dewar. Tissues are stable long-term at ≤ –70°C.

3.1.2. Tissue Disruption and Solubilization

1. Clean the Polytron blade at three-quarter speed in 12% TCA (30 s), then DEPC water, and finally ethanol. Allow to air-dry.
2. Prepare four PLG tubes per 100-mg tissue cube. Centrifuge 3 min at 12,000g to spin the barrier material to the bottom of the tube. Label for the first- and second-round extractions and stand at room temperature.
3. Transfer the 100-mg tissue cube *directly* from the ≤70°C storage into 4 mL cold RNAzol B in a 15-mL polypropylene tube (*see* **Note 2**). Disrupt the tissue completely with the Polytron (15 s at one-third speed, then 5 s at three-quarter speed). Place the homogenate on ice, and dispense into 4 × 1.5-mL microcentrifuge tubes at 1 mL volume per tube. Keep all tubes on ice.
4. Between samples, rinse the Polytron blade in fresh RNAzol B (30 s at three-quarter speed). Repeat the homogenization process from **step 3** for the remaining tissue cubes, remembering that each cube will require four microcentrifuge rotor wells for processing.
5. Proceed to **Subheading 3.2.** Finally, strip down, clean, and sterilize the reassembled Polytron blade before autoclaving and long-term storage.

3.1.3. Cell Solubilization From 60–100 mm Dishes

1. Prepare one PLG tube per cultured dish: Centrifuge (3 min, 12,00g) to spin the barrier material to the bottom of the tube. Also, prepare a suction line (to efficiently and completely remove the culture medium from culture plates/dishes) and place a cell scraper in a 15-mL tube containing 5 mL RNAzol B.
2. Remove the cell culture dishes from the incubator one at a time (*see* **Note 3**). Quickly remove all medium by suction (serum contains RNAse).
3. Add 1 mL cold RNAzol B to the center of the dish. Scrape the cells into the RNAzol B with a scraper by first scraping left to right from top to bottom of dish. Then turn the dish through 90° and repeat the process. Finally, scrape around the outer edge, wipe all liquid to the bottom of the dish, and transfer 1.0–1.1 mL of material to a 1.5-mL microcentrifuge tube, on ice.
4. Shear the cells by aspirating 10–15× with a pipet (1 mL tip, *see* **Note 4**).
5. Discard the used pipet tip and return the scraper to the storage tube (containing RNAzol B). Repeat the scraping/homogenization process from **step 2** for as many culture dishes as can be processed, remembering that each dish will require one microcentrifuge rotor well for processing.
6. Proceed to **Subheading 3.2.**

3.2. Recovery of Total RNA

3.2.1. Phase Separation

1. Add 0.15 vol cold CHCl$_3$ (150 µL) to each microcentrifuge tube. Vortex for 10 s and stand on ice for 5 min. Vortex each tube again for 10s and spin at 12,000g in a microcentrifuge (30 min, 4°C).

3.2.2. Phenol/Chloroform Extraction of Residual Protein From Aqueous Phase Using PLG Tubes

1. Recover up to 550 µL of the upper aqueous phase to a prespun PLG tube (more aqueous solution may be present, but complete recovery increases the risk of RNAse contamination from the protein interphase). Add 500 µL of PCI reagent to each tube, and mix thoroughly by inversion (10×—do *not* vortex). Place on ice for 10 min, and then spin at 4,500g for 5 min at 4°C.
2. Transfer the upper aqueous phase to a fresh prespun PLG tube and repeat the extraction procedure exactly as described above. (This second extraction step is not so necessary for cell extracts, but is for tissue extracts.) Transfer the final aqueous phase to a fresh sterile 1.5-mL tube and stand on ice.

3.2.3. Total RNA Precipitation

During all stages involving the pelleting and washing of RNA, be careful not to disturb the pellet when discarding supernatant. Look for a small brownish disk or smear at the bottom of the tube. Preparations for poly(A+) RNA isolation (**Subheading 3.3.**) can also be made while performing the total RNA precipitation (**step 1** below).

1. Add a small excess (600 µL) of cold isopropanol to each tube containing PCI-purified aqueous phase. Invert each tube several times to ensure thorough mixing of the samples and then move the samples from the ice tray to a dry rack (no ice) before transfer to the −20°C freezer. Place on the bottom (coldest) shelf for 1 h to allow RNA precipitation.
2. During the incubation, set the water bath or block heater to 65°C. Make preparations for poly(A+) mRNA spin column chromatography if required.
3. Remove the precipitated RNA from the −20°C freezer and invert twice. Spin at 12,000*g*, 4°C, for 30 min.

For immediate poly(A+) RNA purification, proceed to **Subheading 3.3.**, and perform **steps 1–3** during centrifugation. Otherwise continue with total RNA solubilization as below.

4. Discard the supernatant (tip swiftly and smoothly in one movement) and add 800 µL of cold 75% ethanol (down the side of the tube so the pellet is not dislodged). Spin the tubes again at 12,000*g*, 10 min, 4°C.
5. Quickly and smoothly tip off the supernatant, and dry the pellets by inverting the tubes on a clean paper towel for 5 min, followed by spinning for 5 min in a vacuum centrifuge, with microcentrifuge tube lids *open*. Do not over dry pellets! (*see* **Note 5**).

For immediate poly(A+) RNA purification, proceed to **Subheading 3.3.** Otherwise continue with total RNA solubilization as below.

6. For cultured cell extracts dedicated to total RNA quantification, add 110 µL MB-grade water to each tube. For tissue extracts, add 27.5 µL MB-grade water to each of the four tubes used to process one tissue cube. To solubilize the RNA completely, transfer the tubes (lids closed) to a water bath at 65°C for 3 min, vortex 10 s, return to the water bath for 2 min, and then place on ice for 3 min. Vortex and centrifuge (300*g*, 5–10 s) each tube briefly to draw all liquid to the bottom of the tube(s). For tissue extraction, pool the four tube contents, mix, and spin briefly (*see* **Note 6**).
7. Transfer 10 µL of the final product to a fresh 1.5-mL tube and add 90 µL MB-grade water. Immediately store the remaining 100 µL undiluted total RNA at ≤ −70°C. Keep the diluted samples on ice for spectrophotometry (*see* **Subheading 3.4.**).

3.3. Poly(A+) RNA Isolation From Total RNA Using Oligo(dT) Spin Columns

Because of the wide demand for high-quality poly(A+) RNA material for demanding applications such as library construction, a large variety of commercial kits are available that have efficiently streamlined this procedure. In general there are two types, those that work from preprepared total RNA (as described above), and those that extract direct from cells or tissue. In general terms, the convenience of a one-step extraction direct from tissue is traded off against a lower percent recovery due to interfering substances from the blood, tissue, or media that may inhibit poly(A) tail binding to the Oligo(dT) capture material. We therefore recommend the prior extraction of total RNA followed *immediately* by the performance of oligo(dT) purification [since poly(A+) tails degrade upon storage once extraction is complete], but the decision can be influenced by tissue abundance, etc. so the final decision should be made with all these factors considered first.

We have reviewed a number of methods for poly(A+) isolation, but at this time one of the easiest and best kits available is that from Qiagen (OligoTex spin column kit). This also has the advantage of exceptionally detailed instructions supplied with the kit. Therefore we have not repeated them here. Suffice it to say, follow the instructions *exactly*, particularly with regard to handling the columns and temperatures of the buffers, and pay particular attention to the capacities of each kit for total RNA loaded, etc.

Once the washing of the poly(A+) RNA on the spin columns is complete, the final elution/recovery is achieved using buffer OEB. The composition of this buffer is 5 mM Tris-HCl, pH 7.5. The decision of what final volume to use is difficult, but bear in mind two sequential small-volume elutions will generally be a better choice than one large-volume elution. We have successfully used two sequential elutions at 25 μL each (*see* **Note 7**). Second, pay attention to making sure that buffer OEB is at the recommended temperature when it is loaded to the column and spin immediately. The end result will be a trade-off between yield and volume. If yield is an issue and the resulting volume is too large, then concentrate the final product by precipitating the poly(A+) RNA as follows. Yield can be maximized by using mussel glycogen as a carrier (detailed below), but be sure it does not interfere with subsequent applications.

1. Be sure the mussel glycogen is at the desired concentration. Use as is or dilute no more than fourfold as required.
2. To each tube of poly(A+) in 100 μL buffer OEB, add 1 μL mussel glycogen solution (20 μg, or if diluted, 5 μg), and 10 μL of 3 M Na-acetate (pH 5.2) solution. Then add 500 μL absolute ethanol. Mix and chill *overnight* at –20°C.
3. Spin 30 min at 12,000g 4°C. Add 800 μL of 75% EtOH (fresh) and spin 10 min at 12,000g, 4°C. Invert on sterile napkin to dry. Vacuum centrifuge 3 min. Add MB-grade water to each tube as required.
4. Transfer to 65°C water bath and hold 3 min. Vortex 10 s. Return to water bath for 2 min. Vortex again. Place on ice for 3 min. Spin briefly to draw the liquid to the bottom of the tube.

5. RNA can either be quantified directly or an aliquot can be diluted and quantified, depending on expected yield (we recommend the latter, but yields of 1 μg or less due to limited starting material force us to perform the former on occasion—be sure the cuvet is clean in this case!).

3.4. Spectrophotometric Quantitation

Measure total RNA or poly(A+) RNA absorbance (A_{260}) against a MB-grade water blank or buffer OEB [if final poly(A+) product was not reprecipitated) as appropriate using a 260-nm light source. Purity can be determined by the A_{260}/A_{280} ratio. A ratio of 1.7 is generally acceptable, with improved purity indicated by ratios up to 2.0:1 (*see* **Note 8**).

1. RNA concentration can be calculated using the equation

   $$μg/μL = (0.04)(A_{260}) (1/n) (DF)$$

   where n is the cuvet path length and DF is the dilution factor (*see* **Note 9**). RNA aliquots measured by spectrophotometry were generally diluted by a factor of 10 [or 100 for quantification of total RNA prior to column loading in the poly(A+) procedure]. Calculate to three decimal places for yields below 1 μg/ μL and to two places for higher yields.

2. Total yield can be calculated by multiplying concentration (μg/μL) by the μL volume in which the RNA was resolubilized.

3. Efficiency of poly(A+) recovery can be determined as a percentage of the total RNA initially recovered [calculated from the aliquot taken prior to oligo(dT) spin column purification]:

   (μg/μL poly(A+) RNA)(110 μL volume) ÷ (μg/μL total RNA aliquot)(990 μL volume)

   Recovery of 5% is normal for single pass column purification (*see* **Note 10**).

4. Do not add diluted spectrophotometry aliquots to undiluted samples. Store concentrated RNA samples at ≤ –70°C.

4. Notes

1. Isoamyl alcohol acts as an antifoaming agent. Several companies also add 8-hydroxyquinoline (an antioxidant) to the PCI reagent, which also imparts a yellow color to the organic phase, making it easier to distinguish from the colorless aqueous phase.

2. This volume is sufficient for most tissues, including liver and kidney, which contain much endogenous RNAse activity. If extracted RNA is consistently degraded, however, reoptimization of this volume may be necessary.

3. Alternatively, all dishes can be removed at once and medium quickly removed by suction before snap-freezing in a shallow tray of N*l* and storage at ≤ –70°C. This gives slightly lower yields but can be useful if running tightly time-controlled experiments. If degradation of the final RNA product is consistently seen,

try also rinsing the dish with serum-free medium before extraction, because serum contains degradative enzymes that may be overloading the extraction reagents and breaking down the RNA.

4. Aspirate smoothly, allowing a small amount of air into the tip on the first few strokes. On subsequent strokes, foaming will occur. This will cause shearing of the cells, but not the RNA, when drawn back and forth through the tip.

5. It is important not to overdry the pellets, because they will then be more difficult to resolubilize.

6. We have frequently observed co-precipitation of a water-insoluble, transparent pellet using this total RNA isolation procedure on some tissues. As the co-precipitate is water-insoluble, RNA can be pipetted away from transparent pellet after heating into a fresh tube, and spectrophotometric quantitation is not affected. Do not attempt to resolubilize by further mixing or aspiration, as RNA will shear. The coprecipitate is removed during passage through oligo(dT) columns when performing the optional poly(A+) RNA isolation procedure. In other tissues, a whitish pellet, probably of polysaccharide composition *(4)*, is coprecipitated with RNA and solubilizes after incubation at 65°C.

7. The first elution recovers approx 90% of column-bound poly(A+) RNA. A second elution will recover all remaining poly(A+) RNA.

8. Nucleic acid and protein absorption spectra overlap, but nucleic acids show a maximum at 260-nm wavelength light while proteins show a maximum at 280 nm. To allow for this, the purity of RNA recovered by the described techniques is traditionally quoted as a ratio of A_{260}/A_{280}. The ratio, without correction, should be 1.5–2.0, with a value of 1.7 and above considered good. However, it is wise initially to check the RNA by Northern analysis, because these values will not reveal whether RNA is intact (it all absorbs the same—intact or degraded), and values can be thrown by contaminating phenol. If a sophisticated spectrophotometer capable of three wavelength measurements, perhaps with automatic correction, is available, the value at A_{320} can be used as background correction for the A_{260} and A_{280} values. The ratio will then be lower (typically 1.45–1.9) but more consistent. Remember also, whichever method you use, the reliability of ratios as a measure of purity decreases with decreasing yields of RNA. Thus for small yields of RNA (<1 µg), it may be best to measure undiluted product. The cuvet should be rinsed thoroughly between samples, however, to ensure no cross-contamination.

9. Given the absorbance of an analyte in solution, concentration can be determined from the equation *(5)*

$$A = (\alpha_s)(c)(n)$$

where *A* is absorbance, or optical density (OD), by analyte at a particular wavelength, α_s is the specific absorbance of the analyte, *c* is the analyte concentration, and *n* is the length (cm) of the light pathway through the solution. Given that the specific absorbance *(6)* of RNA is 0.025 mL·cm^{-1}·µg^{-1} (i.e., 1 OD unit = 40 µg/mL per cm path length), this equation becomes

$$c = (A)\left(\tfrac{1}{\alpha_s}\right)\left(\tfrac{1}{n}\right) = (A)(40)\ \mu g/mL^{-1}/cm^{-1}\left(\tfrac{1}{n}\right)cm = \left(40\right)\left(A\right)\left(\tfrac{1}{n}\right)\mu g/mL^{-1}$$

Taking further into consideration a dilution factor (DF) for spectrophotometry samples and a unit correction factor for concentration expression in μg/ μL, the equation becomes

$$c = \left(40\right)\left(A\right)\left(\tfrac{1}{n}\right)\mu g \cdot mL^{-1}\left(DF\right)\left(\tfrac{1}{1000}\right)mL \cdot \ \mu L^{-1} = \left(0.04\right)\left(A\right)\left(\tfrac{1}{n}\right)\left(DF\right)\mu g \cdot mL^{-1}$$

10. Percentage poly(A+) RNA recovery does not reflect mRNA levels relative to total RNA, as poly(A+) RNA is only mRNA-enriched, with less tRNA and rRNA. Percentage poly(A+) RNA is measured instead to ensure the efficiency and consistency of the method. Typically, poly(A+) RNA should be 2–5% of the total RNA initially applied to the column.

Acknowledgments

The authors would like to thank Masako Ochiai for data concerning poly(A+) isolation and TelTest for reviewing the methods described. This work was supported by National Institutes of Health award HL64601 and HD38843 (Project 1 and Core B).

References

1. Chomczynski, P. and Sacchi, N. (1987) Single-step method of RNA isolation by acid guanidinium thiocyanate-phenol-chloroform extraction. *Anal. Biochem.* **162,** 156–159.
2. Chomczynski, P. (1993) A reagent for the single-step simultaneous isolation of RNA, DNA, and proteins from cell and tissue samples. *Biotechniques* **15,** 532–536.
3. Murphy, N. R. and Hellwig, R. J. (1996) Improved nucleic acid organic extraction through use of a unique gel barrier material. *Biotechniques* **21,** 934–939.
4. Puissant, C. and Houdebine, L. (1990) An improvement of the single-step method of RNA isolation by acid guanidinium thiocyanate-phenol-chloroform extraction. *Biotechniques* **8,** 148–149.
5. Segel, I. H. (1976) Biochemical Calculations, 2nd ed. Wiley, New York.
6. Sambrook, J., Fritsch, E. F., and Maniatis, T. (1989) Appendix E. In *Molecular Cloning, A Laboratory Manual*, 2nd ed. Cold Spring Harbor Laboratory Press, Cold Spring Harbor, NY.

11

Single-Strand Conformational Polymorphism Analysis

Basic Principles and Routine Practice

Yanbin Dong and Haidong Zhu

Summary

Single-strand conformational polymorphism (SSCP) analysis is a simple and sensitive technique for mutation detection and genotyping. The principle of SSCP analysis is based on the fact that single-stranded DNA has a defined conformation. Altered conformation due to a single base change in the sequence can cause single-stranded DNA to migrate differently under nondenaturing electrophoresis conditions. Therefore wild-type and mutant DNA samples display different band patterns.

SSCP analysis involves the following four steps: (1) polymerase chain reaction (PCR) amplification of DNA sequence of interest; (2) denaturation of double-stranded PCR products; (3) cooling of the denatured DNA (single-stranded) to maximize self-annealing; (4) detection of mobility difference of the single-stranded DNAs by electrophoresis under non-denaturing conditions. Several methods have been developed to visualize the SSCP mobility shifts. These include the incorporation of radioisotope labeling, silver staining, fluorescent dye-labeled PCR primers, and more recently, capillary-based electrophoresis. Silver staining is simple, rapid, and cost-effective, and can be routinely performed in clinical laboratories. The use of SSCP analysis to discover and genotype single-nucleotide polymorphisms (SNPs) has been widely applied to the genetics of hypertension, including both monogenic (e.g., Liddle's syndrome) and polygenic disorders (e.g., essential hypertension).

Key Words: Single-strand conformational polymorphism (SSCP); silver staining; mutation discovery.

1. Introduction

Single-strand conformational polymorphism (SSCP) analysis is one of the simplest, most sensitive, and robust techniques for mutation screening and genotyping. Invented more than a decade ago, this technique has been widely applied to detect mutations and polymorphisms in a variety of clinical disorders such as congenital disorders (*1*), cancer (*2,3*), diabetes (*4–6*), and hyper-

From: *Methods in Molecular Medicine, Vol. 108: Hypertension: Methods and Protocols*
Edited by: J. P. Fennell and A. H. Baker © Humana Press Inc., Totowa, NJ

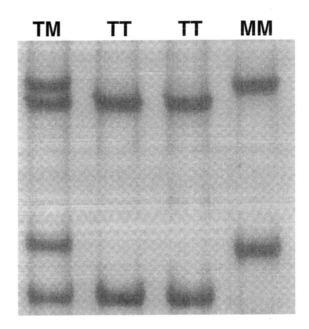

Fig. 1. Silver staining SSCP analysis for detection of the T594M mutation in the epithelial sodium channel β-subunit. The PCR fragment is 245 bp. TM, heterozygous mutant; TT, wild type; MM, homozygous mutant.

tension *(7–13)*. Single-nucleotide polymorphisms (SNPs) account for most of the genetic variability across the human genome. Detection of SNPs in the human genome is thus increasingly important in elucidating the pathogenesis of hypertension.

Under nondenaturing conditions, single-stranded DNA (ssDNA) has a folded conformation, which is determined by its intramolecular interactions and therefore its base sequence. Any single base change can lead to a mobility shift, which can be detected as different band patterns under nondenaturing electrophoresis *(14,15)* (*see* **Fig. 1**).

Based on this basic principle, several techniques have been developed to visualize SSCP mobility shifts, including the incorporation of radioisotope labeling, silver staining, fluorescent dye-labeled primers, and more recently capillary electrophoresis-based methods *(16–19)*. Radioisotope-labeled "hot SSCP" tends to have higher sensitivity but with the disadvantages of safety and hazardous waste management concerns *(20)*. SSCP using fluorescent dye-labeled primers, as well as capillary electrophoresis-based technique, enables higher throughput and lower cost. However, it requires instruments such as an automatic DNA sequencer (ABI377) or a capillary-based genetic analyzer

(ABI3100). The limitation of the high-throughput screening method is the data analysis. The difference between a normal and a mutant sample can be very difficult to register. There is no commercial software available for pattern recognition yet, and therefore the large amount of data has to be reviewed and analyzed manually *(21)*. SSCP-silver staining is a simple, sensitive, and cost-effective technique, which can be routinely performed in clinical laboratories for genetic testing and SNP screening. By using this technique in our laboratory we were able to discover and genotype mutations and SNPs in some candidate genes responsible for essential hypertension and stroke, including the epithelial sodium channels β-subunit (*see* **Fig. 1**) *(10–12)*, aldosterone synthase *(22)*, and CADASIL (cerebral autosomal dominant arteriopathy with subcortical infarcts and leukoencephalopathy) *(23,24)*. The results have been reproducible and reliable. The major procedures involved in SSCP-silver staining are (1) SSCP gel preparation; (2) polymerase chain reaction (PCR) sample preparation; (3) nondenaturing gel electrophoresis; and (4) silver staining. This chapter provides a step-by-step protocol and suggestions to overcome potential problems.

2. Materials

2.1. PCR Amplification

1. Genomic DNA template (50–100 ng).
2. Specific PCR primers (18–21 bp) to amplify a unique region of genome for mutation screening, ideal PCR product size ranges from 100 to 300 bp (*see* **Note 1**).
3. AmpliTaq Gold DNA polymerase (Applied Biosystems).
4. GeneAmp10 PCR buffer: 100 mM Tris-HCl, pH 8.3, 500 mM KCl.
5. 25 mM MgCl$_2$ Solution.
6. 10 mM dNTPs.
7. Deionized water.
8. GeneAmp 9700 PCR thermocycler.

2.2. SSCP and Silver Staining

1. 2 X SequaGel MD (National Diagnostics), stored at room temperature.
2. 0.6 X TBE running buffer (60 mL 10 X TBE stock to 1 L with deionized water).
3. TEMED (Sigma), stored at room temperature.
4. 20% Freshly made ammonium persulfate (Sigma).
5. Denaturing/loading buffer: 95% formamide, 20 mM EDTA, 0.05% bromophenol blue, 0.05% xylene cyanol.
6. Solution 1 (fixing solution): 10% ethanol, 0.5% acetic acid, stable at room temperature (it can be used two to three times).
7. Solution 2: 0.1% freshly made silver nitrate.
8. Solution 3: 6.75 g NaOH, 675 μL formaldehyde in 450 mL deionized water (freshly made).

9. Solution 4: 0.75% freshly made Na_2CO_3.
10. Saran Wrap plastic film.

2.3. Equipment

1. Protean II xi system (Bio-Rad) (*see* **Note 2**).
2. Power supply (Bio-Rad).
3. External recirculating/Chiller (Haake model K20 or Laura model RMS-6) with a temperature range from –20 to 100°C.
4. Orbital shaker for gel staining.

3. Methods
3.1. SSCP Gel Preparation

1. Clean glass plates thoroughly with warm tap water, rinse with tap water, deionized water, and finally ethanol. Wipe dry or air dry.
2. On a clean surface, lay the long plate down first, and then place the left and right spacers along the sides of the long plate. Place the short plate on top of the spacers so that it is even with the bottom edge of the long plate.
3. Loosen the single screw of each sandwich clamp and place each clamp by the appropriate side of the gel sandwich with the locating arrows facing up and toward the glass sandwich.
4. Hold the gel sandwich firmly and fit it into the left and right clamps. Tighten the screws enough to hold the plates in place. Check that the plates and spacers are even at the bottom. If not, realign the plates and spacers to obtain a good seal (*see* **Note 3**).
5. Place the gray sponge onto the front casting slot. Place the sandwich assembly on the sponge with the short glass plate facing forward. Press down the sandwich and turn the handles of the camshaft down to lock the sandwich in place.
6. Make gel solution (*see* **Table 1**): (20 × 20 cm × 0.75 mm, 70 mL for two gels) (*see* **Note 4**).
7. Add 36 μL TEMED and 320 μL of freshly prepared 20% ammonium persulfate to the gel solution, swirl gently, and pour or inject the gel solution into the sandwich.
8. Insert a comb onto the top of the sandwich to form the sample wells and leave to polymerize at room temperature for at least 1 h (*see* **Note 5**).
9. After polymerization, remove the comb by pulling it straight up slowly and gently. Release the gel sandwich from the casting stand and attach the gel sandwich to the core with the short glass plate facing the core. Turn the core to its other side and attach the second gel sandwich (*see* **Note 6**).
10. Fill the upper and lower chambers with 0.6 X TBE buffer and rinse out the wells thoroughly with running buffer using a syringe and needle (*see* **Note 7**).
11. Place the core and the attached gel sandwiches into electrophoresis tank; allow the core to lock in place. Put the lid on and connect the system to an external water chiller, set temperature and prerun for 20 min to reach the desired temperature.

Table 1
SSCP Gel Solution (20 × 20 cm × 0.75 mm, 70 mL for Two Gels)

	0.5X MDE	0.8X MDE
2X MDE stock solution	17.5 mL	28 mL
10X TBE buffer	4.2 mL (0.6X)	4.2 mL (0.6X)
Double-distilled H_2O	48.3 mL	37.8 mL
20% APS (freshly prepared)	320 µL	320 µL
TEMED	36 µL	36 µL

3.2. Sample Preparation

1. Optimize PCR condition for the desired PCR product (*see* **Note 8**).
2. Mix 4 µL PCR product with 4 µL SSCP gel loading buffer and heat it at 95°C for 5 min, and then immediately place on ice (*see* **Note 9**).

3.3. Electrophoresis

1. When the running buffer has reached the desired temperature, stop the prerun, rinse the wells with running buffer again, and load 8 µL of the samples into the wells using "long" tips. Be careful not to pierce the wells during loading.
2. Run the gel at a constant power of 10 W for 10–18 h at 5–15°C (*see* **Note 10**).
3. After electrophoresis is complete, turn the power supply and water chiller system off, disconnect the electrodes, and carefully pull the core out of the electrophoresis tank.

3.4. Silver Staining

1. Lay the core and gel sandwich on a padded surface to absorb buffer spills. Remove the gel sandwich from the core. Carefully remove the gel from the plates and immerse gel in a tray containing solution 1 (10% ethanol and 0.5% acetic acid) and place the tray on top of a shaker to mix for at least 6 min (*see* **Note 11**).
2. Remove solution 1 (this may be saved for reuse) and add freshly made solution 2 (0.1% silver nitrate) for 15 min (*see* **Note 11**).
3. Pour off solution 2 and briefly rinse gel with two changes of deionized water.
4. Add freshly made solution 3 (450 mL: 6.75 g NaOH, 675 µL formaldehyde) for about 20 min (*see* **Note 11**).
5. When band intensity is good enough, pour off solution 3 and add solution 4 (2.25 g Na_2CO_3 in 300 mL deionized water) for 5 min (*see* **Note 11**).
6. Place gel on Saran Wrap, put it on top of the light box, and slide your finger across the gel gently to remove any air bubbles. Read the bands or record the result on Gel Documentation imager.
7. For storage, transfer gel onto filter paper; place it in gel dryer for 60 min. Alternatively, store gel covered in Saran Wrap at 4°C (*see* **Note 12**).

4. Notes

1. Designed primers should be located within introns on either side of splice junctions to detect possible variants of exon–intron boundaries and coding region. The generated PCR product size should range from 100 to 300 bp to maximize the SSCP sensitivity. If an exon is larger than 300 bp, another pair of primers should be designed to amplify overlapped region. The primer design programs can be obtained from the following Websites: http://genome-www2.stanford.edu/cgi-bin/SGD/web-primer and www-genome.wi.mit.edu/cgi-bin/primer/primer3_www.cgi. To check the specificity of primers, go to the Website: www.ncbi.nih.gov/BLAST/.

2. In addition to Protean II xi system, Bio-Rad Dcode system can be used to perform various mutation detection methods including SSCP.

3. Always make sure the plates and spacers are even at the bottom and spacers are parallel to the clamps. Failure to do so can result in gel leakage when casting, as well as buffer leakage during the run.

4. It is important to optimize gel electrophoresis conditions, including gel concentration, to ensure the maximal sensitivity. The most commonly used gel concentrations are between 0.5X (for larger fragments) and 0.8X (for smaller fragments). Be very careful when handling the lower concentration gel (0.5X), because it is very fragile and easily broken.

5. Mix gel solution well before pouring. Inject gel solution gently to avoid bubbles. Cover the wells of the comb with gel solution. Leave gel to polymerize for 2 h for best resolution. Alternatively, cast the gel and leave it to polymerize for 1 h, then cover the top with plastic wrap, leave it in the cool room overnight, and run it the following morning.

6. To avoid buffer leakage, lubricate the entire front of the core gaskets with water or running buffer, or even with white Vaseline, prior to attaching the gel sandwich to the core. This will allow the sandwich to slide onto the gasket properly to achieve a good buffer seal.

7. Before filling the upper chamber with 0.6X TBE buffer, pour 400 mL deionized water into the upper chamber instead, leave it for 1 min, and check whether there is water leakage. If the water appears to be leaking, discard the water, remove the sandwich from the core, relubricate the gasket, and reattach the sandwich to the core. Check the water leakage again until the buffer seal is well achieved. Then fill both the upper and lower chambers with 0.6X TBE buffer. Rinse the wells thoroughly to remove any unpolymerized materials, because they may affect band shapes.

8. It is important to optimize the PCR conditions (primer and magnesium concentration, annealing temperature, and cycle number) for the desired PCR product. The purity of the PCR product is the key factor to obtaining good SSCP results. Check PCR products by agarose gel electrophoresis prior to the SSCP analysis.

9. Samples are heated at 95°C for 5 min to denature the double-stranded DNA into single-stranded DNA, and then rapidly cooled. Rapid cooling favors self-

annealing and prevents complementary strands from forming duplexes. The undenatured PCR products can be run on the same gel for extra control.

10. Running conditions should be optimized for a particular mutation. Running temperature ranges are normally between 5 and 25°C. Each experiment should be run under two different temperatures to achieve the highest sensitivity. Some mutations can be detected at both temperatures; some can only be detected at one temperature. In our laboratory, 5 and 15°C are usually used. Constant power ranges from 10W to 30W. High power may cause uneven electrophoresis, giving rise to "smiling" bands. Running time ranges between 3 and 18 hours, depending on fragment size and constant power.

11. Solution 1 is used to fix the DNA bands. Fixing time can be flexible, from 6 to 15 min. Prepare solutions 2 and 3 during this time period. Solution 2 is for silver staining. Solution 3 is used to wash unstained silver off the gel and manifest bands as dark brown or black regions before significant background develops. This solution needs to be freshly prepared. Do not forget to add formaldehyde; otherwise the bands will not develop. Washing time should be carefully watched. In general it is about 20 min. However, it can be shorter or longer than 20 min, depending on band intensity. If it is too short, bands may not be clear enough. If it is too long, the background may be too strong.

    Solution 4 is used to neutralize of solution 3 and stop bands developing by altering the pH of the gel. Keeping the gel in solution 4 for 3–5 min should be sufficient. Do not leave gel in solution 4 for more than 20 min; otherwise SSCP bands may fade away. SSCP gels are fragile and easily broken, extra care should be taken when handling SSCP gels during the whole process.

12. Gels can be stored at 4°C for up to 2 yr. Dried gels can be kept for even longer. Direct sequencing of samples possessing different band shifts (i.e., wild-type, mutant heterozygote, and mutant homozygote) should be performed in order to confirm and identify sequence alterations. Verified samples can be used as controls for further screening and genotyping.

References

1. Gupta, A. and Agarwal, S. (2003) Efficiency and cost effectiveness: PAGE-SSCP versus MDE and Phast gels for the identification of unknown beta thalassaemia mutations. *Mol. Pathol.* **56**, 237–239.
2. Klumb, C. E., Furtado, D. R., Magalhaes De Resende, L. M., et al. (2003) DNA sequence profile of TP53 gene mutations in childhood B-cell non-Hodgkin's lymphomas: prognostic implications. *Eur. J. Haematol.* **71**, 81–90.
3. Yin, D., Xie, D., Hofmann, W. K., et al. (2002) Methylation, expression, and mutation analysis of the cell cycle control genes in human brain tumors. *Oncogene* **21**, 8372–8378
4. Baroni, M. G., Sentinelli, F., Massa, O., et al. (2001) Single-strand conformation polymorphism analysis of the glucose transporter gene GLUT1 in maturity-onset diabetes of the young. *J. Mol. Med.* **79**, 270–274.

5. Baroni, M. G., Arca, M., Sentinelli, F., et al. (2001) The G972R variant of the insulin receptor substrate-1 (IRS-1) gene, body fat distribution and insulin-resistance. *Diabetologia* **44**, 367–372.

6. Wang, H., Chu, W., Das, S. K., Zheng, Z., Hasstedt, S. J., and Elbein, S. C. (2003) Molecular screening and association studies of retinoid-related orphan receptor gamma (RORC): a positional and functional candidate for type 2 diabetes. *Mol. Genet. Metab.* **79**, 176–182.

7. Hixson, J. E. and Powers, P. K. (1995) Detection and characterization of new mutations in the human angiotensinogen gene (AGT). *Hum. Genet.* **96**, 110–112.

8. Jeunemaitre, X., Bassilana, F., Persu, A., et al. (1997) Genotype-phenotype analysis of a newly discovered family with Liddle's syndrome. *J. Hypertens.* **15**, 1091–1100.

9. Persu, A., Barbry, P., Bassilana, F., et al. (1998) Genetic analysis of the beta subunit of the epithelial Na+ channel in essential hypertension. *Hypertension* **32**, 129–137.

10. Baker, E. H., Dong, Y. B., Sagnella, G. A., et al. (1998) Association of hypertension with T594M mutation in beta subunit of epithelial sodium channels in black people resident in London. *Lancet* **351**, 1388–1392.

11. Dong, Y., Baker, E. H., Sagnella, G. A., Carter, N. D., and MacGregor, G. A. (1998) Use of single-strand conformation polymorphism analysis to screen for the T594M sodium channel mutation. *Biochem. Soc. Trans.* **26**, S393.

12. Dong, Y. B., Zhu, H. D., Baker, E. H., et al. (2001) T594M and G442V polymorphisms of the sodium channel beta subunit and hypertension in a black population. *J. Hum. Hypertens.* **15**, 425–430.

13. Bettinaglio, P., Galbusera, A., Caprioli, J., et al. (2002) Single Strand Conformation Polymorphism (SSCP) as a quick and reliable method to genotype M235T polymorphism of angiotensinogen gene. *Clin. Biochem.* **35**, 363–368.

14. Orita, M., Iwahana, H., Kanazawa, H., Hayashi, K., and Sekiya, T. (1989) Detection of polymorphisms of human DNA by gel electrophoresis as single-strand conformation polymorphisms. *Proc. Natl. Acad. Sci. USA* **86**, 2766–2770.

15. Suzuki, Y., Orita, M., Shiraishi, M., Hayashi, K., and Sekiya, T. (1990) Detection of ras gene mutations in human lung cancers by single-strand conformation polymorphism analysis of polymerase chain reaction products. *Oncogene* **5**, 1037–1043.

16. Makino, R., Yazyu, H., Kishimoto, Y., Sekiya, T., and Hayashi, K. (1992) F-SSCP: fluorescence-based polymerase chain reaction-single-strand conformation polymorphism (PCR-SSCP) analysis. *PCR Meth. Appl* **2**, 10–13.

17. Inazuka, M., Wenz, H. M., Sakabe, M., Tahira, T., and Hayashi, K. (1997) A streamlined mutation detection system: multicolor post-PCR fluorescence labeling and single-strand conformational polymorphism analysis by capillary electrophoresis. *Genome Res.* **7**, 1094–1103.

18. Kukita, Y., Higasa, K., Baba, S., et al. (2002) A single-strand conformation polymorphism method for the large-scale analysis of mutations/polymorphisms using capillary array electrophoresis. *Electrophoresis* **23**, 2259–2266.

19. Andersen, P. S., Jespersgaard, C., Vuust, J., Christiansen, M., and Larsen, L. A. (2003) High-throughput single strand conformation polymorphism mutation detection by automated capillary array electrophoresis: validation of the method. *Hum. Mutat.* **21**, 116–122.
20. Hongyo, T., Buzard, G. S., Calvert, R. J., and Weghorst, C. M. (1993) "Cold SSCP": a simple, rapid and non-radioactive method for optimized single-strand conformation polymorphism analyses. *Nucleic Acids Res.* **21**, 3637–3642.
21. Andersen, P. S., Jespersgaard, C., Vuust, J., Christiansen, M., and Larsen, L. A. (2003) Capillary electrophoresis-based single strand DNA conformation analysis in high-throughput mutation screening. *Hum. Mutat.* **21**, 455–465.
22. Zhu, H., Sagnella, G. A., Dong, Y., et al. (2003) Contrasting associations between aldosterone synthase gene polymorphisms and essential hypertension in blacks and in whites. *J. Hypertens.* **21**, 87–95.
23. Markus, H. S., Martin, R. J., Simpson, M. A., et al. (2002) Diagnostic strategies in CADASIL. *Neurology* **59**, 1134–1138.
24. Dong, Y., Hassan, A., Zhang, Z., Huber, D., Dalageorgou, C., and Markus, H. S. (2003) Yield of screening for CADASIL mutations in lacunar stroke and leukoaraiosis. *Stroke* **34**, 203–205.

12

Single-Nucleotide Polymorphism Genotyping for Disease Association Studies

Myriam Fornage and Peter A. Doris

Summary

The Human Genome Project has led to the discovery of millions of DNA sequence variants in the human genome. The majority of these variants are single-nucleotide polymorphisms (SNPs). Availability of an ultra-high-density SNP map, combined with improvement in genotyping technologies and efficient analytical approaches, opens the possibility of fulfilling the promise of SNP association studies to reveal why some individuals are more susceptible to common chronic diseases such as hypertension and stroke. With millions of SNPs spread throughout the human genome, it is neither practical nor necessary to genotype every single SNP in population samples for association studies. Linkage disequilibrium between sites suggests that it is possible to detect disease association using a relatively sparse collection of SNPs. While the cost associated with assaying a comprehensive set of SNPs is still significant, several technologies show great promise for high-efficiency SNP genotyping. This chapter focuses on two of them: the 5'-nuclease assay and mass spectrometry genotyping.

Key Words: Single-nucleotide polymorphisms; genotyping; mass spectrometry; nuclease assay.

1. Introduction

Identifying the polymorphisms that contribute to disease predisposition and affect drug response is a major goal of the Human Genome Project. Because of their abundance and density, single-nucleotide polymorphisms (SNPs) have been proposed as ideal polymorphic markers in disease association and fine-mapping studies *(1)*. Although to date the use of SNPs has been limited to the analysis of candidate genes and small chromosomal regions *(2,3)*, improvement in genotyping technologies and efficient analytical approaches stemming from the Haplotype Map (HapMap) Project *(4)* may provide a future avenue to fulfilling the promise of SNP studies to reveal why some individuals are more susceptible to common chronic diseases such as hypertension and stroke. With

From: *Methods in Molecular Medicine, Vol. 108: Hypertension: Methods and Protocols*
Edited by: J. P. Fennell and A. H. Baker © Humana Press Inc., Totowa, NJ

millions of SNPs spread throughout the human genome, it is neither practical nor necessary to genotype every single SNP in population samples for association studies. Linkage disequilibrium (LD) between sites suggests that it is possible to detect disease association using a relatively sparse collection of SNPs. For example, Reich et al. *(5)* showed that LD in a US population of Northern European descent extends 60 kb for common alleles, implying that 50,000 SNPs would be needed in genome-wide association study in these populations. In another study, Kruglyak *(6)* proposed that LD is unlikely to extend beyond an average of 3 kb, so that 500,000 SNPs would be required for a genome-wide association study. While the cost associated with assaying a comprehensive set of SNPs is still significant, several technologies show great promise for high-efficiency SNP genotyping. This chapter focuses on two of them: the 5'-nuclease assay and mass spectrometry genotyping.

1.1. Introduction to SNP Genotyping by 5'-Nuclease Assay

The 5'-nuclease assay, commercialized by Applied Biosystems under the registered trademark TaqMan assay, is well suited to large-scale SNP genotyping for several reasons, including automation, accuracy, amenability to high throughput, and reasonable cost efficiency.

The TaqMan assay is a three-step process. First, allele-specific fluorogenic probes, approx 20 bp in length and labeled at the 5'- and 3'-ends with fluorescent reporter and quencher dyes, respectively, hybridize to the target DNA in a sequence-specific manner. When the probes are intact, the proximity of the reporter dye to the quencher dye suppresses the fluorescent activity of the reporter dye. Second, during PCR amplification, flanking PCR primers are extended in the 3'-direction by Taq DNA polymerase activity. The 3'-end of the fluorogenic probes is blocked to prevent extension. Third, as the DNA strand extends from the primer to the bound probe, the 5'-nuclease activity of Taq DNA polymerase cleaves the bound probe at the 5'-end and releases the reporter dye, causing an increase in fluorescent intensity of the reporter dye (*see* Chapter 14). Each allele-specific probe is labeled with a different reporter dye, usually FAM (6-carboxyfluorescein) and VIC (Applied Biosystems proprietary dye). After polymerase chain reaction (PCR) amplification, analysis of fluorescent signals of the distinct reporter dyes leads to automated genotype determination. An increase in only one of the fluorescent signals indicates that the sample is homozygous for either the VIC- or FAM-specific allele, while an increase in both signals indicates that the sample is heterozygous.

1.2. Introduction to Mass Spectrometry as a SNP Genotyping Tool

Mass spectrometry (MS) is a vital tool for the chemical analysis of biological macromolecules. Its introduction to genotyping is relatively recent *(7–12)*.

The most important feature of MS is that it provides a direct measurement of the molecular mass of the analyzed biomolecule. This measurement is highly stable and can be measured with sufficient precision and sensitivity to be a reliable indicator. Numerous technological innovations have dramatically extended the capabilities of mass spectrometry. The most relevant of these in the context of genotyping is the introduction of matrix-assisted, laser desorption ionization *(13)*, which permits large molecules to be ionized with minimal fragmentation and is often used in conjunction with time-of-flight (TOF) spectrometry. DNA molecules to be analyzed are co-crystallized in a matrix comprised of molecules that serve to transfer energy from the laser to the DNA resulting in the surface desorption of DNA ions. These ions are extracted and held in an electric field to permit compensation of initial velocities (this delayed extraction greatly increases the mass accuracy of the method). Finally, mass determination is achieved by measuring time of flight in the spectrometer (**Fig. 1**).

This technique has resulted in sufficient sensitivity to analyze DNA at concentrations typical of those achieved in PCR and post-PCR reactions and with sufficient resolution to readily distinguish mass differences attributable to single-base substitutions in single-stranded DNA from 3 to 28 bases across a mass range of approx 1 to 8 kDa. Although DNA analysis by mass spectrometry is fundamentally a serial process, rapid signal acquisition results in short analysis times, so single samples can be analyzed in a few seconds or less. Furthermore, parallel analysis of more than one DNA sequence variant is possible by designing multiplex genotyping systems in which multiple targets are present in a single genotyping reaction tube.

1.2.1. Direct Analysis of PCR Products

The direct analysis of DNA sequence by MALDI has been demonstrated *(14–16)*. Loss of signal intensity and mass resolution places an upper limit on the size of PCR products that can be analyzed of about 100 nucleotides. Using UV laser ionization/desorption, analysis of sequence has been coupled to both extension termination products, using the same principle as Sanger sequencing, and also to endonucleolytic cleavage to generate small fragments of appropriate range for sequencing *(17,18)* (**Fig. 2**).

1.2.2. Analysis of Chemically Cleaved PCR Products

PCR products amplified in the presence of nucleotide analogs susceptible to postamplification chemical cleavage provide another MS strategy for genotyping *(19)*. The nucleotides used (7-deaza-7-nitro-dATP and -dGTP, 5-hydroxy-dCTP, and 5-hydroxy-dUTP) form standard base pairs that will withstand multiple cycles of PCR, but are readily cleaved (by potassium permanganate and 3-pyrrolidine) post-PCR. Biallelic polymorphisms can be

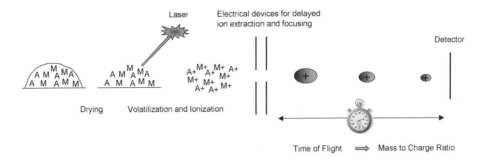

Fig. 1. Principle of MALDI–TOF mass spectrometry (M = matrix; A = analyte). The analyte (PCR product) is embedded in a crystal of matrix molecules at the laser wavelength of the instrument. The matrix is volatilized by energy absorption, entraining the enclosed PCR products in the gas phase where they become ionized. In an electric field, the ions are subsequently accelerated to the detector, which determines the masses according to the time of flight.

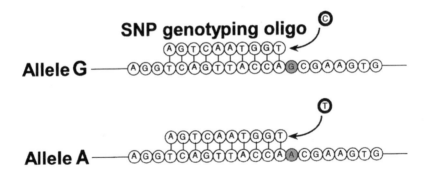

Fig. 2. PCR is used to amplify a short region of genomic DNA containing the target single-nucleotide polymorphism (shaded residues). The PCR product is then annealed to a genotyping oligonucleotide (extension or minisequencing primer) that is extended by a DNA polymerase capable of incorporating terminating dideoxynucleotides. To enhance mass discrimination, deoxynucleotides may be added to the reaction mix. For example, addition of TTP, ddCTP, and ddGTP to the illustrated reaction would result in the immediate termination of the allele G extension primer by the incorporation of ddCTP. However, the A allele would first incorporate the TTP and then be terminated by incorporation of ddGTP. The result is an increased mass difference between the resulting allelic extension products. Although such "tuning" is not essential for single-locus tests, it can be helpful in multiplex reactions to distribute the masses of the reaction components across the mass spectrum.

typed by performing PCR reactions in the presence of one of the modified deoxynucleotide triphosphates (dNTPs). Primers are designed so that they lie close upstream of the polymorphic site. A PCR target sequence that contains a polymorphic base corresponding to the particular modified dNTP that has been used in amplification can be chemically cleaved to form DNA fragments that include a fragment comprised of the forward primer and any bases extended from the primer until the polymorphic site is reached. If an allele is present that does not contain the variant on its forward strand corresponding to the modified dNTP used in amplification, the reaction will extend downstream until the next occurrence of a residue corresponding to the modified dNTP present. Genotype can be assigned by detecting ions corresponding in mass to these two fragments.

2. Materials

2.1. SNP Genotyping by 5'-Nuclease Assay

1. ABI 7700 or 7900 Sequence Detection System or equivalent.
2. Primer Express software (Applied Biosystems) or equivalent.
3. Genomic DNA.
4. Oligonucleotide primers and labeled allele-specific probes.
5. AmpliTaq Gold DNA polymerase (Applied Biosystems).
6. TaqMan Universal PCR Master mix (Applied Biosystems).
7. 96- or 384-well optical PCR plates (Applied Biosystems and others).

2.2. SNP Genotyping by Mass Spectrometry

1. Genomic DNA.
2. Synthetic oligonucleotides for PCR amplification and mini-sequencing.
3. AmpliTaq Gold DNA polymerase (Applied Biosystems).
4. Reaction buffer (Applied Biosystems).
5. 96-well PCR reaction and microtiter plates.
6. Exonuclease I (USB Corporation).
7. Shrimp alkaline phosphatase (Roche Applied Science).
8. Thermosequenase (USB Corporation) or *Tth* polymerase (Roche Applied Science).
9. 96-Well purification spin plates.
10. Poros 50-R1 reversed-phase chromatography matrix (Applied Biosystems).
11. Triethylammonium acetate.
12. Acetonitrile.
13. MALDI matrix consisting of either trihydroxyacetophenone (THAP) or 3-hydroxy-picolinic acid (3-HPA).

3. Methods

3.1. SNP Genotyping by 5'-Nuclease Assay

3.1.1. Probe and Primer Design

The DNA sequence surrounding the polymorphic site dictates probe placement. These guidelines are followed for design of the TaqMan probes: First, the polymorphic site is positioned in the middle third of the sequence, as mismatches at the ends of probes tend not to be as disruptive to hybridization. Second, the 5'-end of a probe cannot be a guanosine residue, as a guanosine adjacent to the reporter dye will partially quench its fluorescence even after cleavage. Third, the T_m of the probe should be between 65 and 67°C (approx 5–7°C higher than the primers). Fourth, runs of four or more identical nucleotides should be avoided. Fifth, the GC content of the probe should be between 30 and 80%, a range were the T_m can be accurately estimated. Sixth, the number of Cs in the probe must be greater than the number of Gs. If the reverse is true, then the complement sequence can be used to design the assay. Finally, the probe should not exceed 30 nucleotides in length. These parameters can be easily manipulated when using the Applied Biosystems proprietary software, Primer Express.

After selecting the probes for the assay, the primers are selected based on the following: First, the estimated *Tm* for the primers should be between 58 and 60°C. Second, runs of three or more identical nucleotides (especially Gs) should be avoided. Third, the GC content should be between 30 and 80%. Fourth, the last five nucleotides at the 3'-end should contain no more than two GC residues. Finally, the ideal size of the amplicon should be maintained between 75 and 150 bp, with primers placed as close to the probe as possible. Primer and probes are ordered from Applied Biosystems or other commercial supplier and should be protected from degradation (*see* **Note 1**).

3.1.2. Assay Optimization

This step ensures that primers produce a robust PCR product prior to their use in the genotyping assay (*see* **Note 2**). Genomic DNA samples (20 ng) are amplified by PCR in a total reaction volume of 25 µL in the presence of reaction buffer (provided in ready-made master mix) and 0.9 µ*M* each of primers. The PCR thermocycle profile consists of a 2-min step at 50°C, a 10-min step at 95°C, and 40 cycles of denaturation (95°C, 15 s) and annealing/extension (62°C, 1 min) steps. PCR products are then analyzed on a 2% agarose gel. PCR conditions are optimized by adjusting annealing/extension temperature or by adjusting primer concentration.

3.1.3. PCR Reaction

PCR amplification is carried out in a final volume of 25 μL containing 20 ng of genomic DNA, 1X TaqMan Universal master mix, and appropriate concentration of primers and probes as determined in the optimization procedure. PCR conditions are those determined from the optimization step. Each amplification series contains negative controls (no DNA) to ensure absence of contamination of the amplification reaction, as well as control samples of known genotype. After amplification, fluorescence analysis of each genotyping plate is performed using the ABI7700 or ABI7900 Sequence Detection System.

3.1.4. Analysis of PCR Products and Production of Genotype Data

Direct detection of PCR product with no downstream processing is accomplished within minutes of PCR completion. The software quantifies a sample's fluorescence by comparing its fluorescent activity to that of a background dye (ROX) present in the reaction buffer, a blank standard containing no DNA, and samples of known genotypes. These comparisons are made in order to normalize the fluorescence readings for variability across samples due to, for example, differences in PCR reactivity or experimental variations. Normalized fluorescence values are then used to perform automated genotype assignment. For each sample, normalized fluorescence value obtained for one of the allele-specific probes is plotted against that obtained for the other allele-specific probe, giving a visual representation of the clustering of the samples in three groups corresponding to the three genotypes. Ambiguous genotypes, which result from poor PCR reactivity, are designated as missing data (*see* **Notes 2–5**). A table recapitulating the fluorescence data for each sample and a matrix of 12 columns and 8 rows, containing the genotype calls for each sample on the plate are also generated. An example of plate read data is given in **Fig. 3**.

3.2. SNP Genotyping by Mass Spectrometry

3.2.1. Oligonucleotide Extension (Minisequencing)

The most widely employed application of mass spectrometry has been the determination of sequence variation at single nucleotide polymorphisms using oligonucleotide extension reactions (minisequencing). This approach requires amplification by PCR of the region containing the variant site(s) followed by a second reaction in which an additional oligonucleotide is annealed upstream of the polymorphic site and extended over it. Use of dideoxynucleotide triphosphates (ddNTPs) and DNA polymerases such as Thermosequenase and *Tth*, which incorporate ddNTPs with high efficiency, results in rapid termination of

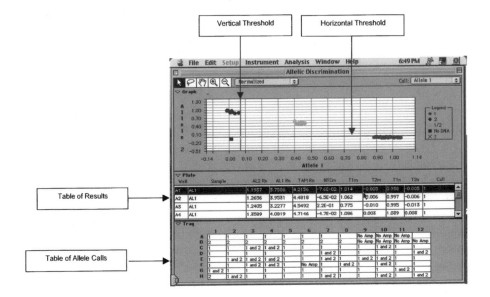

Fig. 3. Example of data generated after analysis of a 96-well genotyping plate using the TaqMan assay. The graphical display (top) represents the normalized fluorescence values detected for allele 1 plotted against those of allele 2, and shows the clustering of the samples into three groups corresponding to the three genotypes. The table (middle) shows the fluorescence values for each dye component (Allele 2 and Allele 1 dyes, TAMRA dye, background for samples with no DNA (NTC)), normalized fluorescence values, and genotype calls. The matrix of calls (bottom) contains the genotype assigned to each sample in the 96-well plate. 1, 1/1 homozygotes; 2, 2/2 homozygotes; 1 and 2, heterozygotes; ?, undetermined; no amp, no amplification (corresponds to no DNA controls).

extension. The resulting extended products will reflect the mass of the incorporated nucleotide at the variant base. Details for genotyping by this method are provided below.

3.2.2. Oligonucleotide Extension Using Modified Extension Primers

A method has been developed to simplify MALDI-TOF analysis of DNA by modifying the chemical properties of the extension oligonucleotide. The phosphate backbone of DNA contains negative charges at each phosphoester bond. These charges reduce the ionization and increase adduct formation, especially of positively charged alkali metal ions present in reaction buffers. Gut and colleagues have reported a series of papers outlining the development of chemically modified extension primers designed to overcome this limitation (7,12,20). In this approach the extension oligo contains two terminal base residues at its 3'-end that are linked together with methylphosphonate linkages that are uncharged and are resistant to digestion by phosphodiesterase. Use of a novel polymerase (*Tma31* FS DNA polymerase) that preferentially incorporates ddNTPs (over dNTPs) into primers containing methylphosphonate linkages results in efficient single-base extension and termination of this oligo. The resulting primer is then digested with phosphodiesterase II and the reaction products loaded directly onto MALDI sample plates without further purification. This approach eliminates the need for alkaline phosphatase denaturation of dNTPs from the PCR amplification reaction and does not require exonuclease digestion of PCR amplification primers because the extension reaction product is considerably smaller than PCR primers and so will not interfere in the MALDI analysis. Further, because of their single negative charge, the oligo 3'-terminals are ionized with high efficiency, providing high signal strength in mass spectrometry.

3.2.3. PCR Conditions

PCR primers are designed to amplify a short sequence, typically from 40 to 100 bp, surrounding the variant sites. In order to reduce cost per test, reaction volumes are minimized. Reactions use 3 ng genomic DNA, 1X PCR buffer, 2.0 m*M* MgCl$_2$, 0.2 m*M* each dNTPs, 1 µ*M* forward and reverse primers, and 0.25 U AmpliTaq Gold DNA polymerase (Applied Biosystems) in a total reaction volume of 4 µL. Further cost reductions can be achieved by multiplexing reactions (*see* **Notes 6** and **7**). Multiplexing can be achieved only at the level of oligo extension or, with more development work, can include multiplexing of PCR amplifications as well. For these multiplex reactions, primers are diluted and mixed in order to simplify PCR cocktail assembly. Reactions are carried out in 96-well PCR plates. To aid in sample tracking, bar-code labels can be placed on each plate to identify the DNA samples and the amplification primer(s) used. Robotic liquid transfer can facilitate throughput and accuracy. For example, we have performed transfer of PCR cocktail to the reaction plates using the Multimek robotic system (Beckman-Coulter).

3.2.4. Extension (Minisequencing) Reaction Conditions

Before performing the minisequencing reactions, 2 µL of a solution containing 2.5 U of exonuclease I (ExoI; Amersham Pharmacia) and 0.25 U of shrimp alkaline phosphatase (SAP; Boehringer Mannheim) are added directly to the PCR reaction and incubated at 37°C for 30 min in order to digest unincorporated dNTPs and PCR primers. Minisequencing reactions are performed in a total reaction volume of 10 µL using: oligonucleotide primers that anneal immediately 5' of each polymorphic site; dideoxynucleotides; and a thermostable polymerase to extend the oligonucleotides. Extension primers and products utilized in multiplexed mini-sequencing reactions are designed so that the masses of unextended and extended oligos can be distinguished from one another. This can be achieved simply by designing a series of extension primers whose masses and whose extension product masses are distributed across a useful range, for example from 3.5 to 6.5 kDa. This can be achieved either by extending the 5'-sequence of the extension oligo to include additional complementary bases or by attaching nonannealing 5'-extension arms (*see* **Notes 8** and **9**).

PCR, ExoI-SAP digestion, and minisequencing extension reactions are all performed in the same vessel, limiting the number of liquid transfers and the possibility of contamination, sample loss, and error. Two different thermostable polymerases, both of which incorporate ddNTPs efficiently, can be utilized in minisequencing reactions: Thermosequenase (Amersham Pharmacia), a highly stable DNA polymerase originally used for Sanger sequencing reactions; and *Tth* polymerase (Applied Biosystems), an RNA polymerase that acts as a DNA polymerase in the presence of manganese chloride. The minisequencing thermal protocol consists of 25 cycles of 20 s at 95°C, 30 s at 54°C, and 40 s at 72°C. Despite the very low T_m of the smaller minisequencing primers, varying annealing temperature has been found to have little or no effect on efficiency of the extension reaction.

3.2.5. Reaction Clean-Up and Plate Spotting

Prior to mass determination, minisequencing reaction products are prepared by mixing each sample with Poros 50-R1 reversed-phase chromatography matrix and centrifuging the samples through 96-well purification spin plates. DNA binds to the reverse-phase media in the presence of triethylammonium acetate, which is then rinsed with aqueous buffer and eluted with either 25% acetonitrile or MALDI matrix consisting of either trihydroxyacetophenone (THAP) or 3-hydroxypicolinic acid (3-HPA) (*see* **Note 10**). Samples eluted with matrix solution can be spotted directly onto the MALDI plates but must be analyzed within approx 24 h. Samples eluted in acetonitrile can be stored frozen for extended periods. After thawing, these samples are mixed with an equal amount of matrix prior to plate spotting. Approximately 400 nL of matrix-sample mixture is spotted onto a 384-well MALDI sample plate manually or using a Symbiot I robotic workstation (Perseptive Biosystems). Bar-code labels are used to verify and record the sample transfer from reaction plates to MALDI plates.

3.2.6. Reaction Product Analysis

Masses of the minisequencing reaction products are assessed using delayed-extraction mass spectrometry. A number of suitable MALDI-TOF MS instru-

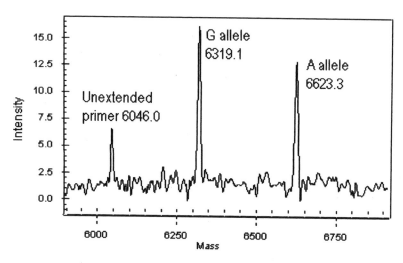

Fig. 4. The mass spectrum is used to detect and to determine the masses of ions generated as a result of matrix-assisted laser desorption ionization (MALDI). The example demonstrated the presence of unextended primers with a mass of 6046.0 Daltons as well as two extended oligos corresponding to the G and A alleles present at the SN locus. These alleles are identified by their expected masses of 6319.1 and 6623.3 Daltons.

ments are available from vendors including Applied Biosystems, Bruker Daltonic, Kratos/Shimadzu, and Micromass/Waters. A turnkey commercial MS genotyping system has been introduced by Sequenom that incorporates most of the elements described above and is extended to facilitate high throughput by including software for design of genotyping systems, allele-calling software to automate extraction of genotype information from mass spectra, and methods to simplify preparation of samples for MS, which is critical in order to achieve high-throughput genotyping. (**Fig. 4**).

4. Notes

1. All primer and probe reagents should be aliquoted to protect from degradation following repeated freeze/thaw and avoid possible contamination.
2. Diffuse distribution of heterozygote normalized results in the plotted data (*see* **Fig. 1**) indicates a weak PCR amplification.
3. Poor discrimination of the genotype group may have several causes: (1) nonspecific binding of the primers—increase of the annealing/extension temperature of the PCR should help; (2) poor quality of the template—high-quality DNA samples are recommended; (3) unequal concentration of the DNA samples—accurate quantitation of DNA concentration and adjustment to equal concentration of the samples are suggested.

4. Absence of the heterozygote category indicates that one probe is not detected. This may be due to probe degradation or poor probe hybridization. Verification of probe sequence and possible redesign may be necessary. This may also indicate that the ratio of FAM/VIC probe is inappropriate. The concentration of each probe in the reaction should be adjusted so as to give equal signal intensity.

5. If more than three genotype clusters are visible, this may indicate that another polymorphic site is present near the polymorphism of interest. Additional measures (e.g., resequencing; database searches) should be used to determine whether this is the case.

6. The inherent simplicity of the oligonucleotide extension approach can be exploited with some simple variations to enhance the power of the technique. Extension oligos can be designed to anneal to either the forward or reverse strands of the PCR product, providing flexibility in assay optimization. While multiplexing from two- to fourfold can be readily accomplished by selecting oligonucleotides for each polymorphic locus that occupy different regions in the mass spectrum, higher levels of multiplex reactions generally require substantial experimentation in order to optimize the PCR amplification reactions. Mass of extension products can be fine-tuned to maximize mass discrimination. For example, extension reaction mixes can be selected so that one allele in a di-allelic system terminates immediately upon incorporation of its complimentary ddNTP, while the alternate allele may first incorporate one or more dNTPs added to the reaction mix before terminating with ddNTP incorporation.

7. In general, the efficiency of multiplex oligo extension reactions is influenced by the abundance of PCR template products. Amplification of short PCR products generally increases the efficiency of the PCR reaction and results in high molar abundance of reaction products. By combining this approach with suitable multiplex PCR design, reactions interrogating 14 allelic variants representing 7 distinct loci have been performed *(8)*. Because PCR and oligo extension enzymes remain the single largest analysis cost components, such multiplexing can provide an important saving essential in large-scale genomics studies. Ultimately, the trade-off between multiplex assay design (assay development and optimization time) and increased throughput and cost efficiency places a ceiling on the ability to exploit multiplexing.

8. Inequality of variant allele extension peaks within a given SNP is a common occurrence in mass detection of minisequencing reactions *(21)*. This inequality is not usually problematic except in extreme cases in which the signal from one allele is less than 10% of the other and falls below the signal-to-noise criterion for allele recognition. Factors contributing to inequality in signal intensity include preferential incorporation of one dideoxynucleotide over the other and sequence-specific differences in desorption and/or ionization of oligonucleotide molecules. Switching the primer sequence to the complementary strand and making modifications to the primer sequence, such as adding a short poly-T tail to one primer, may assist in overcoming these problems *(22)*.

9. As extension primers and products are expanded into the higher mass ranges, some decrease in signal may result from reduced ionization of larger molecules.

This may be due to less efficient desorption and/or decreasing sensitivity of the detector for higher mass molecules. Differences in PCR efficiency as well as competitive ionization in multiplex reactions may also contribute to uneven extension signals. Therefore, it is important to minimize background noise and optimize the concentrations of primers so that primer signal does not mask extension signals. This is especially true in multiplex reactions, where high signal intensities for low-mass primers may result in comparably weak signals for the higher-mass products.

10. The use of THAP matrix can produce substantial depurination peaks that can mask or interfere with detection of extension peak signals in multiplex reactions. Depurination results from MALDI-induced cleavage of the N-β-glucosyl bond by which purines (cytosine and guanine) are attached to the sugar residues of the nucleotide. As a result of partial depurination oligonucleotide peaks will appear in the mass spectrum that correspond to both intact and depurinated, oligonucleotides. Loss of cytosine and guanine by depurination produce characteristic peaks that differ by approx 111 and 151 mass units from the peak produced by the intact oligo. THAP is often used for analysis of oligonucleotides with MALDI-TOF methods because of its even crystallization in the sample well, an especially useful characteristic when sampling in automatic mode. Interference from depurination peaks can make THAP undesirable for high-level multiplexing, however. Because depurination peaks have a predictable mass, careful design of primer and extension masses can help to avoid depurination peak interference when using THAP matrix. An alternative to THAP is the use of 3-HPA, which produces an even baseline and clearly resolved peaks. However, 3-HPA crystallizes in a circular pattern, leaving little material in the center of the well, which can make utilization of automated mass spectroscopy sampling problematic.

References

1. Collins, F. S., Guyer, M. S., and Chakravarti, A. (1997) Variations on a theme: cataloging human DNA sequence variation. *Science* **278**, 1580–1581.
2. Daly, M. J., Rioux, J. D., Schaffner, S. F., Hudson, T. J., and Lander, E. S. (2001) High-resolution haplotype structure in the human genome. *Nat. Genet.* **29**, 229–232.
3. Clark, A. G., Weiss, K. M., Nickerson, D. A., et al. (1998) Haplotype structure and population genetic inferences from nucleotide-sequence variation in human lipoprotein lipase. *Am. J. Hum. Genet.* **63**, 595–612.
4. Couzin, J. (2002) Human genome. HapMap launched with pledges of $100 million. *Science* **298**, 941–942.
5. Reich, D. E., Cargill, M., Bolk, S., et al. (2001) Linkage disequilibrium in the human genome. *Nature* **411**, 199–204.
6. Kruglyak, L. (1999) Prospects for whole-genome linkage disequilibrium mapping of common disease genes. *Nat. Genet.* **22**, 139–144.
7. Sauer, S., Gelfand, D. H., Boussicault, F., Bauer, K., Reichert, F., and Gut, I. G. (2002). Facile method for automated genotyping of single nucleotide polymorphisms by mass spectrometry. *Nucleic Acids Res.* **30**, e22.

8. Bray, M. S., Boerwinkle, E., and Doris, P. A. (2001) High-throughput multiplex SNP genotyping with MALDI-TOF mass spectrometry: practice, problems and promise. *Hum. Mutat.* **17,** 296–304.

9. Tang, K., Fu, D. J., Julien, D., Braun, A., Cantor, C. R., and Koster, H. (1999) Chip-based genotyping by mass spectrometry. *Proc. Natl. Acad. Sci. USA* **96,** 10016–10020.

10. Haff, L. A. and Smirnov, I. P. (1997). Multiplex genotyping of PCR products with MassTag-labeled primers. *Nucleic Acids Res.* **25,** 3749–3750.

11. Ross, P., Hall, L., Smirnov, I., and Haff, L. (1998) High level multiplex genotyping by MALDI-TOF mass spectrometry. *Nat. Biotechnol.* **16,** 1347–1351.

12. Sauer, S., Lechner, D., Berlin, K., et al. (2000) A novel procedure for efficient genotyping of single nucleotide polymorphisms. *Nucleic Acids Res.* **28,** E13.

13. Karas, M. and Hillenkamp, F. (1988) Laser desorption ionization of proteins with molecular masses exceeding 10,000 daltons. *Anal. Chem.* **60,** 2299–2301.

14. Fu, D. J., Tang, K., Braun, A., et al. (1998). Sequencing exons 5 to 8 of the p53 gene by MALDI-TOF mass spectrometry. *Nat. Biotechnol.* **16,** 381–384.

15. Kirpekar, F., Nordhoff, E., Larsen, L. K., Kristiansen, K., Roepstorff, P., and Hillenkamp, F. (1998) DNA sequence analysis by MALDI mass spectrometry. *Nucleic Acids Res.* **26,** 2554–2559.

16. Koster, H., Tang, K., Fu, D. J., et al. (1996) A strategy for rapid and efficient DNA sequencing by mass spectrometry. *Nat. Biotechnol.* **14,** 1123–1128.

17. Nordhoff, E., Luebbert, C., Thiele, G., Heiser, V., and Lehrach, H. (2000) Rapid determination of short DNA sequences by the use of MALDI-MS. *Nucleic Acids Res.* **28,** E86.

18. Kaetzke, A. and Eschrich, K. (2002). Simultaneous determination of different DNA sequences by mass spectrometric evaluation of Sanger sequencing reactions. *Nucleic Acids Res.* **30,** e117.

19. Wolfe, J., Kawate, T., Sarracino, D., et al. (2002) A genotyping strategy based on incorporation and cleavage of chemically modified nucleotides. *Proc. Natl. Acad. Sci. USA* **99,** 11073–11078.

20. Berlin, K. and Gut, I. G. (1999) Analysis of negatively "charge tagged" DNA by matrix-assisted laser desorption/ionization time-of-flight mass spectrometry. *Rapid Commun. Mass Spectrom.* **13,** 1739–1743.

21. Sun, X., Ding, H., Hung, K., and Guo, B. (2000) A new MALDI-TOF based minisequencing assay for genotyping of SNPS. *Nucleic Acids Res.* **28,** E68.

22. Lichtenwalter, K. G., Apffel, A., Bai, J., et al. (2000) Approaches to functional genomics: potential of matrix-assisted laser desorption ionization–time of flight mass spectrometry combined with separation methods for the analysis of DNA in biological samples. *J. Chromatogr. B, Biomed. Sci. Appl.* **745,** 231–241.

13

Denaturing High-Performance Liquid Chromatography Using the WAVE DNA Fragment Analysis System

Elizabeth Donohoe

Summary

Denaturing high-performance liquid chromatography (DHPLC) is a chromatographic mutation analysis technique that is based on temperature-dependent separation of DNA containing mismatched base pairs from polymerase chain reaction (PCR)-amplified DNA fragments. The WAVE system, developed for DHPLC analysis, allows for unattended analysis of 96 samples directly from a PCR plate under a number of different conditions. It utilizes a Peltier cooling platform to maintain sample integrity. Sample detection is achieved via UV absorbance at 260 nm, thereby avoiding the cost, safety, variability, or waste disposal issues associated with radioisotopic, enzyme-linked, or fluorescence detection systems. There are four key aspects to successfully detecting mutations on the WAVE: (1) PCR primer design, (2) PCR protocol, (3) separation gradient, and (4) separation temperature. Provided these procedures are carried out correctly, almost 100% detection of single-nucleotide polymorphisms (SNPs) and small deletion/insertion mutations can be achieved. For this reason, DHPLC is a powerful tool for identifying mutations in candidate genes for hypertension.

Key Words: DHPLC; WAVE; hypertension; mutation detection; ALAP gene; HUT2 gene; chromatography; heteroduplex analysis.

1. Introduction

Denaturing high-performance liquid chromatography (DHPLC) is a novel technology that exploits the differential melting properties of heteroduplex and homoduplex DNA for the detection of mutations (1). The WAVE DNA fragment analysis system provides a rapid, automated scanning method for mutations, even when the nature and location of the mutation is not known. Mutation detection involves four key steps: (1) primer selection and amplicon design, (2) polymerase chain reaction (PCR) amplification, (3) heteroduplex formation, and (4) DHPLC analysis. Its ability to resolve heteroduplex DNA from

From: *Methods in Molecular Medicine, Vol. 108: Hypertension: Methods and Protocols*
Edited by: J. P. Fennell and A. H. Baker © Humana Press Inc., Totowa, NJ

homoduplex DNA in a matter of minutes makes it a powerful tool in the field of mutation detection.

Traditional methods used for DNA mutational analysis, such as single-strand conformational polymorphism (SSCP) and denaturing gradient gel electrophoresis (DGGE), suffer from incomplete detection rates in the range of 70–85% *(2)*. Although DHPLC will not detect large gene deletions and duplications, it has been shown to be a very sensitive method for single-nucleotide polymorphisms (SNPs), small insertions, and deletions with detection rates approaching 100% *(3–7)*. As such, DHPLC is becoming a widely used tool for mutation screening, and already hundreds of known disease genes or candidate disease genes have been screened by this method *(8)*. Of particular relevance to this book, the technique has been applied to both the adipocyte-derived leucine aminopeptidase (ALAP) gene on chromosome 5q15 and the human urea transporter gene (HUT2) in two studies investigating their association with hypertension *(9,10)*.

1.1. Instrumentation

The WAVE DNA fragment analysis system is a fully automated instrument, which utilizes the principles of ion-pair reverse-phase liquid chromatography to perform analytical separations. The system incorporates a 96-well autosampler for high-throughput sample screening and allows the size-based separation of DNA fragments under nondenaturing conditions, or the separation of heteroduplex from homoduplex DNA under partially denaturing conditions.

A DNA sample is injected onto a chromatography column. The stationary phase of the DNASep cartridge is electrically neutral and hydrophobic, and therefore the negatively charged DNA alone cannot adsorb to the column's matrix. An ion-pairing reagent (triethylammonium acetate, TEAA) is used as a bridging molecule to aid the adsorption of DNA fragments to the stationary phase. The hydrophobic interactions between the stationary phase and the bridging molecules are disrupted by an increasing proportion of acetonitrile in the mobile phase, which is driven by high-pressure pumps from the buffer reservoirs through the analytical DNASep cartridge. The DNA is eluted from the column and is detected by a UV detection system *(11)*.

The WAVE system is operated by a combination of two software programs, HSM and WAVEMAKER, where HSM is required to define the location of stored data. Alternatively, the recently released Navigator software package can be used instead of both packages *(12)*, but the HSM and WAVEMAKER software packages will be described here. It should also be noted that there are different instrument models in use. The methods outlined below relate to the 3500HT model, which is equipped with an accelerator for more rapid analysis.

Table 1
Comparison of 3500
and 3500HT WAVE Systems

	3500	3500HT
Cartridge	DNASep	DNA Sep HT
Pump flow rate	0.9 mL/min	1.5 mL/min
Run time	6–7 min	3–4 min
Accelerator	No	Yes
Cartridge	DNASep	DNASep HT

The main differences between the original method, which uses a DNASep cartridge, and the high-throughput (HT) method, which uses a DNASepHT cartridge, are outlined in **Table 1**.

1.2. PCR Considerations for DHPLC Analysis

Template DNA is generated by PCR, the quality of which is an essential factor in DHPLC analysis. Routine optimization of a primer pair for PCR should ensure good purity and yield of the resulting PCR product. However, the melting profile of the amplicon should also be taken into consideration when designing primers for DHPLC (*see* **Subheading 3.2.** and **Note 1**). In addition, the size of the amplicon should be restricted to 150–450 bp, as larger fragments will invariably contain more melt domains and are therefore more difficult to analyze *(13)*. The suitability of DNA polymerases chosen for DHPLC is based on enzyme fidelity and cartridge compatibility. Optimase Polymerase (Transgenomic) is the enzyme of choice for DHPLC, but others, such as Pfu polymerase (Roche) or Amplitaq gold (Applied Biosystems) are also recommended. Other polymerase/buffer systems can be used, but the column warranty relating to the number of injections could be affected. Certain PCR additives such as bovine serum albumin (BSA), dimethyl sulfoxide (DMSO) or formamide are known to adversely affect the column and should not be used *(13,14)*. A list of such additives is available from the manufacturers.

1.3. Temperature-Modulated Heteroduplex Analysis

The DHPLC method is based on temperature-dependent separation of DNA containing mismatched bases from PCR-amplified DNA fragments. The detection of single-nucleotide polymorphisms (SNPs), insertions, and deletions relies on the formation of heteroduplex DNA, which is generated by denaturing and reannealing a mixed population of wild-type and mutant DNA. Individuals who are heterozygous for a single-base-pair mutation or polymorphism

Wild-Type   Mutant   Heteroduplexes   Homoduplexes

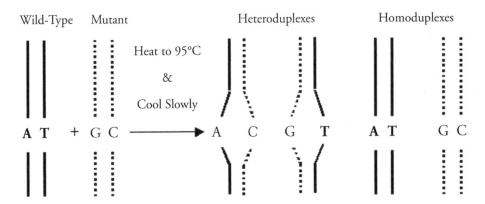

Fig. 1. Heteroduplex formation. When a DNA sample containing wild-type and mutant alleles is heated and then slowly cooled, two homoduplex and two heteroduplex species are formed.

have a 1:1 ratio of wild-type and mutant DNA. By a process often referred to as "heteroduplexing," the PCR products are heated to 95°C and then slowly cooled to form a mixture of heteroduplexes and homoduplexes (*see* **Fig. 1**). The DNA from individuals who carry two mutant alleles must be mixed in equal proportions with wild-type DNA and hybridized to form heteroduplexes *(1)*.

Heteroduplex DNA has different melting characteristics to homoduplex DNA and under partially denaturing conditions, has a reduced retention time on the column. This is due to a bubble formation at the site of the mismatch in the double-stranded DNA heteroduplex, leading to a reduction in the number of charges accessible for the electrostatic interactions between the DNA and the ion-pairing layer of the column matrix. The reduced charge density of the DNA molecule within the single-stranded region results in a shorter retention time on the column. At a temperature approx 1°C below the melting temperature of the fragment, samples carrying a sequence variant will show a significantly different elution profile to wild-type samples. This method of resolving heteroduplexes from the corresponding homoduplexes is known as temperature-modulated heteroduplex analysis (TMHA) *(1,15)*.

1.4. Temperature Optimization/Prediction

For any given sequence, the WAVEMAKER software can predict temperature and gradient conditions that will resolve heteroduplexes on the WAVE system. Sequence variants located at any position in an amplicon are affected by the melting characteristics of the surrounding nucleotides. GC-rich regions lose helicity (i.e., begin to denature) at higher temperatures than AT-rich

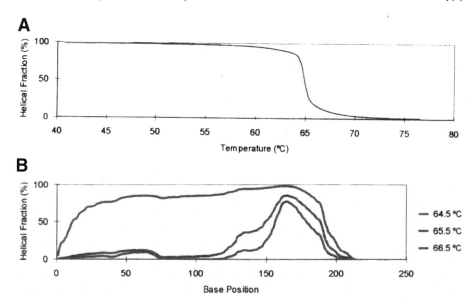

Fig. 2. **(A)** The predicted temperature range for a 214-bp fragment to melt from a double-stranded DNA fragment (100% helical fraction) to a single-stranded fragment (0% helical fraction). **(B)** The pattern of denaturation along the length of the 214-bp fragment at the three temperatures indicated. The predicted temperature for this fragment is 64.5°C (top line). The middle line represents the pattern of denaturation at 65.5°C, and the bottom line at 66.5°C.

domains. The melting characteristics of the DNA fragment will therefore determine the temperature at which a sequence variant located in that particular fragment will resolve using DHPLC *(16)*.

The WAVEMAKER software predicts temperature over a range of 0–100% helical fraction (*see* **Fig. 2**). The optimum melting temperature is at approx 75% helical fraction of the fragment. It is important to input the entire and correct DNA sequence of the fragment in question, because the algorithm used to calculate the melting behavior and to predict the optimum temperature is entirely dependent on the DNA sequence. To select melt temperatures manually, choosing temperatures that give a helical fraction between 50% and 98%, should offer good resolution of heteroduplexes. Ideally, a fragment would have only one melt domain and could therefore be analyzed at just one temperature, but this is rarely the case. Generally, two or even three temperatures are necessary to cover all melt domains in the fragment. When working with difficult templates it is recommended not to rely solely on predicted melting temperatures but to also take into consideration empirical data.

2. Materials

2.1. Equipment

1. Thermocycler (with heated lid).
2. DHPLC WAVE DNA fragment analysis system (Transgenomic).
3. DNA Sep HT cartridge (cat. no. DNA-99-3710, Transgenomic).
4. Transmat silicone sealing mats (*see* **Note 2**) (cat. no. 172024, Transgenomic).
5. PCR plates (*see* **Note 3**) (cat. no. 0030 127307, Eppendorf).
6. Chemical waste container.

2.2. Solutions

1. Optimase polymerase (supplied with Mg^{2+}-free buffer and separate Mg^{2+} solution) (cat. no. 703045, Transgenomic).
2. 100 mM dNTP set, PCR grade (cat. no. 10297-117, Invitrogen).
3. Mutation control standards, low-range mutation standard (cat. no. 560077) and high-range mutation standard (cat. no. 562001, Transgenomic).
4. DNA sizing standard (cat. no. 560078, Transgenomic).
5. Acetonitrile, 99.93+%, HPLC grade (cat. no. 27 071-7, Sigma-Aldrich).
6. WAVE ion-pairing agent, 2 M triethylammonium acetate (TEAA) (cat. no. 553303, Transgenomic).
7. Water (e.g., MilliQ water), use 18 MΩ resistance or better.
8. WAVE optimized buffers (optional): Buffers A, B, D, and syringe solution (cat. nos. 553401, 553402, 553404, and 553403, Transgenomic).

2.3. Software

1. HSM (Hitachi) and WAVEMAKER 4.1 (Transgenomic) software
   Or.
2. Navigator (Transgenomic).

3. Methods

In addition to the following guidelines, refer to the manufacturer's manual outlining in detail the use of the DHPLC system, its software, and maintenance requirements.

3.1. Instrument Operation/Maintenance

Before starting analysis, ensure that the system is functioning properly. The success of a run relies on properly prepared eluents, well-maintained instrument hardware, and a DNASep HT cartridge that is operating within specifications. The prevention and/or removal of contaminants before analysis by flushing the system with the appropriate solvents is essential *(17,18)*.

3.1.1. Buffer/Lines Maintenance

1. Check the level of buffers and make sure that the solvent inlet filters are totally immersed.

Table 2
Constituents Used to Make 1 L of WAVE Buffers

	Buffer A	Buffer B	75% Cleaning solution	8% Cleaning solution
TEAA	50 mL	50 mL	—	—
Acetonitrile (HPLC grade)	250 µL	250 mL	80 mL	750 mL
Water (HPLC or better)	9950 mL	9700 mL	9920 mL	250 mL
Total volume	1 L	1 L	1 L	1 L

2. Check for bacterial growth (*see* **Note 4**).
3. Check level of waste container.

The quality of the buffer solutions for the WAVE is of utmost importance and should be made to analytical chemistry standards, using quality-assured glassware and water of the highest possible quality (minimum standard is HPLC-grade water). Buffers must be made up in a fume hood, using designated volumetric flasks. Bottles must not be washed in washing machines but rinsed thoroughly in water. Make up buffers according to **Table 2**. *Nitrile or butyl gloves should be worn at all times while changing or handling buffers.*

Buffers A, B, and the syringe solution must be made up fresh weekly if not used within this time period, whereas the 75% acetonitrile solution must be changed every 3 wk. After changing the buffers and before beginning analysis, any bubbles that have been introduced must be removed using the "purge" function *(17,18)*. The control panel on the front of the instrument allows the user to select the required supply line.

1. Press "Pump Off."
2. Transfer supply lines to new bottles without touching the inlet filter.
3. Ensure inlet filter is located at the bottom of the bottle.
4. Press "Manual Settings."
5. Adjust settings to Buffer A = 100%, flow rate = 0.9 mL/min.
6. Open purge valve.
7. Switch on pump and press "Purge" for 2–5 min.
8. Repeat for Buffer B and the 75% acetonitrile solution.
9. Press "Purge" again to quit.
10. Switch off pump and close valve.
11. Adjust settings to equilibrating mode (50% A, 50% B, flow rate 0.05 mL/min, oven temperature 50°C) and switch on pump.
12. If the syringe solution has been replaced carry out 20 washes by pressing the "Wash" function.

3.1.2. System Maintenance

1. Injection system washing: The syringe and the injection port must be flushed daily. Press "Wash" on the control panel of the autosampler. Five wash cycles are recommended.
2. Pressure check: Avoid excessive pressure. It is recommended that the pressure be kept below approx 2500 psi (17 *M* Pa). If an increase in pressure occurs, the column should be cleaned with 75% acetonitrile at 80°C for 15 min.
3. Check absorbance on the detector: Press "Auto Zero" on the control panel of the detector. Wait for 2 min and note the value of the absorbance. This must be ±0.002.
4. Accelerator purge: For the 3500HT model, the accelerator must also be purged. Press "Prime" to start and stop the purge. Continue to purge the system as long as air bubbles are visible in the outlet tubing.

3.1.3. Mutation Standards

Once a week, the standards provided by Transgenomics should be run. The 56°C and 70°C mutation standards are used to check the column resolution and oven calibration. Both are PCR fragments of 209 and 219 bp, respectively, with a single-base mutation. Before running standards, run a 75% acetonitrile wash, and then run 5 µL of each standard with a blank or zero injection (set injection volume to 0 µL in sample table) between each one (*see* **Note 5** and **ref. *18***). Ensure the peak profile is of an acceptable standard before proceeding to analyze samples.

3.2. Preparation of Template DNA

It is important to note that the PCR must be oil-free, or serious damage can be caused to the column *(13)*. Typically, the PCR product is checked by agarose gel electrophoresis before DHPLC analysis (*see* **Notes 6–8**). This will ensure that there are no nonspecific products produced in the PCR, that the product is of the required yield, and also that the PCR blank is free from any detectable contamination.

Purification of the PCR product to remove excess reaction components is not necessary for DHPLC (*see* **Note 9**); 5–10 µL of neat PCR product is sufficient for analysis at one temperature. If analysis at a number of temperatures is required, the volume of PCR product prepared must be increased accordingly.

1. Using up to 150 ng genomic DNA (*see* **Note 10**), set up PCR in the usual manner with primers designed specifically for DHPLC analysis of the fragment of interest (*see* **Subheading 3.3.**).
2. Include among your samples enough known wild-type controls for subsequent heteroduplex formation. There are four possible types of samples for analysis on the WAVE:

    a. Unknown—mix with reference DNA.

    b. Known heterozygous mutant—mixing not necessary.

    c. Known homozygous mutant—mix with reference DNA.

    d. Known homozygous wild-type—use as reference DNA.

3. Once PCR is complete, load approximately 5 µL of PCR product and run on an agarose gel to check purity and yield.

4. 10–100 ng Amplified DNA is recommended for DHPLC analysis. Generally, the quality and quantity of amplified fragments should be similar to that suitable for conventional sequencing.

5. Add 10 µL of sample PCR product to 10 µL wild-type PCR product and carry out heteroduplex formation.

6. For efficient heteroduplex formation (*see* **Note 11**), program your thermocycler as follows *(13)*: 95°C for 5 min; 95°C for 22 s; 69 cycles $(T - 1°C)$ for 22 s (where T = temperature of previous cycle).

7. Following formation, run heteroduplexes on the DHPLC system immediately or store at 4°C or at –20°C for maximum 14 d. Heteroduplex formation should be repeated if the storage period is any longer.

3.3. Amplicon and Method Design

Although it is possible to detect SNPs in fragments up to 1.5 kb using the WAVE system, the ideal amplicon size for the detection of unknown mutations is 150–450 bp *(13)*. Primers should ideally be designed to amplify fragments containing only one melting domain. If the entire coding sequence of a gene is to be analyzed, the primers need to cover all exons and intron/exon boundaries. Small exons can be grouped together, but if an exon is too large to analyze in one amplicon or if it contains more than one melting domain, more than one primer pair must be used. Alternatively, the fragment can be analyzed at two or more temperatures.

Primers can be designed manually or with the help of Web-based programs. A collection of primer design sites is available at www.hgmp.mrc.ac.uk/GenomeWeb/nuc-primer.html. It is important to be aware of known polymorphisms when deciding on the location of primer binding sites (*see* **Note 12**). The melting profile of the desired amplicon can then be constructed using WAVEMAKER. Melting profiles can also be obtained from the Web at http://insertion.stanford.edu/melt.html.

3.3.1. Creating an Application Folder

1. Select D-7000 HSM Administration and click "Application Setup."

2. Choose destination drive (usually D).

3. Name the application folder (e.g., username, disease, etc.) and click "Create."

4. Application folder can now be found in the drop-down list on the sample table tab in WAVEMAKER.

3.3.2. Temperature Prediction

1. Obtain a complete and correct sequence of the DNA fragment you wish to analyse, and paste into a Word or Notepad document.
2. Open up WAVEMAKER software, go to File, and select "New project." Immediately save the project in the appropriate application folder
3. Select "Application Type," and choose "Mutation Detection."
3. Select "DNA Sequence" and copy selected DNA sequence; click "Apply."
4. Save and name the DNA sequence, which will now appear in the "Sequence File."
5. Select "Melting Profiles" and "Calculate" to generate the plots.
6. The "Helical Fraction Vs Temperature" displays the predicted temperature range for the melting of the fragment (**Fig. 2A**).
7. The "Helical Fraction Vs Base Position" graph displays the pattern of denaturation along the fragment at the temperatures indicated (**Fig. 2B**).
8. Select melt temperatures, which give a helical fraction between 50 and 98%, for each melt domain in the fragment. Up to three temperatures can be displayed simultaneously.
9. Select the desired temperature and click "Apply" to designate this temperature for analysis. Go to "File" and "Save method."

3.3.3. Gradient Prediction

The WAVEMAKER™ software calculates the correct gradient at the T_m of the fragment *(19)*. For analysis at temperatures other than the T_m, the gradient window should be adjusted to take account of the different elution point due to the change in helicity. This function is dependent on whether the "normal gradient" or the "rapid gradient" is being run. If running a "normal gradient," the "Timeshift" function is used to alter the gradient window by entering a value of 0.5 min/deg different from the T_m. If using the "rapid gradient," it is recommended that the Buffer B window be widened while keeping the time window the same (*see* **Note 13**) *(20)*. If any of the gradient parameters are adjusted, click "Apply" and "Save method." The default gradient parameters for both methods are given in **Table 3**.

3.4. Setting Up a Sample Table

1. Click on the "Sample Table" tab, and open the relevant application folder.
2. Open the required method for the fragment you wish to analyze.
3. Input the required information, e.g., injection volume, sample name, etc.
4. Start and end the project with the "low" and "high" mutation standards.
5. In order to save running time, it is best to group injections with the same screening temperature and to place the injections in increasing order.
6. To run samples, click "Initialize" and then "Run Samples."

Table 3
Default "Normal" and "Rapid" Gradient Parameters

Gradient step	"Normal" conditions	"Rapid" conditions
Loading duration	0.1 min	0.1 min
Loading drop	5%	3%
Gradient slope	2% Buffer B/min	2% Buffer B/min
Gradient duration	4 min	2.5 min
Clean duration	0.5 min	0.1 min
Equilibration duration	0.1 min	0.1 min
Flow rate	0.9 mL/min	1.5 mL/min
Run time	6.3 min	3 min

The "normal" conditions can be run on both DNASep and DNASep HT cartridges, whereas the "rapid" conditions apply only to the HT system.

7. The progress of the run can be viewed by selecting the "Monitor" tab.
8. Results can be viewed while the machine is running or at any time.
9. Click on "Results" tab.
10. To alter the axes or display settings, right-click on the chart.

3.5. Analysis of Results

The signal intensity of DHPLC profiles (for a wild-type peak) should be 2 mV or higher at A260nm *(21)* (*see* **Note 14**). The observation of heteroduplex peaks in a chromatogram (*see* **Figs. 3** and **4**) indicates the presence of a sequence variant, while a homoduplex peak indicates a wild-type sample. Heteroduplex peaks elute earlier from the column than homoduplex peaks and can be observed as either separate peaks or as shoulders on the leading edge of homoduplex peaks (*see* **Note 15**). The manner in which the heteroduplex resolves is influenced by the specific sequence change present and the melting characteristics of the surrounding nucleotides. Any elution profile that differs from the wild-type or reference DNA indicates the presence of a sequence change. Some small "bumps" or peaks may elute earlier in the profile, which must not be confused with mutant peaks (*see* **Note 16**). It is important to note that changes in retention time do not accurately predict the presence of a sequence change. Instead, changes in peak profiles must be used to determine the result.

Trace or peak profiles are not unique for a specific mutation, in that different mutations and polymorphisms can have identical profiles. For this reason, all abnormal chromatogram traces should be investigated by sequencing to verify the presence of a known mutation *(13)*.

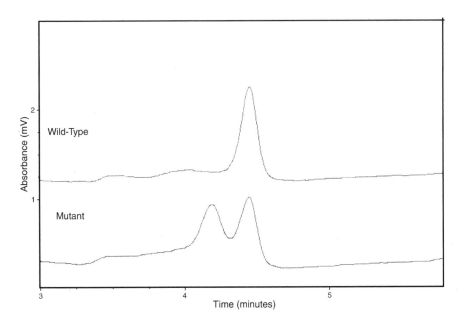

Fig. 3. Example of elution profiles for a wild-type and a mutant sample. The mutant sample contains an insertion/deletion mutation in exon 8 of the *RET* gene.

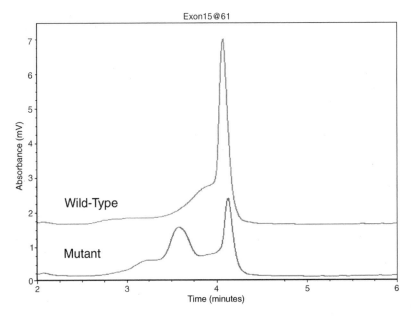

Fig. 4. Example of elution profiles obtained for a wild-type and a mutant sample. The mutant sample contains a stop codon mutation in exon 15 of the *RET* gene.

4. Notes

1. If a sequence variant occurs in a high-melt GC-rich pocket in a fragment with otherwise equal nucleotide ratios, a false negative result may be obtained. It may be necessary to redesign the amplicon, preferably with the GC-rich regions toward the end of the fragment. The use of GC clamps may also be considered *(6)*.

2. Transmat sealing mats were developed to protect samples from contamination and evaporation during storage or analysis in the samples tray of the WAVE system. The design of the mat ensures that the injection needle and port remain free of blockage due to plastic or adhesive contamination *(22)*.

3. Some PCR plates have a tendency to warp in the thermocycler, which can damage the injection needle and compromise the sampling. The problem can be avoided by cutting the plate in two or three places with scissors before placing in the autosampler.

4. Check buffers for bacterial growth. Ensure that they do not present any kind of precipitate or change in color *(18)*.

5. A zero injection step is also recommended when moving between methods at different temperatures on the sample table. Some users report that a slight shift in retention time is observed in the first of a set of samples run at a different temperature. By inserting a zero injection between methods at different temperatures, this problem can be avoided.

6. When checking quality of PCR products, it is important that the intensities of samples and control samples be relatively uniform for efficient heteroduplex formation. Poor-quality and low-yield PCR products can also affect the ability to see mutations *(13)*.

7. Negative controls containing no template DNA should be included for each PCR to check for contamination. Contamination can be excluded by gel electrophoresis or WAVE analysis *(13)*.

8. Ideally, a mutation-positive control should be included for each fragment analysed. If a positive control is not available, a confirmed (e.g., by sequencing) normal control must be included *(13)*.

9. Purification of PCR products is not necessary for DHPLC analysis but if used can actually impair heteroduplex formation.

10. Excess genomic DNA in the PCR reaction can lead to inconsistencies in the WAVE chromatograms. This usually appears as a "bump" after the injection peak.

11. Some published cooling protocols used for heteroduplex formation are too fast and can seriously impair heteroduplex formation *(13)*.

12. A false negative result can be obtained due to allele dropout, caused by sequence variants under the primer binding site, in which case the primers will need to be redesigned *(13)*.

13. Mutations cannot be detected if the sample peak elutes too close to the washoff peak. Adjust percent Buffer B until the sample peak is eluting at a midpoint on the chromatogram. Be careful to ensure the sample peak is not eluting too close to the injection peak either, or mutations can be missed.

14. If no sample peak is obtained, then the PCR has failed. The presence of an injection peak confirms that a sample was injected onto the column.

15. A multiple peak pattern does not necessarily represent the presence of a mutation. This pattern can be easily produced by a combination of poor-fidelity polymerase and high-cycle-number PCR. False positive results can be minimized if a positive result is taken to be a definite change in pattern from the reference sample as opposed to comparing multiple peaks with a single peak *(13)*.

16. If there are primer dimers present in the sample, these will appear as small peaks between the injection peak and the sample peak. A large amount of primer dimer may interfere with the sample peak.

Acknowledgments

I would like to thank my colleagues David Barton, Shirley McQuaid, Seán Ennis, and Brónagh O h'Icí for all their help, and particularly Seán Ennis for providing the WAVE data.

References

1. Taylor, P., Munson, K., and Gjerde, D. Transgenomic, Inc., San Jose, CA. (1999) *Detection of Mutations and Polymorphisms on the WAVE™ DNA Fragment Analysis System.*

2. Solari, V., Ennis, S., Yoneda, L., et al. (2003) Mutation analysis of the RET gene in total intestinal ananglionosis by WAVE™DNA fragment analysis system. *J. Paed. Surg.* **38,** 497–501.

3. Eng, C., Brody, L. C., Wagner, T. M., et al. (2001) Interpreting epidemiological research: blinded comparison of methods used to estimate the prevalence of inherited mutations in BRCA1. *J. Med. Genet.* **38,** 824–833.

4. Oefner, P. J. and Underhill, P. A. (1999) DNA mutation detection using denaturing high-performance liquid chromatography (DHPLC). In *Current Protocols in Human Genetics* (Dracopoli, N. C. and Haines, J., eds.), Wiley-Interscience, New York, pp. 7.10.1–7.10.12.

5. Choy, Y. S., Dabora, S. L., Hall, F., et al. (1999) Superiority of denaturing high-performance liquid chromatography over SSCP for mutation detection in TSC2. *Ann. Hum. Genet.* **63,** 383–391.

6. Narayanaswami, G. and Taylor, P. D. (2001) Improved efficiency of mutation detection by denaturing high-performance liquid chromatography using modified primers and hybridisation procedure. *Genet. Test.* **5,** 9–16.

7. Bunn, C. F., Lintott, C. J., Scott, R. S., and George, P. M. (2002) Comparison of SSCP and DHPLC for the detection of LDLR mutations in a New Zealand cohort. *Hum. Mutat.* **19,** 311.

8. http://insertion.stanford.edu/dhplc-genes1.html.

9. Yamamoto, N., Nakayama, J., Yamakawa-Kobayashi, K., Hamaguchi, H., Miyazaki, R., and Arinami, T. (2002) Identification of 33 polymorphisms in the adipocyte-derived leucine aminopeptidase (ALAP) gene and possible association with hypertension. *Hum. Mutat.* **19,** 251–257.

10. Ranade, K., Wu, K., Hwu, C., Ting, C., Pei, D., and Pesich, R. (2001) Genetic variation in the human urea transporter-2 is associated with variation in blood pressure. *Hum. Mol. Genet.* **19,** 2157–2164.
11. Transgenomic, Inc. (2001) Separation of DNA on the WAVE system in WAVEMAKER™ Software Version 4.1 Manual, pp. 1-7–1-12.
12. Transgenomic, Inc., San Jose, CA. Bioinformatics. www.transgenomic.com.
13. CMGS best practice guidelines for use of the WAVE system in diagnostic service. www.cmgs.org/BPG/Guidelines/2002/DHPLC.htm.
14. Muhr, D., Wagner, T., and Oefner, P. J. (2002) Polymerase chain reaction fidelity and denaturing high-performance liquid chromatography. *J. Chromatogr.* **782,** 105–110.
15. Kaler, S. G., Devaney, J. M., Pettit, E. L., Kirshman, R., and Marino, M. A. (2000) Novel method for molecular detection of the two common hereditary hemochromatosis mutations. *Genet. Test.* **4,** 125–129.
16. Schmitt, T. J., Robinson, M. L., and Doyle, J. Transgenomic, Inc., San Jose, CA. (2000) Single nucleotide polymorphism (SNP), insertion & deletion detection on the WAVE® nucleic acid fragment analysis system. www.transgenomic.com, application note 112.
17. Transgenomic, Inc., San Jose, CA. (2001) Operating the WAVE system. In WAVEMAKER™ Software Version 4.1 Manual, pp. 4-24–4-35
18. Transgenomic, Inc., San Jose, CA. Standard Operating Procedure: Maintenance on the WAVE 3500 Systems. Unpublished material.
19. Transgenomic, Inc., San Jose, CA. (2001) Guided tour of WAVEMAKER™ Software. In WAVEMAKER™ Software Version 4.1 Manual, pp. 3-22–3-30.
20. Transgenomic, Inc., San Jose, CA. Gradient prediction (unpublished material).
21. Matayas, G., De Paepe, A., Halliday, D., Boileau, C., Pals, G., and Steinmann, B. (2002) Evaluation and application of denaturing HPLC for mutation detection in Marfan syndrome: identification of 20 novel mutations and two novel polymorphisms in the FBN1 gene. *Hum. Mutat.* **19,** 443–456.
22. Transgenomic, Inc., San Jose, CA. Bioconsumables. www.transgenomic.com.

14

TaqMan Real-Time PCR Quantification

Conventional and Modified Methods

Michihiro Yoshimura, Shota Nakamura, and Hisao Ogawa

Summary

TaqMan real-time polymerase chain reaction (PCR) is a sensitive and reliable method that is widely used around the world. However, its inability to carry out assays using only small amounts of template DNA represents a serious limitation of the method. Recently, measurement of very small quantities of DNA became possible when a slight modification was applied to the conventional TaqMan real-time PCR method. Using the modified real-time PCR method, we were able to measure very small amounts of DNA template, and succeeded in comparing the levels of aldosterone synthase gene expression in samples of cardiac tissue from patients diagnosed with heart failure and control subjects.

Key Words: TaqMan; real-time PCR; 5'-nuclease assay; fluorescent reporter dye; Taq polymerase; quantitative analysis; aldosterone; CYP11B2; hypertension; heart failure; natriuretic peptide.

1. Introduction

TaqMan real-time polymerase chain reaction (PCR) is a sensitive and reliable method that is widely used around the world. However, its inability to carry out assays using only small amounts of template DNA represents a serious limitation of the method. Recently, measurement of very small quantities of DNA became possible when a slight modification was applied to the conventional TaqMan real-time PCR method. Using the modified real-time PCR method, we were able to measure very small amounts of DNA template, and succeeded in comparing the levels of aldosterone synthase gene expression in samples of cardiac tissue from patients diagnosed with heart failure and control subjects.

From: *Methods in Molecular Medicine, Vol. 108: Hypertension: Methods and Protocols*
Edited by: J. P. Fennell and A. H. Baker © Humana Press Inc., Totowa, NJ

Many methods for measuring the quantity of DNA have been devised. However, a certain amount of template DNA is always required for the measurement using any of the methods. This is a critical situation because, in research on humans, we usually obtain only small extractable amounts of samples.

TaqMan real-time PCR is widely used around the world, but its inability to carry out assays using only small amounts of template DNA represents a serious limitation of the method *(1–3)*, because a certain amount of DNA is required for measurement even using this method. In order to still carry out PCR on a small quantity of template DNA, the only methods are to increase the number of PCR cycles, or the quantity of the tissue samples. However, the trials do not work in many cases. In order to solve this problem, we tried to modify the conventional TaqMan method. As a result, measurement of DNA in very small quantities became possible. This modified real-time PCR method is thought to be the most sensitive one for measuring small quantities of template DNA.

Originally, we devised the conventional TaqMan method for the following situation. Recent animal studies had shown that aldosterone, previously thought to be synthesized solely in the adrenal cortex, was also produced in extraadrenal tissues such as the heart and blood vessels *(4,5)*. In addition, by measuring its levels in plasma samples in the coronary circulation, we were able to show that aldosterone synthesis was elevated in failing human ventricles *(6)*. In order to verify this, we needed to detect the aldosterone synthase gene, CYP11B2, in the human heart. This gene is expressed at low levels in the human heart, and is difficult to detect with conventional real-time PCR, since all the experimental points were so low as to be off the standard curve. This assay system was therefore deemed unsuitable for our purposes, and in order to conquer this problem, the modified method of real-time PCR was devised.

2. Materials

1. TRIzol reagent (Life Technologies, Tokyo, Japan) to obtain RNA from samples.
2. RNeasy minikit along with an RNAse-free DNAse kit (Qiagen, Tokyo, Japan).
3. SuperScript First-Strand Synthesis System protocol (Life Technologies, Tokyo, Japan).
4. The TaqMan Universal PCR Master Mix (P/N 4304437) containing 500 ng of cDNA template, 800 nM each primer, 200 nM TaqMan probe, and 2X TaqMan universal master mix (Perkin-Elmer Applied Biosystems).
5. ABI Prism 7700 sequence detection system (PE Applied Biosystems).

3. Methods

Before explanation of the method, preparation of TaqMan universal PCR master mix, basics of the 5'-nuclease assay, design of primers, probes for real-time PCR, and standard samples are briefly described.

3.1. Preparation of TaqMan Universal PCR Master Mix

The TaqMan Universal PCR Master Mix (P/N 4304437) is a convenient premix of all the components, except for primers and probe, necessary to perform a 5'-nuclear assay. The purpose of this technology is to detect known sequences of genomic, plasmid, or complementary DNA (cDNA). In RNA quantification assays, the TaqMan Universal PCR Master Mix is used in the second step of a two-step reverse transcription-polymerase chain reaction (RT-PCR) protocol. The template is cDNA generated from a reverse-transcription reaction. The TaqMan Universal PCR Master Mix may be used for real-time or plate-read (end-point) detection of DNA. Analysis is performed using the ABI Prism 7700 Sequence Detection System, the ABI Prism 7200 Sequence Detection System, or the TaqMan LS-50B PCR Detection System.

3.2. Basics of the 5'-Nuclease Assay

The mechanism of conventional TaqMan real-time PCR is explained briefly below and in **Fig. 1**. The PCR reaction exploits the 5'-nuclease activity of AmpliTaq Gold DNA polymerase to cleave a TaqMan probe during PCR. The TaqMan probe contains a reporter dye at the 5'-end of the probe and a quencher dye at the 3'-end of the probe. During the reaction, cleavage of the probe separates the reporter and quencher dyes, which results in increased fluorescence of the reporter dye. The accumulation of PCR products is detected directly by monitoring the increase in fluorescence of the reporter dye.

When the probe is intact, the proximity of the reporter dye to the quencher dye results in suppression of the reporter fluorescence primarily by Forster-type energy transfer. During PCR, if the target of interest is present, the probe specifically anneals between the forward and reverse primer sites. The 5'–3'-nucleolytic activity of the AmpliTaq Gold DNA polymerase cleaves the probe between the reporter and quencher dyes only if the probe hybridizes to the target. The probe fragments are then displaced from the target, and polymerization of the strand continues. The 3'-end of the probe is blocked to prevent extension of the probe during PCR. This process occurs in every cycle and does not interfere with the exponential accumulation of the product.

The increase in fluorescence signal is detected only if the target sequence is complementary to the probe and is amplified during PCR. Because of these requirements, no nonspecific amplification is detected.

3.3. Design of Primers, Probes for Real-Time PCR, and Standard Samples

For our studies, oligonucleotide primers and TaqMan probes for human CYP11B2 were designed from the GenBank databases using Primer Express Version 1.0 (Perkin-Elmer Applied Biosystems), as previously described (*1,2*).

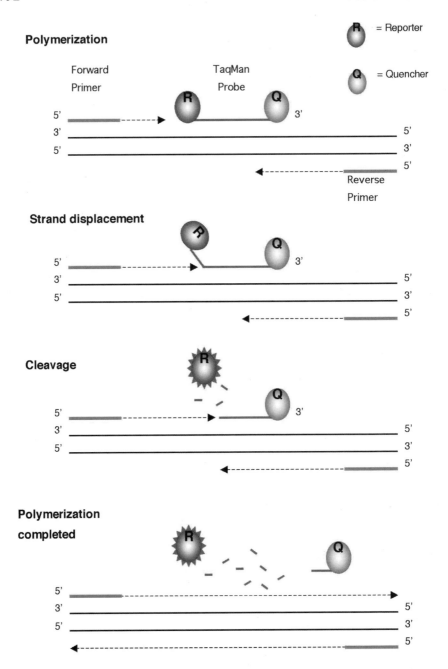

Fig. 1. Amplitaq Gold. The figure depicts the forklike, structure-dependent, polymerization-associated, 5'-3'-nuclease activity of AmpliTaq Gold DNA polymerase during PCR.

The TaqMan probe has a fluorescent reporter dye (FAM; 6-carboxy-fluorescein) covalently linked to its 5'-end and a downstream quencher dye (TAMRA; 6-carboxy-tetramethyl-rhodamine) linked to its 3'-end. Fluorescence quenching depends on the spatial proximity of the reporter and quencher dyes.

Amplification and detection of specific products was carried out in an ABI Prism 7700 sequence detection system (PE Applied Biosystems) using an amplification protocol consisting of 1 cycle at 50°C for 2 min, 1 cycle at 95°C for 10 min, 50 cycles at 95°C for 15 s, and 60°C for 1 min *(1,2)*.

To prepare the template DNA standards, a DNA fragment was fused into a plasmid, amplified, and refined. In the present study, the amount of construct per well was adjusted to 50 pg and then serially diluted, yielding samples containing 50 pg, 5 pg, 5×10^{-1} pg, 5×10^{-2} pg, 5×10^{-3} pg, and 5×10^{-4} pg, which were then used to construct standard plots.

3.4. RT-PCR and Modification of Conventional Real-Time RT-PCR

Samples of total RNA are reverse transcribed according to the SuperScript First-Strand Synthesis System protocol (Life Technologies, Tokyo, Japan) using oligo(dT) as the primer.

3.4.1. The Conventional TaqMan PCR System (*Fig. 2*, Top)

1. Mix a reaction containing 500 ng of cDNA template, 800 n*M* each primer, 200 n*M* TaqMan probe, and 2× TaqMan universal master mix (Perkin-Elmer Applied Biosystems, Tokyo, Japan) *(1,2)*.
2. Assay target and standard samples simultaneously. The critical threshold cycle (C_t), which is defined as the cycle at which the fluorescence from the TaqMan probe becomes detectable above the background, is inversely proportional to the logarithm of the initial number of template molecules.
3. In conventional real-time RT-PCR, C_t = 20–30 cycles, and measurement is difficult if C_t is over 35 *(1,2)*. Consequently, very small amounts of DNA template requiring C_t to be >35 cannot be measured accurately using this approach. In this case, the experiment returns after RT-PCR.

3.4.2. The Modified Conventional TaqMan PCR System (*Fig. 2*, Bottom) (see *Notes 1–4*)

In order to measure very small amounts of DNA template, we modified the conventional real-time PCR method.

1. Subject target gene samples, but not standard samples, to 10 PCR cycles in the absence of the TaqMan probe (protocol: 1 cycle at 50°C for 2 min, 1 cycle at 95°C for 10 min, 10 cycles at 95°C for 15 s, and 60°C for 1 min), which increases the amount of template DNA 1024 (2^{10})-fold.
2. After this preliminary PCR step, add the TaqMan probe to the target samples,

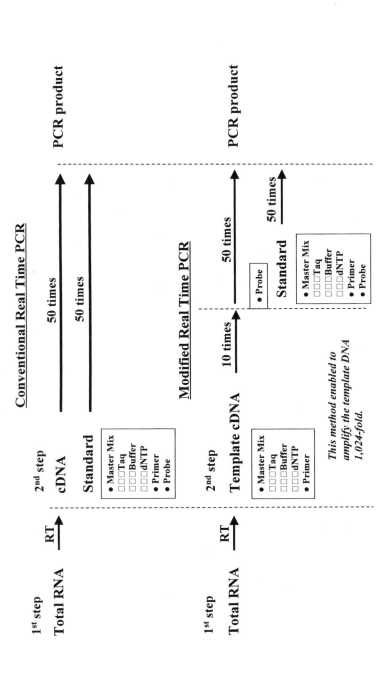

Fig. 2. Protocols of conventional and modified real-time RT-PCR. In the conventional TaqMan PCR system, target and standard samples are assayed simultaneously. When measuring very small amounts of DNA template, it is recommended to use the modified protocol. In this, the target gene samples, but not the standard samples, are subjected to 10 PCR cycles in the absence of the TaqMan probe. After this preliminary PCR step, the TaqMan probe is added to the target samples, and the conventional real-time PCR used with standard samples is applied.

and apply the conventional real-time PCR used with the standard samples (protocol: 1 cycle at 50°C for 2 min, 1 cycle at 95°C for 10 min, 50 cycles at 95°C for 15 s, and 60°C for 1 min). Theoretically, the rate of amplification of the original and the initially amplified samples should be the same, and thus the amount of PCR product ultimately produced from the latter should reflect the original amount of template applied to the assay.

3.5. A Typical Result of Modified Real-Time RT-PCR of the CYP11B2 Gene

Figures 3 and **4** show a typical result of our study, in which we examined the gene expression of CYP11B2 in the human heart. We first performed conventional real-time RT-PCR, but the amount of target gene mRNA in the cardiac tissue proved too small to generate adequate amounts of template DNA for accurate measurement. Therefore, we amplified the target samples by applying 10 PCR cycles without the TaqMan probe, which increased the amount of template DNA 1024 (2^{10})-fold, and only then was the conventional real-time PCR protocol applied (**Fig. 3**).

Theoretically, the rate of amplification of the original and the initially amplified samples should be the same, and thus the amount of PCR product ultimately produced from the latter should reflect the original amount of template applied to the assay. By varying the number of amplification cycles in the initial PCR step, this method should enable quantitative analysis of samples of virtually any size. Using this approach we were able to show that the levels of CYP11B2 expression were significantly higher in the failing heart (**Fig. 4**) *(7)*.

4. Notes

In performing the modified method, being different from conventional real-time RT-PCR, we have to interrupt the PCR reaction once when the first step of the modified real-time PCR method is completed. The following are notes for use at the time of performing this method.

1. Prepare the reaction liquid in which the standard templates are contained just before the initial PCR step is completed.
2. The caps of 96 wells containing unknown templates should be removed quickly.
3. TaqMan probes are subsequently added to all wells containing unknown templates. Following this, standard reactions are set immediately.
4. Since Taq polymerase is continues to react even during the intermission of the PCR reaction, the above-mentioned procedures should be performed as quickly as possible in order to prevent the formation of primer dimers or the inactivation of Taq polymerase. Also, care should be taken to avoid contamination during the procedures.

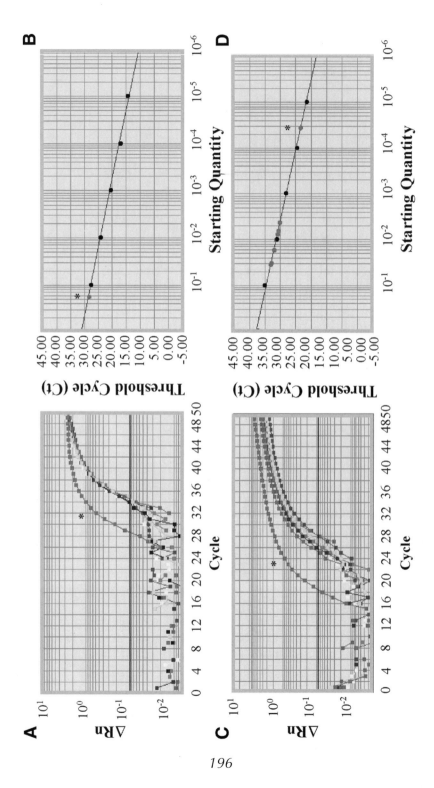

References

1. Heid, C. A., Stevens, J., and Livak K. J. (1996) Real-time quantitative PCR. *Genome Res.* **6,** 986–994.
2. Gibson, U. E. M., Heid, C. A., and Williams, P. M. (1996) A novel method for real-time quantitative RT-PCR. *Genome Res.* **6,** 995–1001.
3. Harada, E., Yoshimura, M., Yasue, H., et al. (2001) Aldosterone Induces Angiotensin-Converting-Enzyme Gene Expression in Cultured Neonatal Rat Cardiocytes. *Circulation* **104,** 137–139.
4. Hatakeyama, H., Miyamori, I., Fujita, T., Takeda, Y., Takeda, R. and Yamamoto, H. (1994) Vascular aldosterone. Biosynthesis and a link to angiotensin II-induced hypertrophy of vascular smooth muscle cells. *J. Biol. Chem.* **269,** 24316–24320.
5. Silvestre J. S., Heymes C., Oubenaissa A., et al. (1999) Activation of cardiac aldosterone production in rat myocardial infarction: effect of angiotensin II receptor blockade and role in cardiac fibrosis. *Circulation* **99,** 2694–2701.

Fig. 3. (*opposite page*) Conventional or modified real-time RT-PCR. (A) Conventional PCR-amplification plot of the target samples. PCR was successfully applied, but Ct was about 34–35 because of the small amounts of template DNA. ΔRn: Normalization is accomplished by dividing the emission intensity of the reporter dye by the emission intensity of the passive reference to obtain a ratio defined as the Rn (normalized reporter) for a given reaction tube. Rn+ is the Rn value of a reaction containing all the components including the template. Rn– is the Rn value of an unreacted sample. This value may be obtained from the early cycles of a real-time PCR run, from those cycles before to a detectable increase in fluorescence. This value may also be obtained from a reaction not containing the template. ΔRn is the difference between the Rn+ value and the Rn– value. The magnitude of the signal generated by the given set of PCR conditions was reliably indicated. (B) shows the typical amplification pattern of the CYP11B2 template standards obtained by serial dilution. Because of the small amounts of template DNA used, the Ct proportional to the amount of DNA template are unevenly distributed in the linear range, with some positioned nearly beyond the range of the standard plots, and all the experimental points, other than the adrenal gland, are so low as to be off the standard curve. This assay system was therefore deemed unsuitable for our purposes. Black dots indicate the standard samples. *(red dot) indicates the adrenal sample. (C) To improve the reliability of our measurements, target gene samples were initially subjected to 10 PCR cycles without the TaqMan probe, after which the protocol for conventional real-time PCR was applied. This initial PCR step increased the amount of template DNA in the target samples. (D) The initial PCR step shifts the Ct into the linear range of the standard curve, making all experimental points, including the adrenal gland, suitable for quantitative analysis. Black dots indicate the standard samples. Red dots indicate the target samples. *(red dot) indicates the adrenal sample.

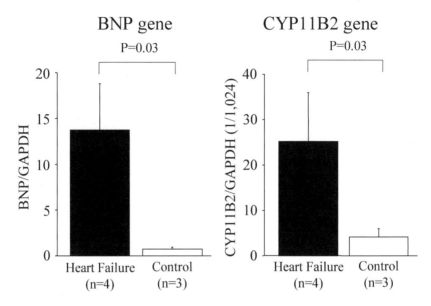

Fig. 4. Quantitative analysis of CYP11B2 or human BNP in samples of human cardiac tissue. We compared the levels of CYP11B2 expression in samples of ventricular tissue from heart failure patients and patients free of cardiovascular disease by our modified real-time PCR method. Whereas the respective CYP11B2/GAPDH ratios for the three patients free of cardiovascular disease are 1.43, 3.45, and 7.57 (×1/1024), they are 8.56, 9.60, 26.15, and 55.70 (×1/1024), in the patients with heart failure. Thus, the indicated levels of CYP11B2 expression in the failing hearts are about six-fold higher than those in the healthy hearts. In addition, we compared the levels of human BNP expression in samples from heart failure patients and patients free of cardiovascular disease by conventional real-time PCR. Whereas the respective BNP/GAPDH ratios for the three patients free of cardiovascular disease are 0.25, 0.61, and 1.18, they are 3.21, 6.65, 22.25, and 22.67 in the patients with heart failure. Therefore, the indicated levels of BNP expression in their failing hearts are about 16-fold higher than those in the control hearts. CYP11B2 was subjected to 10 cycles of PCR before the real-time PCR was run, and so the ratios vs GAPDH were not same between BNP and CYP11B2, and it is ×1/1024 ($1/2^{10}$) for the CYP11B2 gene. BNP, B-type (or brain) natriuretic peptide.

6. Mizuno Y., Yoshimura M., Yasue H., et al. (2001) Aldosterone production is activated in the failing ventricles in humans. *Circulation* **103,** 72—77.
7. Yoshimura M., Nakamura S., Ito T., et al. (2002) Expression of aldosterone synthase gene in the failing human heart: quantitative analysis using modified real-time PCR. *J. Clin. Endocrinol. Metab.* **87,** 3936–3940.

15

Generation of High-Sensitivity Antisense cDNA Probes by Asymmetric PCR

Ian M. Bird

Summary

Monitoring changing levels of mRNA by hybridization analysis relies on the use of labeled probes. The development of antisense single-stranded cDNA probe methodologies (unidirectional polymerase chain reaction [PCR] amplification or asymmetric PCR amplification) allows the production of probes of high sensitivity and low background with excellent linearity of detection. Because the methods are PCR-based, templates do not need extensive modification: selection of oligonucleotide sequences determines the target amplified. Thus such methods are flexible, being successfully achieved on a variety of templates including recombinant plasmids or dsDNA from reverse-transcription PCR (RT-PCR). In addition these probes are relatively easily stripped from hybridization membranes, so allowing repeated probing in Northern analysis.

Key Words: Probe; antisense; CDNA; DCR; asymmetric.

1. Introduction

Monitoring the changing levels of mRNA in cells is often used to determine if changes in protein level may relate to changes in mRNA stability or gene transcription. A commonly used technique by which this can be achieved is Northern analysis, or, for low levels of mRNA, reverse-transcription/polymerase chain reaction (RT-PCR) assay. In both cases, sensitive detection methods still often rely on use of labeled probes. Although olignucleotides have widely been used as probes, their short length and variable GC:AT content contributes to difficulties in consistently achieving sensitivity without high background. Many other improved methods of generating larger probes have been developed over the years, but they can generally be described as three types: double-stranded DNA (dsDNA) generated by random primed or symmetric PCR methods; riboprobes by RNA polymerase generation of antisense copy from target cDNA; and, more recently, antisense single-stranded DNA

From: *Methods in Molecular Medicine, Vol. 108: Hypertension: Methods and Protocols*
Edited by: J. P. Fennell and A. H. Baker © Humana Press Inc., Totowa, NJ

(ssDNA) synthesis by unidirectional or asymmetric PCR. The most commonly used approach is a technique called random priming *(1,2)*, which uses random hexomers or nanomers to prime abundant quantities of purified template to extend into short complementary copies. The advantage is flexibility, because any template can be used without knowledge of sequence, and kits are readily available. However, a limitation of random priming is that product formed is both sense and antisense, so setting up competition between the target membrane and sense products for antisense probe, and this is exacerbated still further by the yield being less than starting template. The result is higher backgrounds and poorer linearity of quantification than with other methods *(3)*. Although symmetric PCR-generated probes offer better results, higher background still occurs *(4)* as a result of equimolar yield of sense strand. Riboprobes offer the other extreme of detection, that is, low backgrounds, high sensitivity, and good linearity, but their setup *(5)* is complicated because dedicated constructs are required to set the probe sequence next to an appropriate priming site for RNA polymerase. The more recent development of antisense single-stranded cDNA probe methodologies (unidirectional PCR amplification or asymmetric PCR amplification) has resolved this dilemma, producing probes of high sensitivity and low background with up to 15 times the sensitivity of random primed probes and excellent linearity of detection even at the lowest levels of target RNA *(3)*. Because the methods are PCR-based, however, templates do not need extensive modification: selection of oligonucleotide sequences determines the target amplified. Thus such methods are flexible, being successfully achieved on a variety of templates including recombinant plasmids or dsDNA from RT/PCR, and the complications of establishing riboprobe methodologies are avoided. In addition, these probes are relatively easily stripped from hybridization membranes, so allowing repeated probing in Northern analysis (up to four times).

Of the two methods for single-stranded antisense probe generation by PCR, we favor asymmetric PCR over unidirectional PCR because it requires less initial template; by providing forward and reverse primers at a 1:100 ratio, double-stranded amplification in the first half of the reaction generates additional sense strand to act as template for an excess of antisense strand generation in later cycles. In this chapter we describe a general protocol for the development of predominantly antisense cDNA probes labeled with [α-^{32}P] dCTP by asymmetric PCR. Using this methodology, probes can be routinely generated in a range of sizes from 200 to 2000 bases, at high specific activity (3.12×10^8 dpm/μg) using a one-step reaction. The resultant product is >90% antisense, exceeds initial template by >20-fold, and does not require cleanup before use. Although these protocols were developed and optimized for Northern analysis, we have found them equally useful in detection of DNA targets such as in RT-PCR product Southern analysis and in screening of isolated clones.

1.1. Recombinant Plasmid Template and Custom Oligonucleotide Primers

Although PCR amplification could be performed using template in the form of a heterogeneous pool of dsDNA, the possibility of spuriously primed products is virtually eliminated by isolation of a cDNA containing the desired probe template within it. Ligation of the dsDNA containing the template region into a plasmid allows improved replication fidelity when cloned in transformed cells over that achieved by pooling symmetrically amplified product (*see* **Note 1**). The region of the insert to be amplified as probe should be specific to your message of interest, not common to a family of proteins. Oligonucleotide primers specific to the region of interest can be designed using software such as Primer, which selects primer sequences based on criteria including melting temperature, GC content, secondary structure potential, and paired primer complementarity. Alternatively, universal plasmid primers may be used, in which case the entire insert and plasmid sequence flanked by the primer pair sequence will be amplified (*see* **Note 2**).

1.2. Thermal Cycling Profiles for Symmetric and Asymmetric Amplification

Each thermal cycle consists of dsDNA template denaturation, primer annealing, and *Taq* DNA polymerization temperature plateaus. The temperature and/or period of each plateau can be suited to probes dependent on their length and on the melting temperatures of the primers. The denaturation of the dsDNA template is consistently performed at 94°C. Annealing can generally be performed at 45°C, 10–15°C below the desired primer melting temperature, to promote greater yield (*see* **Note 3**). *Taq* DNA polymerase synthesizes most efficiently at 72°C, incorporating roughly 1000 bases/min. Maximal symmetric yield occurs before 30 amplification cycles *(6)*, after which free nucleotides and *Taq* activity become limiting. However, because the later cycles of asymmetric amplification are linear, cycle number should be increased to 40 *(7)*. Products of 500 bases or less consume fewer nucleotides, so asymmetric amplification cycle number should be increased still further, to 50.

1.3. Evaluating PCR Parameters by Symmetric Amplification

Template is amplified using abundant forward and reverse primers (30 pmol each). Repeated thermal cycles give rise to an exponential increase of both sense and antisense strand copies of template DNA. If the thermal profile is appropriate, minimal overextension or premature termination will occur and electrophoresed product will appear as a sharp band. If conditions are not optimal, target sequence can be restricted from neighboring sequence to improve product specificity (*see* **Note 2**).

1.4. Agarose/TAE Electrophoresis of Symmetric Products

Symmetric products are size-separated in agarose/TAE and visualized by ethidium bromide staining to confirm amplification efficiency and fidelity. **Figure 1A** shows, left to right, discretely resolved 936-, 1083-, 957-, and 1092-bp bands amplified from different recombinant plasmids, p1–p4, using different custom primer pairs *(3)*. All reactions were performed using the same cycling profile (*see* Profile 1, **Subheading 3.1.2.**) for 750–2000 base templates, demonstrating robust cycling conditions. Cycling Profile 3 for templates ≤ 500 bases was used to amplify 143- and 432-bp templates from plasmids p5 and p6 using custom primer pairs (**Fig. 1B**) (*see* **Note 4**). Separate amplifications with insert intact and excised from plasmid were performed. Ethidium bromide staining does not show improved size specificity using restricted insert as template under these optimized conditions, although overextension is more likely for smaller templates if conditions are not optimized.

1.5. Asymmetric Probe Generation

Having validated cycling conditions, predominantly antisense [α-^{32}P] dCTP-labeled cDNA probes are amplified using a 1:100 forward/ reverse primer asymmetric molar ratio. Exponential amplification occurs until limited forward primers are consumed, after which antisense cDNAs are linearly amplified to a relative abundance over dsDNA in proportion to the remaining number of thermal cycles. To increase specific activity, [dCTP] is reduced to 0.025X the 200 μ*M* concentration each of other nucleotides. **Figure 2** demonstrates typical radiolabel incorporation and mass generation for approx 1000 base probes through a range of [dCTP], which is optimal at 2–5 μ*M*. A >20X yield of probe mass is typically generated from 10 ng dsDNA template at 5 μ*M* dCTP *(3)*.

As shown in **Fig. 3**, although asymmetric PCR yields less product than symmetric amplification because limited forward primer and reduced [dCTP], signal from ssDNA increases to >90% of total signal for asymmetric products, up dramatically from <20% for symmetric products.

1.6. Measurement of Radiolabel Incorporation

Small aliquots of amplified product are dried on ion-exchange filter disks and washed with sodium phosphate buffer to remove unincorporated radiolabel. Percent incorporation is determined by scintillation counting of washed vs unwashed disks in order to determine if sufficient incorporation, and thus sufficient probe mass generation, has occurred. Because of the significant size of

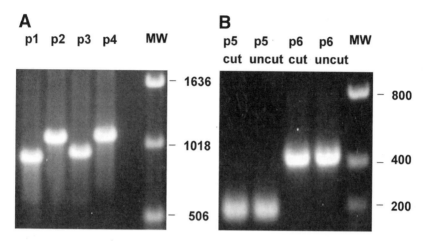

Fig. 1. Ethidium bromide-stained symmetric PCR products amplified using cycling profiles for templates (**A**) 750–2000 bases and (**B**) ≤ 500 bases. Note in (B) that templates were amplified both uncut, and cut by restriction digest.

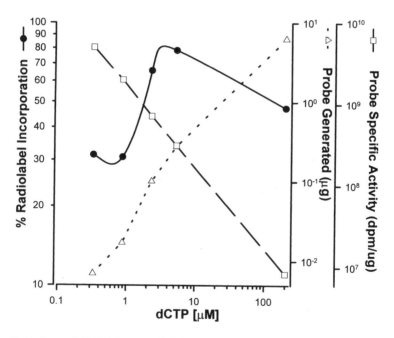

Fig. 2. Effect of [dCTP] on radiolabel incorporation, probe mass, and specific activity. Results were obtained for amplification of a 936-bp target using Protocol 1.

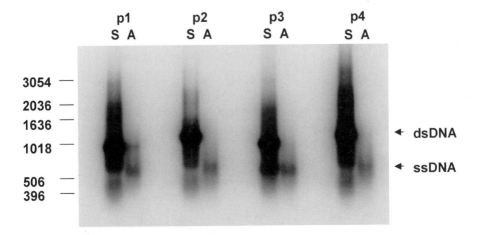

Fig. 3. Determination of single-stranded vs double-stranded product formation under symmetric vs asymmetric amplification conditions. Templates p1–p4 were amplified under symmetric (S) and asymmetric (A) PCR conditions in the absence of radiolabeled dCTP. 10 μL of each reaction product was then resolved in a 1% TAE gel and transferred to nylon membrane before probing with respective symmetrically amplified radiolabeled probes in order to detect both forward and reverse strand products. Note that ssDNA apparent MW is approximately two-thirds that of dsDNA.

these probes compared to unincorporated free nucleotides, membrane washing is relatively easy, so probes can be used without further cleanup, which is a distinct advantage over other conventional probe-generation methods.

2. Materials

2.1. General Reagents

1. Autoclave.
2. NaOH, FW 40.0, Sigma (S0899).
3. HCl, FW 36.46, Sigma (H7020).
4. 0.5-mL Thin-walled reaction tubes, Ambion (12275).
5. Sterile water, molecular-biology grade.
6. *Taq* DNA polymerase, 5 U/μL, Gibco/In Vitrogen (18038042).
7. 10X PCR buffer: 200 m*M* Tris-HCl, pH 8.4, 500 m*M* KCl, provided with *Taq*.
8. 50 mM MgCl$_2$ Provided with *Taq*.
9. 100 m*M* dATP, Amersham Biosciences (27-2035-01).
10. 100 m*M* dCTP, Amersham Biosciences (27-2035-01).
11. 100 m*M* dGTP, Amersham Biosciences (27-2035-01).
12. 100 m*M* dTTP, Amersham Biosciences (27-2035-01).
13. Custom oligonucleotide primers.
14. Recombinant plasmid templates.
15. Mineral oil, Sigma (M5904).

16. Trizma base, FW 121.1, Sigma (T6066).
17. Acetic acid, Sigma (A6283).
18. Kilobase DNA MW ladder, 0.2–12 kb, Gibco/InVitrogen (15615016).
19. [α-^{32}P] dCTP 3000 Ci/mmol, 10 μCi/μL, Amersham Biosciences (PB10205).
20. Aluminum foil.
21. Anion-exchange paper circles, Whatman (DE81).
22. Na$_2$HPO$_4$, FW 142.0, Sigma (S9763).
23. Scintillation vials, suitable for counter.
24. Scintillation fluid, suitable for [^{32}P].
25. PCR cycler, Perkin Elmer (TC1 or 480) or equivalent.
26. Submarine gel apparatus with gel tray and comb, Bio-Rad, or equivalent.
27. Power supply.
28. Transparent Lucite radiation shield.
29. Scintillation counter, Set for [^{32}P] detection.
30. 0.5 M EDTA, pH 8.0: Weigh 16.8 g diSsodium EDTA into 80 mL sterile water, and pH to 8.0 with concentrated or pelleted (approx 2 g) NaOH. Adjust vol to 100 mL and autoclave to sterilize.
31. 10% Sodium dodecyl sulfate (SDS). Dissolve 50 g lauryl sulfate, sodium salt, in 500 mL sterile water and pH to 7.2 with HCl. This solution does not require further sterilization.
32. 20X SSC: 3.0 M NaCl, 0.3 M trisodium citrate, pH 7.0. Weigh out 175.3 g NaCl and 88.2 g Na$_3$-citrate and dissolve in 800 mL molecular-grade water. pH to 7.0, adjust volume to 1 L, and autoclave to sterilize.

2.2. PCR Reagents

1. Recombinant plasmid: Working stocks should be diluted in sterile water to 10 ng/μL and stored in 200-μL aliquots at –20°C.
2. Primers should be least 17 bases, with either a G or C residue in two of the last three bases of the 3'-terminus, with annealing temperatures within 55 to 60°C, with approx 50% GC content (*see* **Note 5**), having no secondary structure and minimal primer dimer formation. Given the mass of primers in optical density units, solubilize in sterile water to 1 μg/μL using an A_{260} of 20 μg/OD unit $\times$ cm (*see* **Note 6**). Using an estimate of 330 g/mol per base, prepare 20 μM working stocks by further dilution as necessary (*see* **Note 6**). Prepare an additional 200 nM stock of forward primer for asymmetric amplification by diluting 1 μL of 20 μM stock to 100 μL with sterile water. Store stocks at –20°C.
3. Step cycle: Holds temperature plateaus for the time interval programmed; should be used for both symmetric and asymmetric amplifications.
4. 2.5 mM dA/C/G/TTP: First dilute the purchased 100 mM nucleotide solutions to 10 mM each with molecular biology-grade water and aliquot for storage. For use in symmetric amplification, combine 20 μL each of 10 mM dATP, dCTP, dGTP, and dTTP. Store this dNTP mix at –20°C in 20-μL aliquots to prevent freeze/thaw degradation of repeatedly used bulk stocks (*see* **Note 7**).
5. 50 mM MgCl$_2$ and 10X PCR buffer. Dispense these reagents, provided with *Taq* DNA polymerase, in 50-μL aliquots and store at –20°C.

6. 5X TAE buffer: 24.2 g Trizma base, 5.71 mL acetic acid, and 10 mL of 0.5 M EDTA, pH 8.0 to 1 L using sterile water (*see* **Note 8**). Store at room temperature.
7. 10-mg/mL ethidium bromide: Dilute ethidium bromide to 10 mg/mL with sterile water and store protected from light at room temperature.
8. 10X sample buffer: To a 1.5-mL Eppendorf tube, add 500 µL glycerol, 200 µL 0.5 M EDTA pH 8.0, 100 µL 10% SDS, 1.0 mg bromophenol blue, and 200 µL sterile water (*see* **Note 9**). Store at room temperature.
9. Sterile 0.5-mL thin-walled tubes. Sterilize tubes with caps open by autoclaving.

2.3. Asymmetric Amplification and Radiolabel Incorporation

1. 2.5 mM dA/G/TTP: Using the 10 mM stocks prepared as under **Subheading 2.1.3.**, combine 20-µL vol each of 10 mM dATP, dGTP, dTTP, and water. Store at –20°C in 20-µL aliquots.
2. 0.25 mM dCTP: Dilute 20 µL 10 mM dCTP stock to 80 µL with sterile water. Then dilute 10 µL of the 2.5 mM dCTP solution to 100 µL with sterile water. Store at –20°C in 10 µL aliquots.
3. 0.5 M Na$_2$HPO$_4$ pH 7.5: 71.0 g Na$_2$HPO$_4$ to 1 L with sterile water and pH to 7.5. Store at room temperature.

2.4. Posthybridization Washing of Membrane

Make up the following buffers (1 L each, prepared from stock 20 X SSC and 10% SDS) for membrane washing.

1. Low-stringency wash buffer: 2X SSC/0.1% SDS.
2. High-stringency wash buffer: 0.1X SSC/0.1% SDS.

3. Methods

3.1. General Methods for Amplification

The following methods apply generally for probes regardless of size, with the exception of thermal cycling profiles and possible restriction digest excision of templates less than 500 bases. Three different cycling profiles are recommended, one for 1000- to 2000-base probes, another for 500- to 1000-base probes, and a third for ≤500-base probes. Size criterion is based on *Taq* incorporation of roughly 1000 bases/min.

3.1.1. Determine Amount of Plasmid to Use as Template

Using a 10-ng/µL working stock, the volume used in µL will equal the size in kilobases of the entire recombinant plasmid (not just the insert, so a 10-ng/µL solution of a 5-kb plasmid including insert would be used at 5 µL-vol).

3.1.2. PCR Cycling Programs

Program the appropriate step cycle thermal profiles into a PCR cycler:

Profile 1: 1000–2000 bases

Symmetric amplification: 94°C 1 min, 45°C 1 min, 72°C 2 min, 30 cycles, linked to 4°C soak.

Asymmetric amplification: 94°C 1 min, 45°C 1 min, 72°C 2 min, 40 cycles, linked to 4°C soak.

Profile 2: 500–1000 bases

Symmetric amplification: 94°C 1 min, 45°C 1 min, 72°C 1 min, 30 cycles, linked to 4°C soak.

Asymmetric amplification: 94°C 1 min, 45°C 1 min, 72°C 1 min, 40 cycles, linked to 4°C soak.

Profile 3: ≤ 500 bases

Symmetric amplification: 94°C 30 s, 45°C 30 s, 72°C 30 s, 30 cycles, linked to 4°C soak.

Asymmetric amplification: 94°C 30 s, 45°C 30 s, 72°C 30 s, 50 cycles, linked to 4°C soak.

3.1.3. Generation of Symmetric Products

1. Thaw PCR reagents, except *Taq* (*see* **Note 10**) on ice. Mix each reagent before use. Aspirate template stock, rather than vortex, to prevent shearing of plasmid. Do not mix *Taq*. Add volumes in order shown to a sterile 0.5-mL tube:

Symmetric PCR Reaction Mix	μL	Final conditions
10X buffer	5.0	10 mM Tris, 50 mM KCl
50 mM MgCl$_2$	1.5	1.5 mM MgCl$_2$
2.5 mM dATP/dCTP/dGTP/dTTP	4.0	10 nmol each
Primer Oligo F (20 pmol/μL)	1.5	30 pmol
Primer Oligo R (20 pmol/μL)	1.5	30 pmol
Sterile H$_2$O	to 50 total	
Plasmid	1 μL/kb	10-ng/kb template
Taq polymerase	1.0	5 U
Mineral oil	25	

2. Cap and transfer tube to cycler. Amplify using appropriate step cycle thermal profile.

3.1.4. Agarose/TAE Separation of Symmetric Products

Cast an agarose/TAE gel (*see* **Note 11**) of sufficient thickness to create well spaces for up to 20-μL loading voll, allowing approx 2 mm between casting tray and bottom of comb.

1. Clean gel casting tray and seal ends with tape. Position comb such that bottom of teeth are approx 2 mm above casting tray.
2. Transfer agarose to microwave-safe glass container and bring to appropriate vol-

ume with 1X TAE. Add 10 μL ethidium bromide solution (*see* **Note 12**). Microwave for 2–3 min with frequent mixing until solution is clear and all agarose is melted. Pour solution into casting tray and allow to cool and harden for 45 min.

3. After 45 min, overlay agarose gel with 1X TAE. Allow 5 min for liquid to soak into wells. Carefully remove comb by lifting straight up. Remove tape and place gel in tank under 1X TAE buffer, oriented such that samples migrate through the length of the gel toward the positive (red) electrode.

4. Thaw Gibco kb DNA ladder on ice and mix. Transfer 4 μL ladder and 5 μL sterile water to fresh 0.5-mL tube and add 1 μL 10X sample buffer.

5. When symmetric amplification is complete, transfer 48-μL aqueous volume to fresh 0.5-mL tube, avoiding mineral oil layer above. Then transfer 10–20 μL of this to fresh tubes containing 1–2 μL 10X sample buffer. Load ladder and samples into wells.

6. To rapidly move DNA into gel, initially run at high voltage (50 V for 30 min on Bio-Rad rigs—*see* **Note 13**). Continue at this voltage until bromophenol dye front migrates halfway to two-thirds of the way down the gel. Alternatively, decrease voltage to as low as 0.5 V/cm for overnight run if desired.

7. Wearing eye protection, view ethidium bromide-stained DNA bands using a short-wave UV wand (*see* **Note 14**). Products should be prominent and discretely resolved into tight bands, with minimal smearing. Estimate size and mass of symmetric product band(s) by comparison to ladder (*see* **Note 15**).

3.1.5. Asymmetric Probe Amplification

1. Thaw radiolabel behind transparent Lucite protective shield. Aspirate but do not vortex.

2. Thaw PCR reagents, except *Taq*, on ice and mix before use. Aspirate template stock, rather than vortex, to prevent shearing of plasmid. Do not mix *Taq*. Add vols in order shown to a sterile 0.5-mL PCR tube (*see* **Note 16**). Work behind Lucite shield during and after addition of radiolabel.

Asymmetric PCR Reaction Mix	μL	Final conditions
10X buffer	5.0	10 mM Tris, 50 mM KCl
50 mM MgCl$_2$	1.5	1.5 mM MgCl$_2$
2.5 mM dATP/dGTP/dTTP	4.0	10 nmol each
0.25 mM dCTP	1.0	0.25 nmol
Primer Oligo F (0.2 pmol/μL)	1.5	0.3 pmol
Primer Oligo R (20 pmol/μL)	1.5	30 pmol
Sterile H$_2$O	to 50 total	
Plasmid	1 μL/kb	10 ng/kb template
[^{32}P]dCTP 3000 Ci/mmol, 10 μCi/μL	5.0	50 μCi, 0.01666 nmol
Taq polymerase	1.0	5 U
Mineral oil	25	

3. Cap and transfer tube to cycler. Amplify using appropriate step cycle thermal profile.

3.1.6. Radiolabel Incorporation Measurement

Work behind Lucite shield. On completion of the reaction, remove 48 µL of the products from below the oil layer into a fresh tube. Dilute to 200 µL with sterile water and mix by aspiration. Check probe incorporation of label as follows.

1. Spot 1 µL of products onto each of three DE81 disks (placed on tin foil) and allow to dry for 5 min.
2. Transfer one disk to a scintillation vial for estimation of total radiolabel.
3. Transfer the two other disks to a 50-mL conical tube. Wash the two disks four times with 0.5 M Na$_2$HPO$_4$, pH 7.5 (10–15 mL), standing for 5 min each time.
4. Finally, rinse the disks in water, methanol (twice), and air-dry for 3–5 min. Transfer disks to separate scintillation vials, add 10 mL scintillation fluid, and count both "washed" and "total" discs in a scintillation counter for 1 min each.
5. Calculate incorporation using the mean of washed counts against total counts. Typical incorporation is 65–70% for all probes. Probe mass should be sufficient to provide 5.0×10^5 to 1.0×10^6 incorporated dpm/mL media used to hybridize probe with membrane-bound RNA.
6. Store in Lucite container at –20°C.
7. At the time of probe use, take the required amount of probe (usually 1×10^6 incorporated dpm/mL hybridization solution) and dilute to at least 100 µL in a PCR tube (*see* **Note 17**). Close lid and heat at 95°C for 5 min on the PCR cycler, then snap-chill on ice 3 min. Briefly spin before opening the lid, then transfer the probe completely to hybridization buffer.

3.1.7. Posthybridization Wash Protocol

We have successfully used these probes in a number of studies for both Northern and Southern analysis using MagnaGraph Membrane from MSI (through Fisher) *(3)*. While the choice of Northern or Southern blot membrane and hybridization buffer are may vary from laboratory to laboratory, the posthybridization washing is very much determined by the probe. Fortunately, probes generated by the above procedures are of significant length and so more consistent composition than oligonucleotide or random primed probes. As such, a standardized highly stringent wash procedure can be used regardless of sequence. Following a minimum 4 h prehybridization and preferably an overnight hybridization with probe, the following wash schedule should be performed, using appropriate radioactivity shields and precautions.

1. Remove the hybridization tube containing the membrane from the oven. Working behind a shield, remove the port cover and tip all the hybridization buffer to a waste beaker. Discard as hot waste.
2. Add 10 mL of 2X SSC/0.1% SDS, to remove excess unbound probe. Then tip off 2X SSC/0.1% SDS to a beaker and discard as radioactive waste.

3. Add 20 mL 2X SSC/0.1% SDS, and incubate for 15–30 min at 42°C. Tip off, and discard as hot waste.
4. Repeat with 20 mL 0.1 X SSC/0.1% SDS for 60 min at 42°C, but discarding waste down radioactive designated sink.
5. Repeat with 20 mL 0.1X SSC/0.1% SDS for 60 min at 42°C.

3.1.8. Autoradiography

Remove the membrane and semi-dry on paper towel. Wrap the blot in Saran Wrap, scan on a direct radioimaging scanner (e.g., Phosphorimager) if required, and then tape down on a film cassette. Keep under film (Amersham Hyperfilm is recommended for [^{32}P] at –70°C). Develop the film after the required time (varies both with probe and tissue mRNA level). Quantify by scanning densitometry.

3.1.9. Probe Stripping and Rehybridization

1. Prepare 1 L of 0.1X SSC/0.5% SDS.
2. Put the membrane in hybridization bottle and set oven to 65°C. Bring 100 mL of 0.1X SSC/0.5% SDS to boil (microwave). Handling the boiling mix with heat-protective/insulated gloves, immediately pour over the membrane and return to hybridization oven. Repeat three more times over 60 min.
3. Check the membrane by overnight exposure or by Geiger counter.
4. Rehybridize as required for other signals and/or "housekeeping" mRNA (*see* **Note 1**). MagnaGraph membrane can be reliably reprobed four times without significant loss of signal.

4. Notes

1. Glycerol stocks of transformed cells (50% glycerol, 50% LB liquid culture) can be stored indefinitely at –70°C for future inoculation of culture media. A variety of commercially available plasmid isolation kits, such as those offered by Qiagen, offer plasmid extracts of purity satisfactory for use as templates in PCR.
2. Universal primers, which anneal to sites on plasmid sequences bordering inserts, are effective for probe generation for use in Northern analysis but, by definition, preclude amplification of a subregion in the cloned insert. Probe use in applications such as cDNA library, genomic, or recombinant plasmid screening is also compromised due to the presence of plasmid sequence in the probe. Additionally, cDNAs amplified from template region of inserts will have discrete 5'-ends but overextended 3'-ends may incorporate neighboring sequence or plasmid linker arm sequence, particularly for small probes. Such additional sequence incorporation in this small fraction of the cDNA pool can be eliminated, as demonstrated in **Fig. 4**, by amplifying template from vector treated with restriction enzymes to release the insert. (The restriction digest reaction mix can be used as template unpurified, because the oligonucleotides will not bind the vector, only the insert, and readthrough is now prevented.)

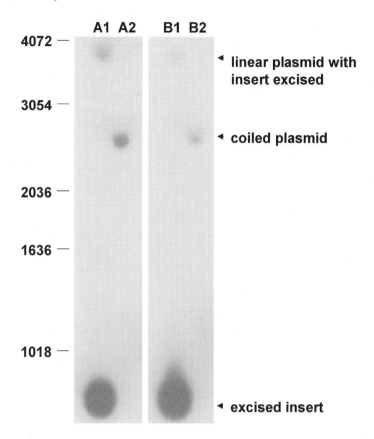

Fig. 4. Plasmid vector detection by probes generated from intact plasmid template and from plasmid with insert excised: 3.9-kb plasmid with 718-bp insert removed by restriction enzyme digestion was resolved alongside intact, coiled recombinant plasmid (lanes A1 and A2, respectively), transferred to membrane, and hybridized with asymmetric PCR probe amplified with primers annealing to the termini of the insert of intact plasmid template. Lanes B1 and B2 contain the same analytes as A1 and A2 but were hybridized with probe amplified with the same primers using restriction enzyme-digested plasmid, i.e., free insert. Signal from linearized host plasmid in A1 is significantly higher than that in B1. Thus, even when using insert specific primers, cutting insert from plasmid template before probe generation will reduce detection of false positives when performing transformed colony screening.

3. Primers designed for use in both asymmetric probe generation and RT-PCR amplification having melting temperatures >60°C will still anneal specifically if template is limited to recombinant plasmid, rather than cDNA library or genomic DNA. The higher melting temperature promotes a greater proportion of binding to available template at 45°C (approx 15°C below the T_m) and so enhances yield.

4. Plasmids p5 and p6, containing partial ovine natriuretic factor clearance receptor and ovine guanylate cyclase type B natriuretic factor receptor cDNAs *(8)*, respectively, were provided by G. Peter Aldred, University of Melbourne, Australia.

5. G and C residues contribute greater hydrogen bonding and thus increase melting temperature. If GC content is low, extending primer length will increase melting temperature.

6. Synthesized primers, commercially available through various vendors such as Midland Certified Reagent Company (Midland, TX), are usually sent at ambient temperature in a lyophilized state. Quantity is given as OD units. We use the specific OD of 20 µg/OD unit · cm, which means the solubilization volume for the oligo is 20 µL molecular-grade water per OD unit. This should be checked on a spectrophotometer. Once the main stock is prepared, store this long-term (so it may be used for other applications) and make a dilution for a working stock for PCR. The dilution requires calculation of molarity and depends on the size/length of the oligo. Assume 330 g/*M* per base and multiply 330 by the number of bases to get the MW. Then calculate the molarity of the 1µg/µL solution. Dilute as directed.

7. Degradation of nucleotides usually occurs after 3–6 mo storage at –20°C. Reactions incorporating [α-^{32}P]dCTP in the presence of diluted dCTP are more sensitive to nucleotide instability and fail before conventional PCR.

8. Resultant 1X TAE solution is 40 m*M* Tris acetate, 1 m*M* EDTA.

9. Resultant 1X concentration is 5% glycerol, 10 m*M* 0.5 *M* EDTA, 0.1% SDS, 0.1-mg/mL bromophenol blue.

10. Remove *Taq* from –20°C immediately prior to adding it to reaction mix and return directly to –20°C storage.

11. Resolve products > 1000 bases in 1% agarose/TAE and those < 1000 bases in 2% agarose/TAE.

12. Alternatively, 10 µL Ethidium bromide/500 mL can be added to submarine tank buffer, which will prevent formation of a gradient formed by migrating ethidium bromide cast into gel. When adding ethidium bromide into buffer rather than casting in gel, allow time for ethidium bromide to penetrate gel and intercalate with DNA samples before viewing with UV light.

13. Voltage conditions will depend on the gel rig, namely, the distance between electrodes. The values given (50 V for 30 min = 25 Vhr) are for a Bio-Rad DNA SubCell with 30 cm between electrodes. Thus the total Vhr will need to be adjusted if your electrodes are at a different distance. Higher voltages should not be used, particularly on small rigs due to excess heating.

14. Negatively charged dsDNA, intercalated with ethidium bromide, migrates downward toward the anode as excess ethidium bromide migrates upward toward cathode.

15. The kb DNA ladder (Gibco) contains 100 ng 1636 bp dsDNA/µL. For low-mass products, use a Low Mass DNA ladder (Gibco), which contains 40 ng 400 bp dsDNA/µL.

16. Equal dpm/µg is incorporated for all probes, but shorter probes incorporate less radiolabel per strand. Specific activity may be further increased by increasing radiolabel added. Further dilution of dCTP to 2 µ*M* will also increase specific activity; however, a small number of reactions may fail to generate product *(3)*.

17. Probe is subaliquoted for each use before heating because repeated heating and cooling of the entire stock promotes breakdown and a rise in background. This way the probe can be used over a period of days to weeks with no degradation of performance each time beyond that of radioactive decay. Probe volume is increased as necessary to 100 µL before heating because there is always some evaporation loss. Heating very small volumes would make it difficult to be sure all probe was transferred to the hybridization tube.

Acknowledgments

This work was supported by National Institutes of Health award HL64601 and HD38843 (Project 1).

References

1. Feinberg, A. P. and Vogelstein, B. (1983) A technique for radiolabeling DNA restriction endonuclease fragments to high specific activity. *Anal. Biochem.* **132,** 6–13.
2. Feinberg, A. P. and Vogelstein, B. (1984) A technique for radiolabeling DNA restriction endonuclease fragments to high specific activity. *Adendum. Anal. Biochem.* **137,** 266–267.
3. Millican, D. S. and Bird, I. M. (1997) A general method for single-stranded DNA probe generation. *Anal. Biochem.* **249,** 114–117.
4. Sturzl, M. and Roth, W. K. (1990) Run off synthesis and application of defined single-stranded DNA hybridization probes. *Anal. Biochem.* **185,** 164–169.
5. Melton, D. A., Krieg, P. A., Rebagliati, M. R., Maniatis, T., Zinn, K., and Green, M. R. (1984) Efficient in vitro synthesis of biologically active RNA and RNA hybridization probes from plasmids containing a bacteriophage SP6 promoter. *Nucleic Acids Res.* **12,** 7035–7056.
6. Linz, U., Delling, U., and Rubsamen-Waigmann, H. (1990) Systematic studies on parameters influencing the performance of the polymerase chain reaction. *J. Clin. Chem. Clin. Biochem.* **28,** 5–13.
7. Gyllensten, U. B. and Erlich, H. A. (1988) Generation of single-stranded DNA by the polymerase chain reaction and its application to direct sequencing of the HLA-DQA locus. *Proc. Natl. Acad. Sci. USA* **85,** 7652–7656.
8. Fraenkel, M. B., Aldred, P. G., and McDougall, J. G. (1994) Sodium status affects GC-B natriuretic peptide receptor mRNA levels, but not GC-A or C receptor mRNA levels, in the sheep kidney. *Clin. Sci.* **86,** 517–522.

16

New Advances in Microarrays

Finding the Genes Causally Involved in Disease

Claudio Napoli, Filomena de Nigris, and Vincenzo Sica

Summary

Much progress has been made in the technologies available to assess global alterations in mRNA levels in clinical research samples. Although such transcript profiling can provide a powerful research tool, the broad range of options can be bewildering for the inexperienced investigator, and more often than not the limitations and pitfalls of this approach are not fully appreciated. It is important to recognize that the major goal of transcript profiling experiments can be to identify novel therapeutic targets or delineate complex patterns of gene expression that provide a potentially pathognomonic phenotype. Microarrays are therefore potentially powerful tools to address the need for high-throughput analysis techniques, but a careful postanalysis follow-up and validation of microarray experiments will be needed soon *(1)*. A projected decrease in cost and complexity may facilitate increased availability of this technology in the physician's office, and future applications may then allow tailoring of clinical diagnosis and targeted therapeutic strategies.

Key Words: Microarray; genomics; expression; atherosclerosis; hypertension.

1. Introduction

In terms of understanding the functions of genes, knowing when, where, and to what extent a gene is expressed is central to investigating the activity and biological roles of its encoded protein. In addition, changes in the multigene patterns of expression can provide clues about regulatory mechanisms and broader bioactivity functions. This knowledge may increase the basic understanding of the cause and consequences of diseases, how drugs and drug candidates work in cells and organisms, and what gene products might have therapeutic uses or may be appropriate targets for therapeutic intervention. Furthermore, profiling genomic transcripts may also assist in the identification

From: *Methods in Molecular Medicine, Vol. 108: Hypertension: Methods and Protocols*
Edited by: J. P. Fennell and A. H. Baker © Humana Press Inc., Totowa, NJ

of diagnostic indicators and prognostic markers that might direct individualized clinical management. Nevertheless, it is important to emphasize that no new approaches replace conventional methods. Indeed, standard methods such as Northern blots, Western blots, and reverse-transcriptase polymerase chain reaction (RT-PCR) are simply used in more targeted fashion to complement the broader measurements and to follow up on the genes, pathways, and mechanisms identified by new techniques such as microarrays. Here, we will illustrate the scientific rationale and new advances of the microarray-based techniques.

The microarray is a new microhybridization-based assay that encodes as many as 20,000 genes and offers the opportunity to make a parallel hybridization of thousands different genes. In analogy to hybridization assays, it involves a microfilter or "chip" made of a porous membrane or material such as glass, plastic, silicon, gold, or gel *(1a–3)*, in which either oligonucleotides or cDNA fragments are spotted or synthesized at high density (e.g., $10,000/cm^2$). Probes for the microarray can be complementary DNA (cDNA), RNA, genomic DNA, or plasmid libraries, which are appropriately labeled and hybridized to the chip *(3–5)*. To measure the resulting hybridization signals, radioactive and fluorescence detection strategies are usually used. The result is an image obtained by fluorescence scanner or phosphorimager that can be processed with computer software to generate a spreadsheet of gene expression values. The application of multiple types of statistical analysis to microarray data allows classification and clustering of genes according to their upregulation or downregulation *(3–5)*. Furthermore, microarrays also can be used to analyze genomic DNA rather than mRNA, to characterize the interactions of proteins, and potentially to characterize other types of molecule with double-stranded DNA *(3–5)*. In the drug discovery and therapeutics arena, microarrays have been used for expression analysis of cells or tissues in different disease states, single-nucleotide polymorphism (SNP) analysis, pharmacogenomics, and toxicogenomics.

1.1. DNA Microarrays

Expression analysis for the quantitative gene expression of many genes can be performed using either one- or two-color fluorescent schemes. One-color analysis is used primarily for arrays prepared by photolithography. Affymetrix patented this process under the trade name GeneChip™ *(6)*. In this method, expression profiles for each sample are generated on a different chip using a single fluorescent label, such as phycoerythin, and the different images are then compared. A two-color analysis protocol has subsequently been developed, whereby two RNA samples are labeled separately with different fluorescent dyes, for example, cyanine 3 and cyanine 5. These labeled probes hybridize to a printed array of cDNA; when the microarray is scanned, the fluorescent signals can be overlaid to visualize genes that have been activated or downregulated.

DNA microarrays can be generated using short oligonucleotides (15–25 nucleotides), long oligonucleotides (50–120 nucleotides) or PCR-amplified cDNA (100–3000 base pairs). *In situ* oligonucleotide synthesis on a solid support involves the use of photolithography to build up each element of the array, nucleotide by nucleotide, up to 20 bases *(7)*. Alternatively, longer nucleotides and cDNA can be spotted directly onto glass slides. Between 10,000 and 30,000 spots can be mechanically deposited onto a single glass slide by robotic instrumentation designed to print from metal pins or inkjets.

1.2. Protein and Peptide Microarrays

DNA arrays are limited to providing information on the identity or amount of RNA or DNA present in a sample, providing that suitable controls are available. Translational products of genes cannot be analyzed on such arrays and therefore require the use of polypeptide-based arrays. To date, such microarrays have not been used to their full potential because of difficulties with the technology *(8)*. An important challenge when producing protein microarrays is maintaining functionality, such as posttranslational modifications and phosphorylation. An important consideration with protein-array surface chemistry is that the chemistry must permit immobilized proteins to retain both secondary and tertiary structure and, thus, biological activity. One of the first technical challenges with protein microarrays is to fix a protein or protein ligand to arrays in a biologically active form. Most arrays are either glass or silicon slides treated with an aldehyde to immobilize the protein *(9)*. Other immobilizing coatings include aluminum or gold, and hydrophilic polymers. Alternatively, proteins can be imprinted on a porous polyacrylamide gel, similar to that used in electrophoresis, and immobilized using a coupling agent that forms a covalent bond with amine groups on the protein molecules *(10)*. The gel provides a biocompatible aqueous three-dimensionl environment, so immobilized proteins can undergo binding reactions in solution.

1.2.1. Alternative Strategies for Protein Microarrays

Alternative strategies involve the use of capture agents. Slides are often imprinted with antibodies, which can be monoclonal, polyclonal, antibody fragments, or synthetic polypeptide ligands. However, the problem with this method is that large numbers of different antibodies are needed. Other options include aptamers—single-stranded oligonucleotides that bind specifically to protein *(11)*. Aptamers have an advantage over antibodies because they can be imprinted using the same technology as mRNA expression arrays. Detection methods currently employed include ELISA-based assays with enzymatic or fluorescent labels, or universal protein stains. There are, however, disadvantages with these methods: ELISA-based assays can yield nonspecific protein–antibody interactions, labeling proteins fluorescently can reduce the quantitative accuracy of assays, and universal protein staining is not an option if the capture molecules are themselves proteins (i.e., antibodies). Other methods of detection that have been optimized for use with protein microarrays include mass spectrometry analysis and surface plasmon resonance *(12)*.

A recent study *(13)* described a novel approach to study protein phosphorylation and its potential inhibition in a peptide microarray format by the quantitative analysis of protein kinase activity. This peptide microarray requires only small quantities of protein and can be used to develop high-throughput assays to monitor the activity of multiple protein kinases. The advantages of protein microarrays over conventional methods, such as ELISA and Western blotting, are that they use less sample and are relatively quick to perform. Protein arrays are thought to be 10–100 times faster than conventional methods (such as two-hydrid systems) *(14)*. The future of protein microarrays could be "custom" arrays designed to capture a few proteins of interest—unlike DNA microarrays, which capture thousands of genes.

1.3. Glycomics

Many proteins and biomolecules are modified by the covalent attachment of sugar residues, known as glycans. Many biological processes involve sugar–receptor binding, and microarrays will become an important tool for the study of such interactions in this rapidly expanding field. Neoglycolipids, spotted onto nitrocellulose and polyvinylpyrrolidone-co-dimethyl maleic acid (PVD), provide an example of a carbohydrate microarray *(15)*. Binding of the carbohydrates to the membranes was verified by the use of fluorescently labeled neoglycolipids or primulin stain for nonfluorescently labeled neoglycolipids. The carbohydrate composition of the bound moieties was identified using *in situ* analysis by mass spectrometry. By binding known oligosaccharide sequences to the membrane, particular lectins or protein motifs can be identified. Alternatively, by binding unknown oligosaccharide structures to the membranes, proteins of known sequence can be screened to investigate which oligosaccharides they bind to. An alternative approach might enable the identification of pathogenic microorganisms through unique glycans expressed on their cell surface *(16)*. Glycans have been spotted to the surface of nitrocellulose membranes and probed using antibodies raised against the microorganisms from which the glycans were derived.

1.4. Tissue and Cell Microarrays

Analysis of gene or protein expression levels can only begin to provide us with relevant information about the biological function of the gene, its potential clinical impact, or its suitability as a drug target. Functional genomics enables the validation of targets that have been identified by microarray screening.

Conventional histological analysis of tissue specimens is a slow and labor-intensive process: tissues are first preserved in formalin before being embedded in paraffin for sectioning, staining, and microscopic analysis on individual glass slides. In 1998 tissue microarrays (TMAs) were developed, whereby an ordered array of tissue samples is placed on a single slide *(17)*. Once constructed, the TMA can be probed with a molecular target (DNA, RNA, or protein) for analysis by immunohistochemistry, fluorescence *in situ* hybridization (FISH), or other molecular detection methods *(18)*, enabling high-throughput *in situ* analysis of specific molecular targets in hundreds or even thousands of tissue specimens *(19)*. Only small amounts of reagent (microliter volumes) are required to analyze an entire array, offering greater consistency at reduced cost.

1.4.1. Advantages

The advantage of this technique is, because the cell microarrays are printed with the same robotic microarrayer device as is used to print conventional DNA microarrays, a similar magnitude of density can be achieved (i.e., approx 6000–10,000 spots per slide). And because such small quantities are used, potentially rare cell lines or biological samples can be used to assay many genes simultaneously. These transfected-cell microarrays can be used to identify potential drug targets *(20)*. These cell microarrays can also be used in loss-of-function analysis using plasmid-based small interfering RNAs (siRNAs). RNA interference is a useful genetic tool for the rapid and systematic silencing of genes of interest in mammalian cells (reviewed in **ref. *21***). By printing siRNA-plasmid constructs on slides in a manner analogous to cDNA constructs, it is possible to create cell microarrays in which each cluster of cells is deficient in a defined gene product *(22)*.

Another, different approach for generating cell microarrays has been described *(23)* and is used for the rapid screening of cell surface-specific antibodies to determine selectivity and cross-reactivity. High-density cell suspensions are directly printed onto glass slides using a robotic microarrayer device; glycerol is added to prevent complete dehydration of the printed cells, to conserve native protein structures, and to ensure retention of the antigenicity of the cell surface molecules; and the interactions of the antibodies subsequently bound to the cell microarrays are analyzed via immunofluorescence.

Table 1
Microarrays on the Web

General links

Lab-on-a-chip, www.lab-on-a-chip.com
Genomics Proteomics, www.genomicsproteomics.com
Bio-IT World, www.bio-itworld.com
BioArray Software Environment—*BASE*, http://base.thep.lu.se
Pharmocogenomics Online, www.pharmacogenomicsonline.com

DNA microarrays

Affymetrix, www.affymetrix.com
Rosetta Inpharmatics, www.rii.com
The Brown Lab, Stanford University, cmgm.stanford.edu/pbrown
Silicon Genetics Genespring, www.sigenetics.com

Protein microarrays

ESF Programme on Integrated Approaches for Functional Genomics;
  www.functionalgenomics.org.uk/sections/resources/protein_arrays.htm

Glycomics

NIGMS Consortium for Functional Glycomics, http://web.mit.edu/glycomics/
  consortium
Glycominds, www.glycominds.com
University of New Hampshire Center for Structural Biology,
www.glycomics.unh.edu
Oxford Glycobiology Institute list of publications, http://www.bioch.ox.ac.uk/
  glycob/publications.html

Tissue arrays and cell microarrays

Whitehead Institute, www.wi.mit.edu/nap/features/nap_feature_sabatiniappt.html
NHGRI Tissue Microarray Project, www.nhgri.nih.gov/DIR/CGB/TMA
UCLA Tissue Array Core Facility, www.genetic.ucla.edu/tissuearray

1.5. Data Analysis: Many Options

Once data are collected, correct analyses have to be applied. Outputs can be displayed as lists, but are more typically visualized by some variation of the red/green light, originally introduced by Eisen and colleagues *(24)*. Many computational analysis tools and new microarray packages are now available on the Web for data analysis of microarray-derived data (some examples are listed in **Table 1**). The statistical analysis is important to detect whether there are reliable biologically relevant differences in the expression level. The statistical analysis is usually done using either clustering algorithms or conventional sta-

Table 2
Analysis Techniques for Microarray Expression Profiling

Nome	Description
Hierarchical agglomerative	Forms clusters starting at lowest level
Hierarchical divisive	Forms clusters starting at highest level
Self-organizing maps	Partitions genes/experiments into a prespecified number of groups by mapping onto nodes
K-means	Partitions genes/experiments into a prespecified number of groups by finding centroids
Quality cluster algorithm	Forms groups based on diameter quality measure and jackknife correlations
Super vector machines	Machine learning process that incorporates nonarray information
Gene shaving	Seeks groups of genes that maximize variation among experiments
Class prediction	Identifies genes whose behavior predicts defined classes

tistical tests. A selection of published clustering techniques for expression profile data analysis is listed in **Table 2** (*24–30*). The processing of data includes background subtraction, normalization, and detection of outliers.

The difficulties of data analysis derive from the myriad of potential sources of random and systematic measurement error in the microarray process and from the small number of samples relative to the large number of variables. This issue complicates data analysis and interpretation and jeopardizes the validity of many of the microarray findings reported to date (*3,31*). For example, statistically significant differences in gene expression may reflect the biasing effects of extraneous factors rather than the biology. Lack of statistical significance can indicate low experimental sensitivity rather than absence of biological effect, while low sensitivity can be caused by an inadequate number of replicates or failure to control extraneous factors that contribute to random error. When analyzing gene expression data, it is also necessary to evaluate the error derived from measurements. Random error is minimized by repeating the measurements. Systematic error (bias) is controlled experimentally as far as possible, although additional statistical correction is invariably necessary with current microarray technology. Extraneous factors that contribute to random error or bias of microarray expression values include target accessibility, which is affected by variation in absorbency of discrete nylon membrane, target fixation on membrane, and variation in washing procedures (*3*).

1.5.1. Quality Control for Hybridization

Multiple spotting of target DNA on a slide provides a means of assessing the quality of data for a gene on that slide. The coefficient of variation (CV) is defined as the standard deviation divided by the mean of the spot intensity for each gene *(32,33)*. The quality of data on the expression level is inversely correlated with its CV. When a CV for one gene is greater than 10% among genes used as internal controls, the data for that gene are considered unreliable. In calibration experiments the same sample is labeled with two different dyes and hybridized to the same slide. The calibration experiment provides a control to investigate possible systemic errors, such as slide effect, dye effect, and gene label effect *(32,33)*. The slide effect is caused by variation in imaging between slides hybridized with the same probe. Factors affecting hybridization may include the amount of probe DNA immobilized on the slide during array fabrication and the amount of labeled cDNA added to the slide and the local environment in each hybridization chamber. Fluorescent dyes have different efficiency incorporation during the labelling, and they are detected by the scanner with different efficiencies *(32)*. The effect of these factors is accounted for by the normalization curve in normalization experiments, in which two differentially expressed mRNA pool are separately labelled with two dyes and are cohybridized to the same slide defining the curve calibration *(32)*. Comparison of expression levels across different cDNA microarray experiments is easier when a common reference is cohybridized to every microarray. A mix of the products that are printed and their subsequent amplification toward either sense or antisense cRNA provides an excellent alternative common reference *(33)*.

1.5.2. Bootstrapping Cluster Analysis

Statistical inferences are based on the application of a complicated randomization technique called bootstrapping (reviewed in **ref. *26***). The bootstrapping procedure, based on the reliability of clustering algorithm analysis (various simulated datasets based on the statistical models are created), relies on experimental replication and good design in microarray experiments. When accuracy is high, the bootstrap estimates of relative expression will be more like the original estimates and the bootstrap clustering will be more like the original clustering. Without an assessment of the clusters, one cannot make valid inferences about genes that show similar behavior.

1.6. The Future of Microarray-Based Technologies

DNA-, protein-, glycomic-, and cell-based microarrays continue to be developed to extract more data from smaller sample volumes. New technologies are now emerging to improve their overall design, to increase the speed of

Table 3
Novel Microarray-Based Technologies

Chips in space for microgravity functional genomics

CombiMatrix Corporation (www.combimatrix.com) has developed a patented array
 processor system for the production of cost-effective custom oligonucleotide
 arrays using electrochemistry. The array is manufactured in a porous, three-
 dimensional layer that sits on top of a semiconductor chip.

In situ synthesized peptide assays on microfluidic chips

Xeotron Corporation (www.xeotron.com) has developed peptide/peptidomimetics
 arrays on a microfluidic platform (XeoChip™) using digital photolithography for
 the rapid screening of high-affinity binding sequences.

4-D Flow-Thru Chip™ for chemiluminescence detection of biomolecules

MetriGenix (www.metrigenix.com) has developed a patented, automated
 microfluidic biochip for the spotting and analysis of nucleic acids, RNA, DNA,
 proteins, or cells in one-quarter of the time of conventional flat-bed microarray
 systems.

Multiplexed biomolecular analysis using microcantilever arrays

The University of California, Berkeley (www.berkeley.edu) has developed a label-
 free technique based on a microcantilever that can be used to quantitatively detect
 DNA hybridization, protein–protein, protein–ligand, and possibly DNA–protein
 interactions.

Resonance light scattering on protein microarrays

Genicon Sciences Corporation (www.geniconsciences.com) has developed an
 application for resonance light-scattering particles (RLS Particles™) in protein
 microarrays for high-sensitivity signal generation without enzymatic signal
 amplification to enable detection down to the femtomolar range.

---

analysis, and to reduce sample size even further. **Table 3** indicates commercially available microarray technologies that use novel platform technologies.
There is a significant requirement for integration of a suitable chemometric
data analysis and an information management system that can permit a measured data reduction, enabling the analyst to make the necessary key decisions
(34,35). At present, this is an area where microarray technology is still in its
relative infancy—the link between the micro- and macrosensor devices must
be strengthened, with better integration of chemistry and electronics *(36)*. In
fact, future requirements will also involve a much closer marriage of data
acquisition and data management and a greater all-encompassing linkage of
individual components of any standard analysis. Fundamentally, for the pharmaceutical sciences, this needs to be in a form that can be validated clearly.

Validation and global customer buy-in could be presently considered "sticking" points in the wider application and acceptance of microtechnology. Application will undoubtedly expand to include diagnostic testing and to encompass wider biotechnological applications (in environmental monitoring and identification of structural motifs relevant to the use and verification of genetically modified crops and foods *[36]*).

1.6.1. Microfluidics

Microfluidic device (MFD) technology—typically used to move small volumes of both liquids and gases—is a dynamic branch of analytical science with huge possibilities for bioanalysis *(36)*. Possibly the most assured application of microarray and MFD hybridization will be the creation of specific and adaptable "micro total analytical systems" (μTAS)—MFDs will not be used simply as alternatives to microarrays but will be fused with them to produce fully integrated modular microfluidic microarrays *(35,36)*. This would enable tailoring of a whole series of subtasks within an analysis and also coupling of this technology to microarray-based identification.

Structured MFDs are currently available that can involve microporous structure or fabricated channels on a scale of micrometers or submicrometers *(37)*. The formation of monolithic structures from resinous, polymeric, or mineral matter, such as silicon and silicates or calixarenes *(38)*, could be useful in ion exchange, adsorption chromatography, microcapillary electrophoresis *(39)*, and flow cytometry. Other possibilities for these devices include uses in sample cleanup, such as that undertaken in solid-phase extraction (SPE).

Chromatography *(40)*, amperometric, and ion-selective solid-state electrode sensors are potential applications for MFDs. In itself, this has spin-off use in the production of artificial organs and microimplants, and in molecular pharmacology. In this case, the use of nanoarchitectured devices or lithographic networks might provide a possibility for further miniaturization and provide a route for inclusion of multiple-module analytical devices and so-called nanobots (nanometer-sized robots) in the body *(34)*. Other possibilities for future MFD technologies are metering devices for nano- or picoliter dispensing systems *(41)*. This would again be possible by mass manufacture of rigidly controlled etching and deposition of nanofeatures (chemical mosaics) and potential reagents, perhaps by using micro- or nanoparticles or molecular imprintation. **Table 4** indicates the interrelationships of microfluidics and microarray technology.

1.6.2. Molecular Imprintation

Molecular imprintation involves fabrication of a sensitized molecular layer. The technology has scope for use in many analytical systems but has received

Table 4
Interrelationships of Microfluidics and Microarray

Microfluidic system

Exists as micro-total analytical system (μTAS) with
    combined modules engineered to incorporate
    microarray mosaics
Exist as a separate entity
Used where little sample is available
When combined with microarrays:

Advantages

Labor-saving and cost-effective
In situ, in vivo analysis system
Miniaturization of total analytical system,
    specificity

Problems

Multiple use and recycling
Inhibitory development and unit cost
Analytical validation concerns
Reliability under mass manufacture

much attention for its use with piezoelectric technology, such as the quartz crystal resonance sensor (QCRS) or surface plasmon resonance (SPR) analysis. These techniques are considered useful in biofluid, environmental monitoring, and quantitative gene and proteome profiling *(42)*. A possible use of molecular imprintation is in a polymerization process (MIP), in which polymeric material is chemically sculpted into the shape of the target analyte molecule based on poly[meth(acrylate)] or poly(pyrrole) formation around molecular templates *(43,44)*. The ultimate application is the creation of synthetic biocatalysts for reaction engineering *(45)*, affinity ligands, for use in flow-based systems, such as MFDs and biosensors. The potential selectivity of molecularly imprinted components means that they are often perceived as "synthetic antibodies" that can be targeted directly at cell interiors and subcellular structures, for further use in techniques such as scintillation assay and magnetic resonance imaging (MRI) *(46)*.

1.7. Limitations of Microarray-Based Analysis

One of the most important problems in microarray experiments is the reproducibility in interpreting data. Several reports have already appeared identifying changes in classes and clusters of genes whose expression changes during cardiac remodeling hypertrophy or heart failure *(47,48)*. Collectively, these studies represent a major leap forward in sorting out the different pathways in the heart or isolated cardiac myocytes, where changes in gene expression and very probably in protein expression have occurred. However, it is necessary to consider several important issues pertinent to data analysis and interpretation. To have good-quality data, it is mandatory at the outset to produce high-quality labeled RNA or cDNA.

For the data analysis, it is necessary to consider several issues, the first being the volume of data. For storage and manipulation of data, gigabytes of computer storage and a fast network connection are required. Second, we need to consider the magnitude of changes in gene expression that should be considered significant. Another approach is to conduct multiple statistical tests and bootstrapping on the same data (*see* **Subheading 1.5.**). In this case, the usual error rates applied to each test are no longer valid. Whereas some theoretical work has been done along these lines, it has not yet been extended to the microarray problem to any great extent *(49)*. However, the numbers of original studies employing microarray expression profiling and the availability of computational tools for analysis of large datasets increase every year. The power of these studies is to produce vast quantities of data that represent the changes in transcription profile of cells or biopsy tissues from selected patients. However, this power is also a limitation of the arrays technique *(50)*, as one of the most challenging aspects of gene expression analysis is the selection among the vast quantities of data those genes that could have a real causal role. Indeed, the change in the transcriptional level of a gene is not correlated with the causal role of that gene. Sometimes small changes in a key gene can produce a large biological effect. Moreover, when considering microarray data few studies address the combinatorial nature of transcription, a well-established phenomenon in eukaryotes *(51)*. In addition, changes in gene expression are not invariably associated with changes in protein synthesis, in which case the significance of altered gene expression may be questionable. Furthermore, rather than altered expression, subcellular translocalization or posttranslational modifications of proteins are also considerably meaningful for their biological effects, but would not be disclosed by microarray techniques. Thus the microarray techniques may be viewed as guiding tools to point the investigator in the right direction, with more conclusive functional information collected in subsequent complementary studies.

1.8. Examples of Microarray Application to Some Cardiovascular Diseases

The microarray technique has been important in investigating cellular mechanisms of vascular physiology and pathophysiology (reviewed in **ref. 3**). The DNA microarray approach was used to investigate the gene expression profile in cultured endothelial cells exposed for 24 h to shear stress *(52,53)*. Similarly, it was shown that mechanical stimuli induced changes in transcription profile of smooth muscle cells *(54)*. Endothelial cells exposed to shear stress for 7 d increase the expression of several genes, but in particular a unique endothelial transcription factor, Kruppel-like factor (KLF-2) *(55)*, a target for angiotensin II signaling and an essential regulator of cardiovascular remodeling. The biological response of human endothelial cells to Gram-negative lipopolysaccharide has also been assessed by microarray *(56)*. These studies led through genomic investigation to the identification of molecules downstream of transforming growth factor-b and tumour necrosis factor-a signaling, and clarified the chemotactic pathways that participate in infection-related vascular dysfunction *(57)*.

Atherosclerosis is a multifactorial and temporally dynamic disease *(58,59)* that can be modulated by a large number of environmental and genetic factors. The microarray technique is therefore particularly suitable for sifting through the spectrum of candidate genes in an attempt to focus on specific culprits and identify novel pathways associated with atherogenesis. For example, it was demonstrated that homocysteine can activate 3-hydroxy 2-methylglutayl coenzyme reductase in vascular endothelial cells, thereby promoting atherogenesis *(60)*. In smooth muscle cells, a new gene pathway participating in vascular inflammation was identified that involved the eotaxin gene and its receptor CCR3 *(61)*. Chip experiments on high-density lipoprotein-deficient mice revealed several novel genes involved in oxidative processes, vascular dysfunction, and sterol metabolism *(62)*. Recently, we have described a large list of early genes involved in vascular dysfunction and atherogenesis in hypercholesterolemic mice *(63)*. The microarray has also been used more recently to study vascular function in a murine model of hypertension. It has been used in rats that had quantitative trait loci (QTL) for blood pressure to characterize their related phenotypes on every chromosome *(64)*. New information on gene expression profiles in spontaneously hypertensive rats and Wistar-Kyoto rats is now also available *(65)*.

2. Materials

1. RNeasy kit (QIAGEN).
2. Ice-cold RNAse-free phosphate-buffered saline, pH 7.4.
3. Oligo dT primer with a T7 RNA polymerase promoter site added to its 3'-end.
4. Biotin-labeled cRNA (Enzo Diagnostics kit).
5. Qiagen's RNeasy minicolumns.
6. Affymetrix Mu11k subA and subB chips.
7. SuperScript RT (Life Technologies).
8. Taq polymerase (Qiagen).
9. AlphaImager 2000 software (Alpha Innotech Corporation), or equivalent.

3. Methods: Worked Example Using Affymetrix Mu11k subA and subB Chips

3.1. Tissue Preparation

1. At 3 mo of age, euthanize mice by an overdose of anesthetic.
2. Perfuse aortas for 10 min under physiological pressure with ice-cold RNAse-free phosphate-buffered saline, pH 7.4, through a cannula inserted into the left ventricle.
3. Quantify lesion sizes in the aortic origin by computer-assisted imaging analysis (e.g., in **ref. 63**). The rest of the aorta is used to determine gene expression.
4. Blot-dry aortic segments, flash-freeze, and stored in liquid nitrogen until further processing. To assess the absence or presence of lesions in the aortic tree, two entire aortas from each group are fixed, paraffin-embedded, and serially dissected from the heart to the iliac bifurcation.
5. Stain every tenth section with haematoxylin and eosin and examine microscopically.

3.2. Determination of Aortic Gene Expression by cDNA Microarray

A total of 12 Mu11k chip sets (subA and subB, each) are used to compare normo- and hypercholesterolemic groups and for comparisons between different arterial segments within groups. Pooled tissues of three mice each, as well as equally pooled samples of all mice in the 0.075% cholesterol and control groups, are used.

1. Extract total tissue RNA using an RNeasy kit (Qiagen).
2. Determine RNA using spectrophotometry.
3. Synthesis double-stranded cDNA using 50 ng of total RNA and an oligo-dT primer with a T7 RNA polymerase promoter site added to its 3'-end, following the protocol recommended by Affymetrix.
4. Use this cDNA for in vitro transcription in the presence of biotin-labeled ribonucleotides to yield biotin-labeled cRNA (Enzo Diagnostics kit).
5. Clean cRNA using Qiagen's RNeasy minicolumns and protocols.
6. Assess RNA integrity by 1% agarose gel electrophoresis and optical density determined at 260 and 280 nm.
7. Fragment cRNA (15 μg) and use in a hybridization mix.
8. Hybridize an aliquot of the mix containing at least 10 μg cRNA to the Affymetrix Mu11k subA and subB chips.
9. Wash the chips, stain, and scan.

3.3. Secondary Analysis by Semiquantitative Polymerase Chain Reaction Analysis

Genes exhibiting significant increases by microarray analysis should be subjected to secondary analysis by semiquantitative polymerase chain reaction (PCR) (*63*).

1. Perform reverse-transcription (RT)-PCR by converting 150 ng of total RNA to cDNA using oligo-dT priming and SuperScript RT (Life Technologies) as directed.
2. Amplify cDNA in a 50-µL reaction containing 100 ng of each primer and 1X Master Mix Taq polymerase (Qiagen). Cycle conditions are 94°C, 5 min; 45 cycles (94°C, 30 s; 58°C, 30 s; 72°C, 90 s); 72°C, 5 min; 4°C. Block temperature is decreased to 20°C and 5-µL aliquots taken after cycles 29, 32, 35, 38, 41, and 45.
3. Visualize by gel electrophoresis and quantitate using AlphaImager 2000 software. Carry out PCR by denaturing at 95°C for 5 min, followed by 25 (GAPDH) cycles followed by extension at 72°C for 10 min. PCR products are separated on a 1% agarose gel and imaged by UV luminescence.

3.4. Data Analysis

Gene-chip output files should be inspected for artifacts and proper array grid alignment. Data of all experiments are globally normalized using The Equalizer, an application for Windows NT written in Microsoft Visual Basic 6 *(63)*. Normalization includes linearizing the expression and background correction (98.5% > background). Genes are prioritized according to the difference between the calculated metric $P(g,c)$ and 100 random permutations of classification. Genes for which significant differences ($p < 0.05$) are detected between control and hypercholesterolemic groups by nearest-neighbors analysis and/or Student's t-test are then further analyzed with GeneSpring 3.2.8 (Silicon Genetics) *(63)*. Data are expressed as mean ± SEM.

References

1. Chuaqui, R. F., Bonner, R F., Best, C. J. M., et al. (2002) Post-analysis follow-up and validation of microarray experiments. *Nat. Genet.* **32,** 509–514.
1a. Chese, M., Yang, R., Hubbell, E., et al. (1996) Accessing genetic information with high-density DNA array. *Science* **224,** 610–614.
2. Schena, M., Shalson, D., Davis, R. W., et al. (1995) Quantitative monitoring of gene expression patterns with a complementary DNA microarray. *Science* **270,** 467–470.
3. Napoli, C., Lerman, L. O., Sica, V., Lerman, A., Tajana, G., and de Nigris, F. (2003) Microarray analysis: a novel reasearch tool for cardiovascular scientists and physicians. *Heart* **89,** 597–604.
4. Roth, F. P., Hughes, J. D., Estep, P. W., et al. (1998) Finding DNA regulatory motifs within unaligned noncoding sequences clustered by whole-genome mRNA quantification. *Nat. Biotechnol.* **16,** 939–945.
5. Tavazoie, S., Hughers, J. D., Campbell, M.J., et al. (1999) Systematic determination of genetic network architecture. *Nat. Genet.* **22,** 281–285.
6. Fodor, S. P. A., et al. (1995) Array of oligonucleotides on a solid substrate. U.S. Patent 5445934.
7. Lipshutz R. J., et al. (1999) High density synthetic oligonucleotide arrays. *Nat. Genet.* **21,** S20–S24.

8. Dalton R. and Abbott A. (1999) Can researchers find recipe for proteins and chips? *Nature* **402,** 718–719.

9. MacBeath G. and Schreiber S. L. (2000) Printing proteins as microarrays for high-throughput function determination. *Science* **289,** 1760–1763.

10. Arenkov P., et al. (2000) Protein microchips: use for immunoassay and enzymatic reactions. *Anal. Biochem.* **278,** 123–131.

11. Lee, M. and Walt D. R. (2000) A fiber-optic microarray biosensor using aptamers as receptors. *Anal. Biochem.* **282,** 142–146.

12. Nedelkov D., et al. (2002) Design of buffer exchange surfaces and sensor chips for biosensor chip mass spectrometry. *Proteomics* **2,** 441–446.

13. Houseman, B. T. et al. (2002) Peptide chips for the quantitative evaluation of protein kinase activity. *Nat. Biotechnol.* **20,** 270–274.

14. Mitchell P. A perspective on protein microarrays. (2002) *Nat. Biotechnol.* **20,** 225–229.

15. Fukui, S., et al. (2002) Oligosaccharide microarrays for high-throughput detection and specificity assignments of carbohydrate-protein interactions. *Nat. Biotechnol.* **20,** 1011–1017.

16. Wang, D., et al. (2002) Carbohydrate microarrays for the recognition of cross-reactive molecular markers of microbes and host cells. *Nat. Biotechnol.* **20,** 275–281.

17. Konone, J., et al. (1998) Tissue microarrays for high-throughput molecular profiling of tumour specimens. *Nat. Med.* **4,** 844–847.

18. Kallioniemi, O. P., et al. (2001) Tissue microarray technology for high-throughput molecular profiling of cancer. *Hum. Mol. Genet.* **10,** 657–662.

19. Rimm, D. L. et al. (2001) Amplification of tissue by construction of tissue microarrays. *Exp. Mol. Pathol.* **70,** 255–264.

20. Bailey, S. N., et al. (2002)Applications of transfected cell microarrays in high-throughput drug discovery. *Drug Discov. Today* **7,** S113–S118.

21. Hannon, G. J. (2002) RNA interference. *Nature* **418,** 244–251.

22. Wu R. Z., et al. (2002) Cell-biological applications of transfected-cell microarrays. *Trends Cell Biol.* **12,** 485–488.

23. Schwenk, J. M., et al. (2002) Cell microarrays: an emerging technology for the characterisation of antibodies. *Biotechniques* **33** (Suppl.), 54–61.

24. Eisen, M. B., Spellman, P. T., Brown, P. O., et al. (1998) Cluster analysis and display of genome wide expression patterns. *Proc. Natl. Acad. Sci. USA* **95,** 14863–14868.

25. Stoeckert, C. J., Causton, H. C., and Ball, C. A. (2002) Microarray databases: standards and ontologies. *Nat. Genet.* **32,** 469–473.

26. Kerr, M. K. and Churchill, G. A. (2001) Bootstrapping cluster analysis: assessing the reliability of conclusions from microarray experiments. *Proc. Natl. Acad. Sci. USA* **98,** 8961–8965.

27. Brown, M. P., Grundy, W. N., Lin, D., et al. (2000) Knowledge-based analysis of microarray gene expression data by using support vector machines. *Proc. Natl. Acad. Sci. USA* **97,** 262–267.

28. Holter, N. S., Mitra, M., Maritan, A., et al. (2000) Fundamental patterns underlying gene expression profiles: simplicity from complexity. *Proc. Natl. Acad. Sci. USA* **97,** 8409–8414.

29. Alter, D., Brown, P. O., and Botstein, D. (2000) Singular value decomposition for genome wide expression data processing and modeling. *Proc. Natl. Acad. Sci. USA* **97,** 10,101–10,106.

30. Bittnerr M, Meltzer P, Trent J. (1999) Data analysis and integration: of steps and arrows. *Nat. Genet.* **22,** 213–215.

31. Miller, R. A., Galecki, A., and Shmookler-Reis, R. J. (2001) Interpretation, design, and analysis of gene array expression experiments. *J. Gerontol.* **56,** B52–B57.

32. Tseng, G. C., Oh, M. K., Rohlin, L., et al. (2001) Issues in cDNA microarray analysis: quality filtering, channel normalization, models of variations and assessment of gene effects. *Nucleic Acid Res.* **29,** 2549–2557.

33. Sterrenburg, E., Turk, R., Boer, J. M., et al. (2002) A common reference for cDNA microarray hybridization. *Nucleic Acid Res.* **30,** e116.

34. Schulte, T. H., et al. (2002) Microfluidic technologies in clinical diagnostics. *Clin. Chim. Acta* **321,** 1–10.

35. Berry, S. (2002) Honey, I've shrunk biomedical technology! *Trends Biotechnol.* **20,** 3–4.

36. Khandurina J. and Guttman A. (2002) Bioanalysis and microfluidic devices. *J. Chromatogr. A* **943,** 159–183.

37. Kuo, T.-C., et al. (2003) Hybrid three-dimensional nanofluidic/microfluidic devices using molecular gates. *Sensors Actuators A* **102,** 223–233.

38. Dickert F. L. and Sikorski R. (1999) Supramolecular strategies in chemical sensing. *Mater. Sci. Eng. C* **10,** 39–46.

39. Schweitz, L. (2002)Molecularly imprinted polymer coatings for open-tubular capillary electrochromatography prepared by surface initiation. *Anal. Chem.* **74,** 1192–1196.

40. Chovan, T. and Guttman, A. (2002) Microfabricated devices in biotechnology and biochemical processing. *Trends Biotechnol.* **20,** 116–122.

41. Ellson, R. (2002) Picoliter: enabling precise transfer of nanoliter and picoliter volumes. *Drug Discov. Today* **7,** S32–S34.

42. Huang, N.-P., et al. (2002) Biotin-derivatised poly(l-lysine)-g-poly(ethylene glycol): a novel polymeric interface for bioaffinity sensing. *Langmuir* **18,** 220–230.

43. Okuno, H., et al. (2002) Characterisation of overoxidised polypyrrole colloids imprinted with l-lactate and their application to enantioseparation of amino acids. *Anal. Chem.* **74,** 4184–4190.

44. Nicholls, I. A., et al. (2001) Can we rationally design molecularly imprinted polymers?. *Anal. Chim. Acta* **435,** 9–18.

45. Bruggemann, O. (2001) Chemical reaction engineering using molecularly imprinted polymeric catalysts. *Anal. Chim. Acta* **435,** 197–207.

46. Ye, L., et al. (2002) Scintillation proximity assay using molecularly imprinted microspheres. *Anal. Chem.* **74,** 959–964.

47. Stanton, L. W., Garrard, L. J., Damm, D., et al. (2000) Altered patterns of gene expression in response to myocardial infarction. *Circ. Res.* **86,** 939–945.
48. Friddle, C. J., Koga, T., Rubin, E. M., et al. (2000) Expression profiling reveals distinct sets of genes altered during induction and regression of cardiac hypertrophy. *Proc. Natl. Acad. Sci. USA* **97,** 6745–6750.
49. Rao, J. S. and Bond, M. (2001) Microarrays managing the data deluge. *Circ. Res.* **88,** 1226–1227.
50. Butte, A. (2002) The use and analysis of microarray data. *Nat. Rev Drug Discov.* **1,** 951–960.
51. Pilpel, Y., Sudarsanam, P., and Church, G. M. (2001) Identifying regulatory networks by combinatorial analysis of promoter elements. *Nat. Genet.* **29,** 153–159.
52. Chen, B. P., Lii, Y. S., Zhao, Y., et al. (2001) DNA microarray analysis of gene expression in endothelial cells in response to 24-h shear stress. *Physiol. Genomics* **7,** 55–63.
53. Garcia-Gardena, G., Comander, J., Anderson, K. R., et al. (2001) Biochemical activation of vascular endothelium as determinant of its function and phenotype. *Proc. Natl. Acad. Sci. USA* **98,** 4478–4485.
54. Feng, Y., Yang, J. H., Huang, H., et al. (1999) Transcriptional profile of mechanically induced genes in human vascular smooth muscle cells. *Circ. Res.* **5,** 1118–1123.
55. Dekker, R J., van Soest, S., Fontijn, R. D., et al. (2002) Prolonged fluid shear stress induces a distinct set of endothelial cell genes, most specifically lung Kruppel-like factor (KLF2). *Blood* **100,** 1689–1698.
56. Zhao, B., Bowden, R. A., Stavchansky, S. A., et al. (2001) Human endothelial cell response to Gram-negative lipopolysaccharide assessed with cDNA microarrays. *Am. J. Physiol. Cell Physiol.* **281,** C587–C595.
57. Haley, K. J., Lilly, C. M., Yang, J H., et al. (2000) Overexpression of eotaxin and CCR3 receptor in human atherosclerosis: using genomic technology to identify a potential novel pathway of vascular inflammation. *Circulation* **102,** 2185–2189.
58. Ross, R. (1999) Atherosclerosis—an inflammatory disease. *N. Engl. J. Med.* **340,** 115–126.
59. Palinski, W. and Napoli, C. (2002) The fetal origins of atherosclerosis: maternal hypercholesterolemia, and cholesterol-lowering or antioxidant treatment during pregnancy influence in utero programming and postnatal susceptibility to atherogenesis. *FASEB J.* **16,** 1348–1360.
60. Li, H., Lewis, A., Brodsky, S., et al. (2002) Homocysteine induces 3-hydroxy 3-methylglutaryl coenzyme a reductase in vascular endothelial cells: a mechanism for development of atherosclerosis? *Circulation* **105,** 1037–1043.
61. Haley, K. J., Lilly, C. M., Yang, J. H., et al. (2000) Overexpression of eotaxin and the CCR3 receptor in human atherosclerosis: using genomic technology to identify a potential novel pathway of vascular inflammation. *Circulation* **102,** 2185–2189.
62. Callow, M. J., Dadoit, S., Gong, E. L., et al. (2000) Microarray expression profiling identifies genes with altered expression in HDL-deficient mice. *Genome Res.* **110,** 2022–2029.

63. Napoli, C., de Nigris, F., Welch, J. S., et al. (2002) Maternal hypercholesterolemia during pregnancy promotes early atherogenesis in LDL receptor-deficient mice and alter aortic gene expression determined by microarray. *Circulation* **105**, 1360–1367.

64. Kwitek-Black, A. E. and Jacob, H. J. (2001) The use of designer rats in the genetic dissection of hypertension. *Curr. Hypertens. Rep.* **3**, 12–18.

65. Okuda, T., Sumiya, T., Iwai, N., et al. (2002) Difference of gene expression profiles in spontaneous hypertensive rats and Wistar-Kyoto rats from two sources. *Biochem. Biophys. Res. Commun.* **296**, 537–543.

17

Pharmacogenetics and Pharmacogenomics

Klaus Lindpaintner

1. Introduction

The advances made over the last 30 yr in molecular biology, molecular genetics, and genomics, and the development of associated methods and technologies, have had a major impact on our understanding of biology, including the action of drugs and other biologically active xenobiotics. The tools that have been developed and the knowledge of the fundamental principles underlying cellular function have become indispensable for almost any field of biological research, including biomedicine and health care.

It is important to realize that, with regard to pharmacology and drug discovery, these accomplishments have in the last 30 yr led gradually to a rather fundamental shift from the "chemical paradigm" to a "biological paradigm." Where previously medicinal chemistry drove new developments in drug discovery, with biology almost an ancillary service that examined new molecules for biological function, biology, based on a new-found understanding of physiological effects of biomolecules and pathways, has now taken the lead. Biology is now requesting from the chemist compounds that modulate the function of these biomolecules or pathways, with (at least theoretically) a predictable functional impact in the setting of integrated physiology.

One particular aspect of the progress in biology, namely, our understanding of genetics and especially the cataloging of genome sequences, has uniquely captured the imagination of both scientists and the public. The austere beauty of Mendel's laws, the compeling esthetics of the double-helix structure, and the awe-inspiring accomplishment coupled with an unprecedented public relations campaign of the Human Genome Project have combined to generate public excitement and almost certainly unrealistically high expectations regarding the impact that genetics/genomics will have on the practice of health care. The

From: *Methods in Molecular Medicine, Vol. 108: Hypertension: Methods and Protocols*
Edited by: J. P. Fennell and A. H. Baker © Humana Press Inc., Totowa, NJ

interface between genetics/genomics and pharmacology, pharmacogenetics, and pharmacogenomics (usually in the most loosely defined terms) is commonly touted as heralding a "revolution" in medicine, yet as soon as one begins to probe more carefully, little substance is yet to be found to support these enthusiastic claims.

As pointed out above, the major change in how we discover drugs—from the chemical to the biological paradigm—had already occurred some time ago; current advances, in due time, are promising to move us from a physiology-based to a (molecular) pathology-based approach to drug discovery, allowing advancement from a largely palliative to a more cause/contribution-targeting pharmacopeia.

This chapter is intended to provide a (somewhat subjective) view of what the disciplines of genetics and genomics have and will contribute to drug discovery and development, and more broadly to the practice of health care. Particular emphasis will be placed on examining the role of genetics—acquired or inherited variations at the level of DNA-encoded information—in "real life," that is, with regard to common complex diseases such as hypertension. A realistic understanding of this role is absolutely essential for a balanced assessment of the impact of "genetics" on health care in the future. Definitions of some of the terms that are in wide and often unreflected use today (almost always sorely missing from both academic and public policy-related documents on the topic) will be provided, with an understanding that much of the field is still in flux, and that these may well change. Particular emphasis will be given to pharmacogenetics, where a more systematic classification than is generally found will be attempted. It is important to remain mindful that what will be discussed is to a large extent still uncharted territory, so by necessity many of the positions taken, reasoned on today's understanding and knowledge, must be viewed as somewhat speculative in nature. Where appropriate and possible, select examples will be provided, although it should be pointed out that much of the literature in the area of genetic epidemiology and pharmacogenetics lacks the stringent standards normally applied to peer-reviewed research, and replicate data are generally absent.

2. Definition of Terms

There is widespread indiscriminate use of, and thus confusion about, the terms "pharmacogenetics" and "pharmacogenomics." Although no universally accepted definition exists, there is an emerging consensus on the differential meaning and use of the two terms (*see* **Table 1**).

Table 1
Terminology

Pharmacogenetics

   Differential in vivo effects of a drug in different patients, dependent on the
      presence of inherited gene variants
   Assessed primarily genetic (SNP) and genomic (expression) approaches
   A concept to provide more patient/disease-specific health care
   One drug, many genomes (i.e., different patients)
   Focus: patient variability

Pharmacogenomics

   Differential effects of compounds—in vivo or in vitro—on gene expression,
      among the entirety of expressed genes
   Assessed by expression profiling
   A tool for compound selection/drug discovery
   Many "drugs" (i.e., early-stage compounds), one genome (i.e., "normative"
      genome [database, technology platform])
   Focus: compound variability

2.1. Pharmacogenetics

The term *genetics* relates to the presence of individual properties, and interindividual differences in these properties, as a consequence of having inherited (or acquired) them. Thus, the term *pharmacogenetics* describes the interactions between a drug and an individual's (or perhaps more accurately, groups of individuals') characteristics as they relate to differences in the DNA-based information. Pharmacogenetics, therefore, refers to the assessment of clinical efficacy and the safety and tolerability profile, that is, the pharmacological, or response phenotype of a drug in groups of individuals who differ with regard to certain DNA-encoded characteristics. It tests the hypothesis that these differences—if indeed associated with a differential response phenotype—may allow prediction of individual drug response. The DNA-encoded characteristics are most commonly assessed based on the presence or absence of polymorphisms at the level of the nuclear DNA, but may be assessed at different levels when such DNA variation translates into different characteristics, such as differential mRNA expression or splicing, protein levels or functional characteristics, or even physiological phenotypes—all of which would be seen as surrogate, or more integrated markers of the underlying genetic variant. It should be noted that some authors continue to subsume all applications of expression profiling under the term *pharmacogenomics*, in a definition of the terms that is more driven by the technology used rather than by their functional context.

2.2. Pharmacogenomics

In contrast, the term *pharmacogenomics*, and its close relative, *toxicogenomics*, are linked to *genomics*, the study of the genome and the entirety of expressed and nonexpressed genes in any given physiological state. These two fields of study are concerned with a comprehensive, genome-wide assessment of the effects of pharmacological agents, including toxins/toxicants, on gene expression patterns. Pharmacogenomic studies are thus used to evaluate the differential effects of a number of chemical compounds—in the process of drug discovery commonly applied to lead selection with regard to inducing or suppressing the expression of transcription of genes in an experimental setting. Except for situations in which pharmacogenetic considerations are "frontloaded" into the discovery process, interindividual variations in gene sequence are not usually taken into account in this process. In contrast to pharmacogenetics, pharmacogenomics does not focus on differences between individuals with regard to the drug's effects, but rather examines differences among several (prospective) drugs or compounds with regard to their biological effects using a "generic" set of expressed or nonexpressed genes. The bases of comparison are quantitative measures of expression, using a number of gene-expression profiling methods, commonly based on microarray formats. By extrapolation from the experimental results to (theoretically) desirable patterns of activation or inactivation of gene expression in the setting of integrative pathophysiology, this approach, it is hoped, will provide a faster, more comprehensive, and perhaps even more reliable way to assess the likelihood of finding an ultimately successful drug than previously available methods, which involved mostly in vivo animal experimentation.

Thus, although both pharmacogenetics and pharmacogenomics refer to the evaluation of drug effects using (primarily) nucleic acid markers and technology, the directionalities of their approaches are distinctly different: pharmacogenetics represents the study of differences among a number of individuals with regard to clinical response to a particular drug ("one drug, many genomes"), whereas pharmacogenomics represents the study of differences among a number of compounds with regard to gene expression response in a single (normative) genome/expressome ("many drugs, one genome"). Accordingly, the fields of intended use are distinct: the former will help in the clinical setting to find the medicine most likely to be optimal for a patient (or the patients most likely to respond to a drug), the latter will aid in the setting of pharmaceutical research to find the "best" drug candidate from a given series of compounds under evaluation.

3. Pharmacogenomics: Finding New Medicines More Quickly and Efficiently

Once a screen (assay) has been set up in a drug discovery project, and lead compounds are identified, the major task becomes the identification of an optimized clinical candidate molecule among the many compounds synthesized by medicinal chemists. Conventionally, such compounds are screened in a number of animal or cell models for efficacy and toxicity, experiments that, while having the advantage of being conducted in the in vivo setting, commonly take significant amounts of time and depend entirely on the similarity between the experimental animal condition/setting and its human counterpart, that is, the validity of the model.

Although such experiments will never be entirely replaced by expression profiling on either the nucleic acid (genomics) or the protein (proteomics) level, these technique offers powerful advantages and complimentary information. First, efficacy and profile of induced changes can be assessed in a comprehensive fashion (within limitations—primarily sensitivity and completeness of transcript representation of the technology platform used). Second, these assessments of differential efficacy can be carried out much more expeditiously than in conventionally used, pathophysiology-based animal models. Third, the complex pattern of expression changes revealed by such experiments may provide new insights into possible biological interactions between the actual drug target and other biomolecules, and thus reveal new elements, or branch points of a biological pathway that may be useful as surrogate markers, novel diagnostic analytes, or as additional drug targets. Fourth, increasingly important, these tools serve to determine specificity of action among members of gene families that may be highly important for both efficacy and safety of a new drug. It must be borne in mind that any and all such experiments are limited by the coefficient of correlation with which the expression patterns determined are linked to the desired in vivo physiological action of the compound.

A word of caution regarding microarray-based expression profiling appears to be in order: the power of comprehensive (almost) genome-wide assessment of expression patterns has led to what may justly be described as somewhat of an infatuation with this technology that at times leaves a certain degree of critical skepticism to be desired. In particular, the pairwise comparison algorithms used in much of this work (competition staining of a case and a control sample on the same physical array) raise a number of questions regarding selection bias, which take on particular significance because the overall sample sizes are commonly (very) small. Biostatistical analytical approaches are commonly less than sophisticated, if used at all. Additionally, it is important to remain aware of the fact that all microarray expression data are of only associative character, and must be interpreted mindful of this limitation.

As a subcategory of this approach, toxicogenomics is increasingly evolving as a powerful adjuvant to classic toxicological testing. As pertinent databases are being created from experiments with known toxicants, revealing expression patterns that may potentially be predictive of longer-term toxic liabilities of compounds, future drug discovery efforts should benefit by insights allowing earlier rejection of compounds likely to cause such complications.

When using these approaches in drug discovery—even if implemented with proper biostatistics and analytical rigor—it is imperative to understand the probabilistic nature of such experiments: a promising profile on pharmacogenomic and toxicogenomic screens will enhance the likelihood of having selected an ultimately successful compound, and will achieve this goal more quickly than conventional animal experimentation, but will do so only with a certain likelihood of success. The less reductionist approach of the animal experiment will still be needed. It is to be anticipated, however, that such approaches will constitute an important time- and resource-saving first evaluation or screening step that will help to focus and reduce the number of animal experiments that will ultimately need to be conducted.

4. Pharmacogenetics: More Targeted, More Effective Medicines for Our Patients

4.1. Genes and Environment

It is common knowledge that today's pharmacopeia—inasmuch as it represents enormous progress compared with what our physicians had only 15 or 20 yr ago—is far from perfect. Many patients respond only partially, or fail to respond altogether, to the drugs they are given, and others suffer adverse events that range from unpleasant to serious and life-threatening.

There is an emerging consensus that all common complex diseases—i.e., the health problems that are by far the main contributors to society's disease burden as well as to public and private health spending—are "multifactorial" in nature. In other words, they are brought on by the coincidence of certain intrinsic (inborn or acquired) predispositions and susceptibilities on the one hand, and extrinsic, environment-derived influences on the other, with the relative importance of these two influences varying across a broad spectrum. In some diseases, external factors appear to be more important; while in others, intrinsic predispositions prevail. In most cases, a number of both intrinsic (genetic) as well as extrinsic factors appear to contribute, although it is not presently clear how much this reflects the requirement of several intrinsic and extrinsic factors to coincide in any one individual, or how much this reflects the causative heterogeneity of each of today's conventional, clinical diagnoses—a fact for which there is similar consensus. In either case, the disease-contributing role that intrinsic, genetically encoded properties play with regard to the occurrence of the disease is fundamentally different in these common, complex diseases as compared to the classic, monogenic, "Mendelian" diseases. In the latter the impact of the genetic variant is typically categorical in nature—i.e., deterministic—in the former case the presence of a disease-associated genetic variant is merely of probabilistic influence, raising (or lowering) the likelihood of disease occurrence to some extent, but never predicting it in a black-and-white fashion.

If we regard a pharmacological agent as an extrinsic, environmental factor with a potential to affect the health status of the individual to whom it is administered, then individually differing responses to such an agent would—under the paradigm just elaborated—be expected to be based on differences regarding the "intrinsic" characteristics of these patients, as long as we can exclude variation in the exposure to the drug (this is important, as in clinical practice nonadherence to prescribed regimens of administration, or drug–drug interactions interfering with bioavailability of the drug, are perhaps the most likely culprits when such differences in response phenotype are observed). The influence of such intrinsic variation on drug response may be predicted to be more easily recognizable, and more relevant, the steeper the dose–response curve of a given drug is. The argument for the greater likelihood of observing environmental factor/gene interactions with drugs as compared to, say, foodstuffs, goes along the same lines.

Clearly, a better, more fundamental and mechanistic understanding of the molecular pathology of disease and of the role of intrinsic, biological properties regarding the predisposition to contract such diseases, as well as of drug action on the molecular level, will be essential for future progress in health care. Current progress in molecular biology and genetics has indeed provided us with some of the prerequisite tools that should help us reach the goal of improved understanding.

4.2. An Attempt at a Systematic Classification of Pharmacogenetics

Two conceptually quite different scenarios of interindividually differential drug response may be distinguished on the basis of the underlying biological variance (*see* **Table 2**):

1. In the first case, the underlying biological variation is *in itself not disease-causing* or -contributing, and becomes clinically relevant *only* in response to the exposure to the drug in question ("classical pharmacogenetics").

Table 2
Pharmacogenetics Systematic Classification

"Classical" pharmacogenetics
   Pharmacokinetics
      Absorption
      Metabolism
         Activation of prodrugs
         Deactivation
         Generation of biologically active metabolites
      Distribution
      Elimination
   Pharmacodynamics
      Palliative drug action (modulation of disease symptoms or disease signs by
         targeting physiologically relevant systems, without addressing those
         mechanisms that cause or causally contribute to the disease)
"Molecular differential diagnosis-related" pharmacogenetics
   Causative drug action (modulation of actual causative pathway of contributory
      mechanisms)

2. In the second case, the biological variation is *directly disease-related*, is per se of
pathological importance, and represents a sub-group of the overall clinical dis-
ease/diagnostic entity. The differential response to a drug is thus related to how
well this drug addresses, or is matched to, the presence or relative importance of
the pathomechanism it targets, in different patients—i.e., the "molecular differential diagnosis" of the patient ("disease mechanism-related pharmacogenetics").

Although these two scenarios are conceptually rather different, they result in
similar practical consequences with regard to the administration of a drug,
namely, stratification based on a particular, DNA-encoded marker. It seems
therefore legitimate to subsume both under the umbrella of "pharmacogenetics."

4.3. "Classical Pharmacogenetics"

This category includes differential *pharmacokinetics* and *pharmacodynamics*.
Pharmacokinetic effects are due to interindividual differences in absorption,
distribution, metabolism (with regard to both activation of prodrugs, inactivation of the active molecule, and generation of derivative molecules with biological activity), or excretion of the drug. In any of these cases, the differential
effects observed are due to the presence at the intended site of action either of
inappropriate concentrations of the pharmaceutical agent, or of inappropriate
metabolites, or of both, resulting either in lack of efficacy or toxic effects.
Pharmacogenetics, as it relates to pharmacokinetics, has been recognized as an
entity for more than 100 years, going back to the observation, commonly cred-

ited to Archibald Garrod, that a subset of psychiatric patients treated with the hypnotic, sulphonal, developed porphyria. We have since then come to understand the underlying genetic causes for many of the previously known differences in enzymatic activity, most prominently with regard to the P-450 enzyme family, and these have been the subject of recent reviews *(1,2)* (*see* **Table 3**). However, such pharmacokinetic effects are also seen with membrane transporters, such as in the case of differential activity of genetic variants of MDR-1 that affects the effective intracellular concentration of antiretrovirals *(3)*, or of the purine-analog-metabolizing enzyme, thiomethyl-purine-transferase *(4)*.

Notably, despite the widespread recognition of isoenzymes with differential metabolizing potential since the middle of the 20th century, the practical application and implementation of this knowledge has been minimal so far. This may be the consequence, on one hand, of the irrelevance of such differences in the presence of relatively flat dose–effect curves (i.e., a sufficiently wide therapeutic window), as well as, on the other hand, the fact that many drugs are subject to complex, parallel metabolizing pathways, where in the case of underperformance of one enzymes, another one may compensate. Such compensatory pathways may well have somewhat different substrate affinities, but allow plasma levels to remain within therapeutic concentrations. Thus, the number of such polymorphisms that have found practical applicability is rather limited and, by and large, restricted to determinations of the presence of functionally deficient variants of the enzyme, thiopurine methyltransferase, in patients prior to treatment with purine-analog chemotherapeutics.

Pharmacodynamic effects, in contrast, may lead to interindividual differences in a drug's effects despite the presence of appropriate concentrations of the active drug compound at the intended site of action. Here, DNA-based variation in how the target molecule, or another (downstream) member of the target molecule's mechanistic pathway can respond to the medicine modulates the effects of the drug. This will apply primarily to palliatively working medicines that improve a condition symptomatically by modulating disease-phenotype-relevant (but not disease-cause-relevant) pathways that are not dysfunctional but can be used to counterbalance the effect of a dysfunctional, disease-causing pathway, and therefore allow mitigation of symptoms. A classical example of such an approach is the acute treatment of thyrotoxicity with β-adrenergic-blocking agents: even though the sympathetic nervous system does in this case not contribute causally to tachycardia and hypertension, dampening even its baseline tonus through this class of drugs relieves the cardiovascular symptoms and signs of this condition, before the causal treatment (in this case available through partial chemical ablation of the hyperactive thyroid gland) can take effect. Notably, the majority of today's pharmacopeia actually belongs to this class of palliatively acting medicines.

Table 3
Pharmacogenetics: Chronology and Systematics

Pharmacogenetic phenotype	Described	Underlying gene/mutation	Identified
Sulphonal porphyria	ca. 1890	Porphobilinogen deaminase?	1985
Suxamethonium hypersensitivity	1957–60	Oseudocholinesterase	1990–92
Primaquin hypersensitivity; favism	1958	G-6-PD 1988	
Long QT syndrome	1957–60	*Herg*, etc. 1991–97	
Isoniazid slow/fast acetylation	1959–60	N-acetyltranferase	1989–93
Malignant hyperthermia	1960–62	Ryanodine receptor	1991–97
Fructose intolerance	1963	Aldoalse B1988–95	
Vasopressin insensitivity	1969	Vasopressin receptor2	1992
Alcohol susceptibility	1969	Aldehyde dehydrogenase	1988
Debrisoquine hypersensitivity	1977	CYP2D6 1988–93	
Retinoic acid resistance	1970	PML-RARA fusion gene	1991–93
6-Mercaptopurin toxicity	1980	Thiopurine methyltransferase	1995
Mephenytoin resistance	1984	CYP2C19 1993–94	
Insulin insensitivity	1988	Insulin receptor	1988–93

Phase I enzyme	Testing substance
Aldehyde dehydrogenase	Acetaldehyde
Alcohol dehydrogenase	Ethanol
CYP1A2	Caffeine
CYP2A6	Nicotine, coumarin

	Testing substance
CYP2C9	Warfarin
CYP2C19	Mephenytoin, omeprazole
CYP2D6	Dextromethorphan, dbrisoquine, sparteine
CYP2E1	Chloroxazone, caffeine
CYP3A4	Erythromycin
CYP3A5	Midazolam
Serum cholinesterase	Benzoylcholine, butyrlcholine
Paraoxonase/arylesteraseP	Paraoxon

Phase II enzyme	Testing substance
Acetyltransferase (NAT1)	*para*-Aminosalizylsäure
Acetyltransferase (NAT2)	Isoniazid, sulfamethazine, caffeine
Dihydropyrimidin dehydrogenase	5-Fluorouracil
Glutathione transferase (GST-M1)	*trans*-Stilbene-Oxid
Thiomethyltransferase	2-Mercaptoethanol, D-penicillamine, captopril
Thiopurine methyltransferase	6-Mercaptopurine, 6-thioguanine, 8-azathioprine
UDP-glucuronosyl-transferase (UGT1A)	Bilirubin
UDP-glucuronosyl-transferase (UGT2B7)	Oxazepam, ketoprofen, estradiol, morphine

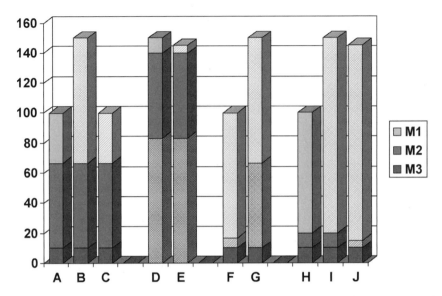

Fig 1. **(A)** Normal physiology: three molecular mechanisms (M1, M2, M3) contribute to a trait. **(B)** Diseased physiology D1: derailment (cause/contribution) of molecular mechanism 1 (M1). **(C)** Diseased physiology D1: causal treatment T1 (aimed at M1). **(D)** Diseased physiology D3: derailment (cause/contribution) of molecular mechanism 3 (M3). **(E)** Diseased physiology D3, treatment T1: treatment does not address cause. **(F)** Diseased physiology D1, palliative treatment T2 (aimed at M2). **(G)** Diseased physiology D1, palliative treatment T2; T2-refractory gene variant in M2. **(H)** Normal physiology variant: differential contribution of M1 and M2 to normal trait. **(I)** Diseased physiology D1-variant: derailment of mechanism M1. **(J)** Diseased physiology D1-variant: treatment with T2. Solid colors indicate normal function, stippling indicates pathological dysfunction, hatching indicates therapeutic modulation.

A schematic (**Fig. 1**) is provided to help clarify these somewhat complex concepts, in which a hypothetical case of a complex trait/disease is depicted where excessive, dysregulated function of one of the trait-controlling/contributing pathways (**Fig. 1A,B**) causes symptomatic disease—the example used refers to blood pressure as the trait, and hypertension as the disease in question, respectively (for the case of a defective or diminished function of a pathway, an analogous schematic could be constructed, and again for a deviant function). A palliative treatment would be one that addresses one of the pathways that—while not dysregulated—contributes to the overall deviant physiology (**Fig. 1F**), while the respective pharmacogenetic-pharmacodynamic scenario would occur if this particular pathway was, due to a genetic variant, not responsive to the drug chosen (**Fig. 1G**). A palliative treatment may also be ineffective if the particular mechanism targeted by the palliative drug (due to the presence of a molecular variant) provides less than the physiologically expected baseline contribution to the relevant phenotype (**Fig. 1H**). In such a case, modulating an *a priori* unimportant pathway in the disease scenario will not yield successful palliative treatment results (**Fig. 1I,J**).

One of the most persuasive examples we have accumulated to date for such palliative drug-related pharmacogenetic effects has been observed in the field of asthma. The treatment of asthma relies on an array of drugs aimed at modulating different "generic" pathways, thus mediating bronchodilation or anti-inflammatory effects, often without regard to the possible causative contribution of the targeted mechanism to the disease. One of the mainstays of the treatment of asthma is activation of the β-2-adrenoceptor by specific agonists, which leads to relaxation of bronchial smooth muscles and, consequently, bronchodilation. Recently, several molecular variants of the β-2-adrenoceptor have been shown to be associated with differential treatment response to such β-2-agonists *(5,6)*. Individuals carrying one or two copies of a variant allele that contains a glycine in place of arginine in position 16 were found to have a three- and fivefold reduced response to the agonist, respectively. This was shown in both in vitro *(7,8)* and in vivo *(8)* studies to correlate with an enhanced rate of agonist-induced receptor downregulation, but not with any difference in transcriptional or translational activity of the gene, or with agonist binding. In contrast, a second polymorphism affecting position 19 of the β upstream peptide was shown to affect translation (but not transcription) of the receptor itself, with a 50% decrease in receptor numbers associated with the variant allele—which happens to be in strong linkage disequilibrium with a variant allele position 16 in the receptor. The simultaneous presence of both mutations would thus be predicted to result in low expression and enhanced downregulation of an otherwise functionally normal receptor, depriving patients carrying such alleles of the benefits of effective bronchodilation as a "palliative" (i.e., noncausal) countermeasure to their pathological airway hyper-reactivity. Importantly, there is no evidence that any of the allelic variants encountered are associated with the prevalence or incidence, and thus potentially the etiology, of the underlying disease *(9,10)*. This would reflect the scenario depicted in **Fig. 1H**.

Inhibition of leukotriene synthesis, another palliative approach to the treatment of asthma, proved clinically ineffective in a small fraction of patients who carried only non-wild-type alleles of the 5-lipoxygenase promoter region *(11)*. These allelic variants had previously been shown to be associated with decreased transcriptional activity of the gene *(12)*. It stands to reason—consistent with the clinical observations—that in the presence of already reduced 5-lipoxygenase activity, pharmacological inhibition may be less effective (**Fig. 1H–J**). Of note, again, there is no evidence for a primary, disease-causing or -contributing role of any 5-lipoxygenase variants; all of them were observed at equal frequencies in disease-affected and non-affected individuals *(12)*.

Pharmacogenetic effects may not only account for differential efficacy, but also contribute to differential occurrence of adverse effects. An example of this scenario is provided by the well-documented "pharmacogenetic" association between molecular sequence variants of the 12S rRNA, a mitochondrion-encoded gene, and aminoglycoside-induced ototoxicity *(13)*. Intriguingly, the mutation that is associated with susceptibility to ototoxicity renders the sequence of the human 12S rRNA similar to that of the bacterial 12S rRNA gene, and thus effectively turns the human 12S rRNA into the (bacterial) target for aminoglycoside drug action—presumably mimicking the structure of the bacterial binding site of the drug *(14)*. As in the other examples, presence of the 12S rRNA mutation *per se* has no primary, drug treatment-independent pathological effect.

One may speculate that, analogously, such "molecular mimicry" may occur within one species: adverse events may arise if the selectivity of a drug is lost because a gene that belongs to the same gene family as the primary target loses its "identity" vis-à-vis the drug and attains, based on its structural similarity with the principal target, similar or at least increased affinity to the drug. Depending on the biological role of the "imposter" molecule, adverse events may occur—even though the variant molecule, again, may be quite silent with regard to any contribution to disease causation. Although we currently have no obvious examples for this scenario, it is certainly imaginable for various classes of receptors and enzymes.

4.4. Pharmacogenetics as a Consequence of Molecular Differential Diagnosis

As alluded to earlier, there is general agreement today that any of the major clinical diagnoses in the field of common complex disease, such as hypertension, diabetes, or cancer, are comprised of a number of etiologically (i.e., at the molecular level) more or less distinct subcategories. In the case of a causally acting drug this may imply that the agent will only be appropriate, or will work best, in the fraction of all the patients who carry the clinical diagnosis in whom the dominant molecular etiology, or at least one of the contributing etiological factors, matches the mechanism of action of the drug in question (**Fig. 1C**). If the mechanism of action of the drug addresses a pathway that is not disease-relevant—perhaps already downregulated as an appropriate physiological response to the disease, then the drug may be expected to be ineffective (**Fig. 1D,E**).

Thus, unrecognized and undiagnosed disease heterogeneity—disclosed indirectly by presence or absence of response to a drug targeting a mechanism that contributes only to one of several molecular subgroups of the disease—

provides an important explanation for differential drug response and likely represents a substantial fraction of what we today somewhat indiscriminately subsume under the term "pharmacogenetics."

Currently, the most frequently cited example for this category of "pharmacogenetics" is trastuzamab (Herceptin®), a humanized monoclonal antibody directed against the *her*-2-oncogene. This breast cancer treatment is prescribed based on the level of *her*-2-oncogene expression in the patient's tumor tissue. Differential diagnosis at the molecular level not only provides an added level of diagnostic sophistication, but also represents a prerequisite for choosing the appropriate therapy. Because tastuzamab specifically inhibits a "gain-of-function" variant of the oncogene, it is ineffective in the two-thirds of patients who do not "overexpress" the drug's target, whereas it significantly improves survival in the one-third of patients who constitute the "subentity" of the broader diagnosis "breast cancer" in whom the gene is expressed *(15)*. Some have argued against this being an example of "pharmacogenetics," because the parameter for patient stratification (i.e., for differential diagnosis) is the somatic gene expression level rather than a particular "genotype" data *(16)*. This is a difficult argument to follow, because in the case of a treatment effect-modifying germline mutation it would obviously not be the nuclear gene variant *per se*, but its specific impact on either structure–function or on expression of the respective gene–gene product that would represent the actual physiological corollary underlying the differential drug action. Conversely, an *a priori* observed expression difference is highly likely to reflect a—potential but as yet undiscovered—sequence variant. As pointed out earlier, there are a number of examples in the field of pharmacogenomics where the connection between genotypic variant and altered expression has already been demonstrated *(12,17)*.

Another example, although still hypothetical, of how proper molecular diagnosis of relevant pathomechanisms will influence drug efficacy, is in the evolving class of anti-AIDS/HIV drugs that target the CCR5 cell-surface receptor *(18–20)*. These drugs would be predicted to be ineffective in those rare patients who carry the delta-32 variant, but who nevertheless have contracted AIDS or test HIV-positive (most likely due to infection with an SI-virus phenotype that utilizes CXCR4) *(21,22)*.

It should be noted that the pharmacogenetically relevant molecular variant need not affect the primary drug target, but may equally well be located in another molecule belonging to the system or pathway in question, both up- or downstream in the biological cascade with respect to the primary drug target.

4.5. Different Classes of Markers

Pharmacogenetic phenomena need not be restricted to the observation of a direct association between allelic sequence variation and phenotype, but may extend to a broad variety of indirect manifestations of underlying, but often (as yet) unrecognized sequence variation. Thus, differential methylation of the promoter-region of O6-methylguanine-DNA-methylase has recently been reported to be associated with differential efficacy of chemotherapy with alkylating agents. If methylation is present, expression of the enzyme that rapidly reverses alkylation and induces drug resistance is inhibited, and therapeutic efficacy is greatly enhanced *(23)*.

4.6. Complexity Is To Be Expected

In the real world, it is likely that combination of several of the scenarios depicted may be present. This will affect how well the patient responds to a given treatment, or the likelihood of suffering an adverse event. Thus, a fast-metabolizing patient with poor-responder pharmacodynamics may be particularly unlikely to gain any benefit from taking the drug in question, while a slow-metabolizing status may counterbalance in another patient the same inopportune pharmacodynamics, while a third patient, who is a slow metabolizer and displaying normal pharmacodynamics, may be more likely to suffer adverse events. In all these patients, both the pharmacokinetic and pharmacodynamics properties may result from the interaction of several of the mechanisms described above. In addition, the co-administration of other drugs, or even the consumption of certain foods, may affect and further complicate the picture for any given treatment.

5. Incorporating Pharmacogenetics into Drug Development Strategy

It is important to note that despite the public hyperbole and the high-strung expectations surrounding the use of pharmacogenetics to provide "personalized care," these approaches are likely to be applicable to only a fraction of medicines that are being developed. If and when such approaches will be used, they will represent no radical new direction or concept in drug development, but simply a stratification strategy as has been used all along.

A more precise diagnosis of disease, arising from a better understanding of pathology at the molecular level, will increasingly subdivide today's clinical diagnoses into molecular subtypes and will foster medical advances. If considered from the viewpoint of today's clinical diagnosis, these advances will appear as "pharmacogenetic" phenomena, as described above. However, the sequence of events that is today often presented as characteristic for a "pharmacogenetic scenario" (namely, exposing patients to the drug, recognizing a differential (i.e., quasi-bimodal) response pattern, discovering a marker that predicts this response, and creating a diagnostic product to be co-marketed with the drug henceforth) is likely to be reversed. Rather, in the case of "pharmacogenetics" due to a match between drug action and dysregulation of a disease-contributing mechanism, we will likely search for a new drug specifically, based on a new mechanistic understanding of disease causation or contribution (i.e., a newly found ability to diagnose a molecular subentity of a previously broader and less precise clinical disease definition). Thus, pharmacogenetics will not be so much about finding the "right medicine for the right patient," but about finding the "right medicine for the disease subtype." This is, in fact, good news: the conventional "pharmacogenetic scenario" would invariably present major challenges from both a regulatory and a business development and marketing standpoint, as it will confront development teams with a critical change in the drug's profile at a very late point during the development process. In addition, the timely development of an approvable diagnostic in this situation is difficult at best, and it's marketing as an "add-on" to the drug a less than attractive proposition to diagnostics business. Thus, the "practice" of pharmacogenetics will, in many instances, be marked by progress along the same path that has been a source of medical progress for the last several hundred years: differential diagnosis first, followed by the development of appropriate, more specific treatment modalities.

Thus, the sequence of events in this case would likely involve the development of an in vitro diagnostic test as a standalone product that may be marketed on its own merits, allowing the physician to establish an accurate, state-of-the-art diagnosis of the molecular subtype of the patient's disease. Such a diagnostic may prove helpful even in the absence of specific therapy by guiding the choice of existing medicines and/or of nondrug treatment modalities such as specific changes in diet or lifestyle. Availability of such a diagnostic—as part of the more sophisticated understanding of disease—will undoubtedly foster and stimulate the search for new, more specific drugs. Once such drugs are found, availability of the specific diagnostic will be important for carrying out appropriate clinical trials. This will allow a prospectively planned, much more systematic approach toward clinical and business development, with a greater chance of success.

In practice, some extent of guesswork will remain, due to the nature of common complex diseases. First, all diagnostic approaches—including those based on DNA analysis in common complex diseases, as stressed above—will ultimately only provide a measure of probability, not of certainty. Although the variances of drug response among patients who do (or do not) carry the drug-specific subdiagnosis will be smaller, there will still be a distribution of differential responses. In general, the drug will work better in the "responder" group, but there will be some patients among this subgroup who will respond less or not at all. Conversely, not everyone belonging to the "nonresponder" group

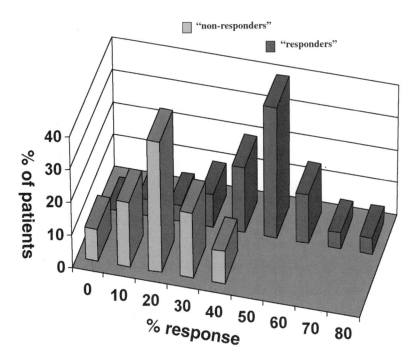

Fig. 2. Hypothetical example of bimodal distribution according to marker that indicates "nonresponder" or "responder" status. Note that in both cases a distribution is present, with overlaps, thus, the categorization into "responders" or "nonresponders" based on the marker must be understood to convey only the probability to belong to one or the other group.

will completely fail to respond, depending perhaps on the relative magnitude with which the particular mechanism contributes to the disease. It is important to bear in mind, therefore, that even in the case of fairly obvious bimodality, patient responses will still show distribution patterns, and that all predictions as to responder or nonresponder status will only have a certain likelihood of being indeed accurate (**Fig. 2**). The terms "responder" and "nonresponder" applied to patients stratified based on a DNA marker represent Mendelian thinking-inspired misnomers that should be replaced by more appropriate terms that reflect the probabilistic nature of any such classification, such as "likely (non)responder."

Based on our current understanding of the polygenic and heterogeneous nature of these disorders, we will—even in an ideal world where we would know about all possible susceptibility gene variants for a given disease and have treatments for them—only be able to exclude, in any one patient, those that do not appear to contribute to the disease, and therefore deselect certain treatments. We will most likely find ourselves left with a small number—two to four, perhaps—of potentially disease-contributing gene variants whose relative contribution to the disease will be difficult, if not impossible, to rank in an individual patient. It is likely that trial and error and that great intangible quantity, "physician experience," will still play an important role, albeit on a more limited and subselective basis.

The alternative scenario, where differential drug response and/or safety occurs as a consequence of a pathologically irrelevant, purely drug response-related pharmacogenetics scenario, is more likely to present greater difficulty in planning and executing a clinical development program because, presumably, it will be more difficult to anticipate or predict differential responses *a priori*. When such a differential response occurs, it will also potentially be more difficult to find the relevant marker(s), unless it happens to be among the "obvious" candidate genes implicated in the disease physiopathology or the treatment's mode of action. Although screening for molecular variants of these genes, and testing for their possible associations with differential drug response, is a logical first step, if unsuccessful, it may be necessary to embark on an unbiased genome-wide screen for such a marker or markers. Despite recent progress in high-throughput genotyping, the obstacles that will have to be overcome on the technical, data analysis, and cost levels are formidable. They will limit the deployment of such programs, at least for the foreseeable future, to select cases in which there are very solid indications for doing so, based on clinical data showing a near-categorical (e.g., bimodal) distribution of treatment outcomes. Even then, we may expect to encounter for every success—which will be owed to a favorably strong linkage disequilibrium across considerable genomic distance in the relevant chromosomal region—as many or more failures, in cases where the culpable gene variant cannot be found due to the higher recombination rate or other characteristics of the stretch of genome on which it is located.

6. Regulatory Aspects

Regulatory agencies in both Europe and the United States are beginning to show keen interest in the potential role that pharmacogenetic approaches may play in the development and clinical use of new drugs, and the potential challenges that such approaches present to the regulatory approval process. While no formal guidelines have been issued, the pharmaceutical industry has already been reproached—albeit in a rather nonspecific manner—for not being more proactive in the use of pharmacogenetic markers. It will be of key importance for all concerned to engage in intensive dialogue, at the end of which will hopefully emerge a joint understanding that stratification according to DNA-based markers is fundamentally nothing new, and no different from stratification according to any other clinical or demographic parameter, as has been used all along.

Still, based on the (in the case of common complex diseases, scientifically unjustified) perception that DNA-based markers represent a different class of stratification parameters, a number of important questions will need to be addressed and answered. Among the most important ones are questions concerning:

1. The need and/or ethical justification (or lack thereof) to include likely nonresponders in a trial for the sake of meeting safety criteria, which, given the restricted indication of the drug, may indeed be excessively broad
2. The need to use active controls if the patient/disease stratum is different from that in which the active control was originally tested
3. The strategies to develop and gain approval for the applicable first-generation diagnostic, as well as for the regulatory approval of subsequent generations of tests to be used to determine eligibility for prescription of the drug
4. A number of ethical-legal questions relating to the unique requirements regarding privacy and confidentiality for "genetic testing" that may raise novel problems with regard to regulatory audits of patient data (see below)

A concerted effort to avoid what has been termed "genetic exceptionalism"—the differential treatment of DNA-based markers as compared with other personal medical data—should be made so as to not further complicate the already very difficult process of obtaining regulatory approval. This seems, justified based on the recognized fact that in the field of common complex disease, DNA-based markers are not at all different from "conventional" medical data in all relevant aspects—namely, specificity, sensitivity, and predictive value.

7. Pharmacogenetic Testing for Drug Efficacy vs Safety

By stratifying patient eligibility for a drug according to appropriate markers, pharmacogenetic approaches may be useful both to raise efficacy and to avoid adverse events. In both cases, clinical decisions and recommendations must be supported by data that have undergone rigorous biostatistical scrutiny. Based on the substantially different prerequisites for and opportunities to acquire such data, and to apply them to clinical decision making, we expect the use of pharmacogenetics for enhanced efficacy to be considerably more common than for the avoidance of adverse events.

The likelihood that adequate data on efficacy in a subgroup may be generated is reasonably high, given the fact that unless the drug is viable in a reasonably sizable number of patients, it will probably not be developed due to lack of a viable business case, or at least only under the protected environment of orphan drug guidelines. Implementation of pharmacogenetic testing to stratify for efficacy, provided that safety in the nonresponder group is not an issue, will primarily be a matter of physician preference and sophistication, and potentially of third-party-payer directives. This would appear less likely to become a matter of regulatory mandate, unless a drug has been developed selectively in a particular stratum of the overall indication (in which case a contra-indication label for other strata is likely to be issued). An argument can be made against depriving those who carry the "'likely' nonresponder" genotype regarding eligibility for the drug, but who individually, of course, may respond to the drug with a certain, albeit lower probability. From a regulatory aspect, use of pharmacogenetics for efficacy, if adequate safety data exist, appears largely unproblematic—the worst-case scenario (a genotypically inappropriate patient receiving the drug) would result in treatment without expected beneficial effect, but with no increased risk of adverse effects—i.e., what one would expect under conventional paradigms.

The utility and clinical application of pharmacogenetic approaches toward improving safety, in particular with regard to serious adverse events, will meet with considerably greater hurdles and is therefore less likely to become reality. A number of reasons are cited for this: first, in the event of serious adverse events associated with the use of a widely prescribed medicine, withdrawal of the drug from the market is usually based almost entirely on anecdotal evidence from a rather small number of cases—in accordance with the Hippocratic mandate, *"primum non nocere."* If the sample size is insufficient to demonstrate a statistically significant association between drug exposure and event, as is typically the case, it will most certainly be insufficient to allow meaningful testing for genotype–phenotype correlations; the biostatistical hurdles become progressively more difficult as many markers are tested and the number of degrees of freedom applicable to the analysis for association continues to rise. Therefore, the fraction of attributable risk shown to be associated with a given at-risk (combination of) genotype(s) would have to be very substantial for regulators to accept such data. Indeed, the low prior probability of the adverse event, by definition, can be expected to yield an equally low positive (or negative) predictive value. Second, the very nature of safety issues raises the hurdles substantially because in this situation the worst-case scenario—administration of the drug to the "wrong" patient—will result in higher odds of harm to the patient. Therefore, it is likely that the practical application of successfully investigating and applying pharmacogenetics toward limiting adverse events will likely be restricted to diseases with dire prognosis, where a high medical need exists, where the drug in question offers unique potential advantages (usually bearing the characteristics of a "life-saving" drug), and where the tolerance even for severe side effects is much greater than for other drugs. This applies primarily to areas such as oncology or HIV/AIDS. In most other indications, the sobering biostatistical and regulatory considerations discussed represent barriers that are unlikely to be overcome easily; and the proposed, conceptually highly attractive, routine deployment of pharmacogenetics as a generalized drug surveillance or pharmaco-vigilance practice following the introduction of a new pharmaceutical agent *(24)* faces these scientific as well as formidable economic hurdles.

8. Ethical-Societal Aspects of Pharmacogenetics

No discussion about the use of genetic/genomic approaches to health care can be complete without considering their impact on the ethical, societal, and legal level.

Much of the discussion about ethical and legal issues relating to pharmacogenetics is centered on the issue of "genetic testing," a topic that has recently also been the focus of a number of guidelines, advisories, white papers, and so on, issued by a number of committees in both Europe and the United States. It is interesting to note that the one characteristic that almost all these documents share is a studious avoidance of defining what exactly a "genetic test" is. Where definitions are given, they tend to be very broad, including not only the analysis of DNA but also of transcription and translation products affected by inherited variation. Inasmuch as the most sensible solution to this dilemma will hopefully be a consensus to treat all personal medical data in a similar fashion regardless of the degree to which DNA-encoded information affects it (noting that there really isn't any medical data that are not to some extent affected by intrinsic patient properties), it may, for the time being, be helpful to let the definition of what constitutes "genetic data" be guided by the public perception of "genetic data"—inasmuch as the whole discussion of this topic is prompted by these public perceptions.

In the public eye, "genetic test" is usually understood either as (1) any kind of test that establishes the diagnosis (or predisposition) of a classic monogenic, heritable disease, or (2) as any kind of test based on nucleic acid analysis. This includes the (non-DNA-based) Guthrie test for phenylketonuria as well as forensic and paternity testing, as well as a DNA-based test for Lp(a), but not the plasma protein-based test for the same marker (even though the information derived is identical). Since monogenic disease is, in effect, excluded from this discussion, it stands to reason to restrict the definition of "genetic testing" to the analysis of (human) DNA sequence.

Based on the perceived particular sensitivity of "genetic" data, institutional review boards commonly apply a specific set of rules to granting permission to test for DNA-based markers in the course of drug trials or other clinical research, including (variably) separate informed consent forms, the anonymization of samples and data, specific stipulations about availability of genetic counseling, provision to be able to withdraw samples at any time in the future, and so on.

Arguments have been advanced *(24)* that genotype determinations for pharmacogenetic characterization, in contrast to "genetic" testing for primary disease risk assessment, are less likely to raise potentially sensitive issues with regard to patient confidentiality, misuse of genotyping data or other nucleic acid-derived information, and the possibility of stigmatization. Although this is certainly true when pharmacogenetic testing is compared to predictive genotyping for highly penetrant Mendelian disorders, it is not apparent why in common complex disorders issues surrounding predictors of primary disease risk would be any more or less sensitive than those pertaining to predictors of likely treatment success/failure. Indeed, two lines of reasoning may actually indicate an increased potential for ethical issues and complex confrontations among the various stakeholders to arise from pharmacogenetic data.

First, while access to genotyping and other nucleic acid-derived data related to disease susceptibility can be strictly limited, the very nature of pharmacogenetic data calls for a rather more liberal position regarding use: if this information is to improve the patient's chance of successful treatment, then it is essential that it is shared among at least a somewhat wider circle of participants in the health care process. Thus, the prescription for a drug that is limited to a group of patients with a particular genotype will inevitably disclose the receiving patient's genotype to any one of a large number of individuals involved in the patient's care at the medical and administrative level. The only way to limit this quasi-public disclosure of this patient's genotype data would be if he or she were to sacrifice the benefits of the indicated treatment for the sake of data confidentiality.

Second, patients profiled to carry a high disease probability along with a high likelihood for treatment response may be viewed, from the standpoint of, for instance, insurance risk, as quite comparable to patients displaying the opposite profile, that is, a low risk of developing the disease, but a high likelihood of not responding to medical treatment if the disease indeed occurs. For any given disease risk, then, patients who are less likely to respond to treatment would be seen as a more unfavorable insurance risk, particularly if nonresponder status is associated with chronic, costly illness rather than with early mortality, the first case having much more far-reaching economic consequences. The pharmacogenetic profile may thus, under certain circumstances, even become a more important (financial) risk-assessment parameter than primary disease susceptibility, and would be expected—inasmuch as it represents but one stone in the complex disease mosaic—to be treated with similar weight, or lack thereof, as other genetic and environmental risk factors.

Practically speaking, the critical issue is not only about the sensitive nature of the information, and if and how it is disseminated and disclosed, but how and to what end it is used. Obviously, generation and acquisition of personal medical information must always be contingent on the individual's free choice and consent, as must be all application of such data for specific purposes. There is today an urgent need for the requisite dialogue and discourse among all stakeholders within society to develop and endorse a set of criteria by which the use of genetic, indeed of all personal medical information should occur. It will be critically important that society as a whole endorses, in an act of solidarity with those destined to develop a certain disease, guidelines that support the beneficial and legitimate use of the data in the patient's interest while at the same time prohibiting their use in ways that may harm the individual, personally, financially, or otherwise. As long as we trust our political decision processes to reflect societal consensus, and as long as such consensus reflects the principles of justice and equality, the resulting set of principles should assert such proper use of medical information. Indeed, both aspects—data protection and patient/ subject protection, are seminal components of the mandates included in the World Health Organization's "Proposed International Guidelines on Ethical Issues in Medical Genetics and Genetic Services" *(25)*, which mandate autonomy, beneficence, no maleficence, and justice.

9. Summary

Pharmacogenetics, in the different scenarios included in this term, will represent an important new avenue toward understanding disease pathology and drug action, and will offer new opportunities of stratifying patients to achieve optimal treatment success. As such, it represents a logical, consequent step in the history of medicine—evolution, rather than revolution. Its implementation will take time, and will not apply to all diseases and all treatments equally. If society finds ways to sanction the proper use of this information, thus allowing and protecting its unencumbered use for the patient's benefit, important progress in health care will be made.

References

1. Dickins, M. and Tucker, G. (2001) Drug disposition: To phenotype or genotype. *Int. J. Pharm. Med.* **15,** 70–73. Also see: www.imm.ki.se/CYPalleles.
2. Evans, W. E. and Relling, M. V. (1999) Pharmacogenomics: Translating functional genomics into rational therapies. *Science* **206,** 487–491. Also see: www.sciencemag.org/feature/data/1044449.shl.

3. Fellay, J., Marzolini, C., Meaden, E. R., Back, D. J., Buclin, T., and Chave, J. P. (2002) Response to antiretroviral treatment in HIV-1-infected individuals with allelic variants of the multidrug resistance transporter 1: a pharmacogenetics study. *Lancet* **359,** 30–36.

4. Dubinsky, M., Lamothe, S., Yang, H. Y., Targan, S. R., Sinnett, D., Theoret, Y. (2000) Pharmacogenomics and Metabolite Measurement for 6-Mercaptopurine Therapy in Inflammatory Bowel Disease. *Gastroenterology* **118,** 705–713.

5. Martinez, F. D., Graves, P. E., Baldini, M., Solomon, S., Erickson, R. (1997) Association between genetic polymorphisms of the beta2-adrenoceptor and response to albuterol in children with and without a history of wheezing. *J. Clin. Invest.* **100,** 3184–3188.

6. Tan, S., Hall, I. P., Dewar, J., Dow, E., and Lipworth, B. (1997) Association between beta 2-adrenoceptor polymorphism and susceptibility to bronchodilator desensitisation in moderately severe stable asthmatics. *Lancet* **350,** 995–999.

7. Green, S. A., Turki, J., Innis, M., and Liggett, S. B. (1994) Amino-terminal polymorphisms of the human beta 2-adrenergic receptor impart distinct agonist-promoted regulatory properties. *Biochemistry* **33,** 9414–9419.

8. Green, S. A., Turki, J., Bejarano, P., Hall, I. P., and Liggett, S. B. (1995) Influence of beta 2-adrenergic receptor genotypes on signal transduction in human airway smooth muscle cells. *Am. J. Respir. Cell. Mol. Biol.* **13,** 25–33.

9. Reihsaus, E., Innis, M., MacIntyre, N., and Liggett, S. B. (1993) Mutations in the gene encoding for the beta 2-adrenergic receptor in normal and asthmatic subjects. *Am. J. Respir. Cell. Mol. Biol.* **8,** 334–349.

10. Dewar, J. C., Wheatley, A. P., Venn, A., Morrison, J. F. J., Britton, J., Hall, I. P. (1998) Beta2 adrenoceptor polymorphisms are in linkage disequilibrium, but are not associated with asthma in an adult population. *Clin. Exp. Allergy* **28,** 442–448.

11. Drazen, J. M., Yandava, C. N., Dube, L., et al. (1999) Pharmacogenetic association between ALOX5 promoter genotype and the response to anti-asthma treatment. *Nat. Genet.* **22,** 168–170.

12. In, K. H., Asano, K., Beier, D., et al. (1997) Naturally occurring mutations in the human 5-lipoxygenase gene promoter that modify transcription factor binding and reporter gene transcription. *J. Clin. Invest.* **99,** 1130–1137.

13. Fischel-Ghodsian, N. Genetic factors in aminoglycoside toxicity. (1999) *Ann. NY Acad. Sci.* **884,** 99–109.

14. Hutchin, T. and Cortopassi, G. (1994) Proposed molecular and cellular mechanism for aminoglycoside ototoxicity. *Antimicrob. Agents Chemother.* **38,** 2517–2520.

15. Baselga, J., Tripathy, D., Mendelsohn, J., et al. (1996) Phase II study of weekly intravenous recombinant humanized anti-p185(HER2) monoclonal antibody in patients with HER2/neu-overexpressing metastatic breast cancer. *J. Clin. Oncol.* **14,** 737–744.

16. Haseltine, W. A. (1998) Not quite pharmacogenomics (letter; comment). *Nat. Biotechnol.* **16,** 1295.

17. McGraw, D. W., Forbes, S. L., Kramer, L. A., and Liggett, S. B. (1998) Polymorphisms of the 5' leader cistron of the human beta2-adrenergic receptor regulate receptor expression. *J. Clin. Invest.* **102,** 1927–1932.

18. Huang, Y., Paxton, W. A., Wolinsky, S. M., et al. (1996) The role of a mutant CCR5 allele in HIV-1 transmission and disease progression. *Nat. Med.* **2,** 1240–1243.

19. Dean, M., Carrington, M., Winkler, C., et al. (1996) Genetic restriction of HIV-1 infection and progression to AIDS by a deletion of the CKR5 structural gene. *Science* **273,** 1856–1862.

20. Samson, M., Libert, F., Doranz, B. J., et al. (1996) Resistance to HIV-1 infection in Caucasian individuals bearing mutant alleles of the CCR-5 chemokine receptor gene. *Nature* **382,** 722–725.

21. O'Brien, T. R., Winkler, C., Dean, M., et al. (1997) HIV-1 infection in a man homozygous for CCR5 32. *Lancet* **349,** 1219.

22. Theodorou, I., Meyer, L., Magierowska, M., Katlama, C., and Rouzious, C. (1997) Seroco Study Group. HIV-1 infection in an individual homozygous for CCR5 32. *Lancet* **349,** 1219–1220.

23. Esteller, M., Garcia-Foncillas, J., Andion, E., et al. (2000) Inactivation of the DNA-repair gene mgmt and the clinical response of gliomas to alkylating agents. *N . Engl . J . Med .* **343,** 1350–1354.

24. Roses A. Pharmacogenetics and future drug development and delivery. (2000) *Lancet* **355 ,** 1358–1361.

25. WHO Expert Advisory Group. (2000) Proposed international guidelines on ethical issues in medical genetics and genetic services. World Health Organisation, http://whqlibdoc.who.int/hq/1998/WHO_HGN_GL_ETH_98.1.pdf.

IV

PROTEINS AND PROTEOMICS

18

Determination of the Endogenous Nitric Oxide Synthase Inhibitor Asymmetric Dimethylarginine in Biological Samples by HPLC

Tom Teerlink

Summary

Asymmetric dimethylarginine (ADMA) is an endogenous inhibitor of all isoforms of nitric oxide synthase, the enzyme that synthesizes nitric oxide from arginine. Elevated plasma concentrations of ADMA are associated with hypertension and other risk factors for cardiovascular disease. Symmetric dimethylarginine (SDMA), a stereoisomer of ADMA that does not inhibit nitric oxide synthase, is also present in plasma in concentrations that are almost equal to ADMA concentrations. Any analytical method used for the determination of ADMA should therefore be able to discriminate between ADMA and SDMA. In this chapter a high-performance liquid chromatography (HPLC) method for the simultaneous analysis of arginine, ADMA, and SDMA is described. Solid-phase extraction is used to isolate all basic amino acids. Subsequently, amino acids are converted into relatively stable adducts by derivatization with o-phthalaldehyde reagent containing mercaptopropionic acid. Derivatives are then separated by reversed-phase HPLC using isocratic elution and fluorescence detection. The method requires only 0.05–0.2 mL of sample, allowing the analysis of plasma from small laboratory animals. Because of its high precision, this method is particularly suited to detect small concentration differences between samples, e.g., in the assessment of ADMA metabolism at the organ level by measurement of arterio–venous concentration differences.

Key Words: Asymmetric dimethylarginine; ADMA; symmetric dimethylarginine; SDMA; arginine; nitric oxide; nitric oxide synthase; cardiovascular disease; hypertension; HPLC; derivatization. .

1. Introduction

Nitric oxide (NO) is synthesized from arginine by nitric oxide synthases, a family of enzymes with endothelial, neuronal, and inducible isoforms (1). The arginine–NO pathway has been recognized to play a crucial role in neurotransmission, host defense, and the regulation of vascular tone. NO produced by the vascular endothelium is an important player in the regulation of blood flow

From: *Methods in Molecular Medicine, Vol. 108: Hypertension: Methods and Protocols*
Edited by: J. P. Fennell and A. H. Baker © Humana Press Inc., Totowa, NJ

and pressure by inducing relaxation of smooth muscle cells in the vascular wall. In addition, it decreases the adhesiveness of the endothelium for circulating cells, inhibits platelet aggregation, and suppresses the proliferation of smooth muscle cells. Therefore, the basal production of NO by the endothelium is generally considered to be antiatherogenic. In 1992 Vallance et al. reported that NO synthesis in humans can be inhibited by the endogenous compound asymmetric dimethylarginine (ADMA) *(2)*. They demonstrated that local infusion of ADMA into the brachial artery caused a dose-dependent fall in forearm blood flow. Moreover, they showed that in patients with end-stage renal failure, plasma levels of ADMA were significantly elevated. This landmark publication has initiated rapidly expanding research into the role of ADMA in the regulation of NO synthesis in health and disease. Several studies have shown an association between elevated plasma concentrations of ADMA and hypertension *(3–6)*. Accumulating evidence suggests that ADMA plays an important role in cardiovascular disease *(7)*. ADMA has been shown to be inversely correlated with flow-mediated vasodilation *(8)* and to be an important determinant of carotid artery intima-media thickness *(9)*. ADMA is a risk factor for acute coronary events in middle-aged men *(10)* and for overall mortality and cardiovascular events in patients with end-stage renal disease *(11)*. In addition, we have recently shown that in critically ill patients on a surgical intensive care unit, high plasma concentrations of ADMA were associated with high mortality *(12)*. ADMA is formed by enzymatic methylation of arginine residues in proteins, a process that probably plays a role in the modulation of protein–nucleic acid interactions *(13)*. Other protein methylating enzymes can lead to the formation of symmetric dimethylarginine (SDMA). Upon intracellular proteolysis of these methylated proteins, free ADMA and SDMA are released. The chemical structures of ADMA and SDMA are shown in **Fig. 1**. It should be noted that in contrast to ADMA, SDMA does not inhibit NO synthesis. There are two major mechanisms for disposal of free ADMA. First, it can be removed from the circulation by renal excretion, a pathway shared by SDMA. Second, ADMA can be degraded by the enzyme dimethylarginine dimethylaminohydrolase (DDAH), an enzyme present in many organs *(14,15)*. The latter pathway is unique for ADMA, as SDMA is not a substrate for DDAH. Several conditions may thus lead to elevated plasma levels of ADMA, that is, increased methylation of proteins, enhanced proteolysis of methylated proteins, reduced renal excretion, and decreased activity of DDAH. In diseased states, any of these conditions, acting either alone or in concert, may lead to increased ADMA levels.

High-performance liquid chromatography (HPLC) is the method of choice for the analysis of ADMA. Because SDMA is structurally very similar to ADMA and the concentrations of both compounds in plasma are almost equal,

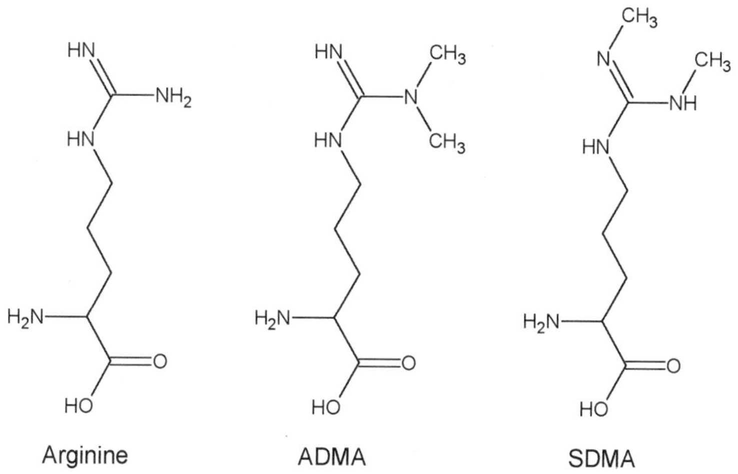

Fig. 1. Structure of arginine, asymmetric dimethylarginine (ADMA), and symmetric dimethylarginine (SDMA).

it is imperative that any chromatographic method for the analysis of ADMA be capable of adequately separating both compounds. The methodology described in this chapter is based on the simultaneous analysis of arginine, ADMA, and SDMA by HPLC (*16*). Sample pretreatment consists of isolation of basic amino acids by solid-phase extraction on polymeric cation-exchange columns, followed by derivatization with *o*-phthalaldehyde reagent containing 3-mercaptopropionic acid (**Fig. 2**). The resulting derivatives are separated by reversed-phase chromatography with fluorescence detection. The method is routinely used for the analysis of plasma samples using a 0.2-mL sample volume. The high sensitivity of the method also allows the determination of very low ADMA levels in cerebrospinal fluid (*17*) and the analysis of 0.05-mL plasma samples obtained from experimental animals. The method has high precision, making it a valuable tool for the measurement of arterio-venous concentration differences in experimental studies (*18*) and changes in plasma ADMA concentrations after pharmacological intervention (*19,20*). In addition, the method is suited for the analysis of tissue samples or the determination of ADMA in protein hydrolysates.

2. Materials

2.1. Equipment

1. Vacuum manifold for use with solid-phase extraction (SPE) cartridges (Waters Corporation, Milford, MA).
2. 1-mL (30-mg) Oasis MCX SPE cartridges (Waters cat. no. 186000252).

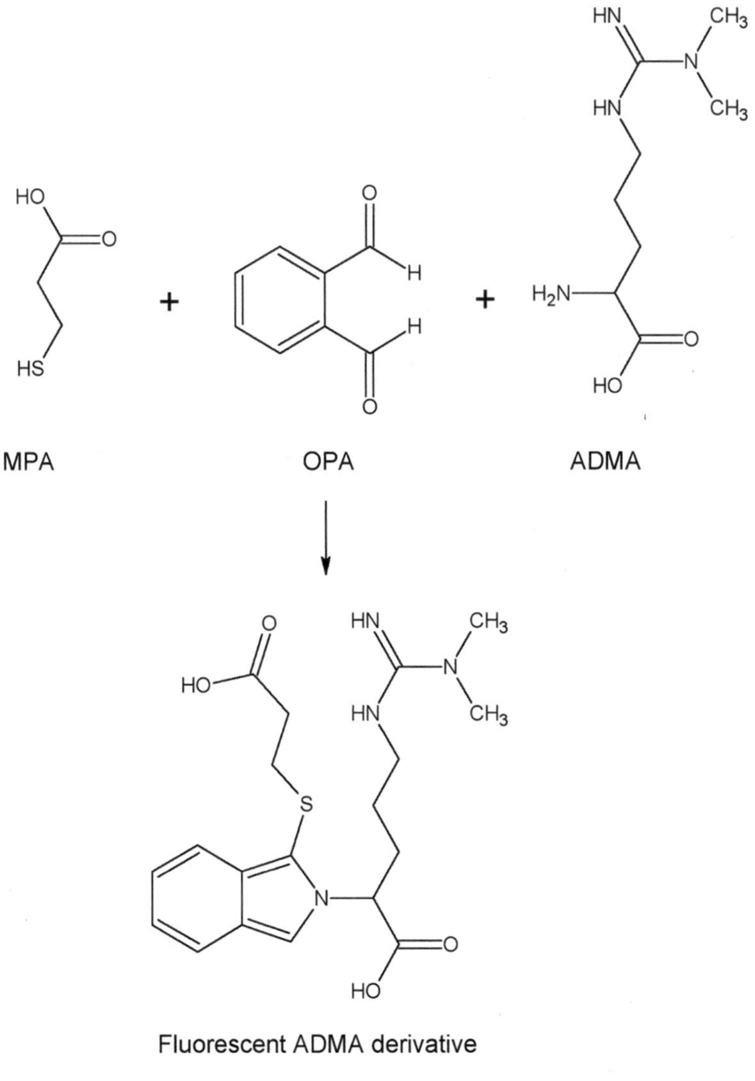

Fig. 2. Reaction of ADMA with the *o*-phthalaldehyde (OPA) reagent containing 3-mercaptopropionic acid (MPA). Note that a ternary adduct between ADMA, OPA, and MPA is formed.

3. Equipment for evaporation of solvents (such as Reacti-Therm heating module combined with Reacti-Therm evaporator; Pierce, Rockford, IL).
4. Glass tubes (11 × 75 mm).
5. Analytical HPLC system (Waters Corporation, Milford, MA).
   a. Alliance 2695 separations module.
   b. Model 474 fluorescence detector.

   c. Millennium 32 version 3.0 chromatography software.

   d. Symmetry C18 column, 3.9 × 150 mm, 5-µm particle size (Waters cat. no. WAT046980).

   e. Symmetry Sentry C18 guard column, 3.9 × 20 mm, 5-µm particle size (Waters cat. no. WAT054225). This column requires a universal Sentry guard holder (Waters cat. no. WAT046910).

   f. Autosampler vials (conical, 0.3 mL) with caps and PTFE/silicone septa (Waters cat. no. 186000852).

2.2. Reagents

1. Asymmetric dimethylarginine (ADMA; N^G,N^G-dimethylarginine) supplied as dihydrochloride salt (e.g., Sigma D4268).
2. Symmetric dimethylarginine (SDMA; $N^G,N^{G'}$-dimethylarginine) supplied as di-(p-hydroxyazobenzene-p'-sulfonate) salt (e.g., Sigma D0390).
3. Monomethylarginine (MMA; N^G-methylarginine) supplied as acetate salt (e.g., Sigma M7033).
4. Homoarginine supplied as hydrochloride salt (e.g., Sigma H9141).
5. Arginine (e.g., Merck 101542).
6. Boric acid (e.g., Merck 100165).
7. Potassium dihydrogen phosphate (e.g., Merck 104873).
8. Concentrated (25%) ammonia (e.g., Merck 105432).
9. Concentrated (37%) hydrochloric acid (e.g., Merck 113386)
10. HPLC-grade acetonitrile and methanol (e.g., Hipersolv HPLC grade from BDH, Poole, England).
11. Phthaldialdehyde, o-phthalaldehyde, OPA (e.g., Fluka 79760).
12. 3-Mercaptopropionic acid, MPA (e.g., Fluka 63770).
13. Phosphate-buffered saline (PBS): 1 mM NaH_2PO_4, 9 mM Na_2HPO_4, and 137 mM NaCl, adjusted to pH 7.0.

3. Methods

3.1. Preparation of Standards

Individual calibration standards of 1 mM for arginine, homoarginine, ADMA, and SDMA are prepared by dissolving accurately weighed amounts of the compounds in 10 mM HCl using volumetric glassware (*see* **Note 1**). Concentration and purity of these stock solutions is checked by derivatization and chromatography (*see* **Note 2**). The standard solutions are stable at 4°C for more than a year. A combined standard solution is prepared by mixing appropriate volumes of the individual standard solutions using 10 mM HCl as diluent. Final concentrations are 100 µM for arginine and 10 µM for homoarginine, ADMA, and SDMA. This combined stock solution is aliquoted in cryovials and stored at –20°C. A stock solution of the internal standard MMA (1 mM dissolved in 10 mM HCl) is prepared and stored in aliquots at –20°C (*see* **Note 3**).

3.2. Sample Clean-Up by Solid-Phase Extraction

1. Plasma samples are thawed and briefly centrifuged to remove any debris. A vial with the combined standard solution stored in the freezer is allowed to thaw and then thoroughly mixed. A vial with internal standard is thawed and diluted with PBS to a final concentration of 40 μ*M*.
2. Load the SPE vacuum manifold with 20 SPE cartridges (*see* **Note 4**) and put 10-mL plastic tubes in the collection rack.
3. Pipet 0.2 mL of plasma (*see* **Note 5**) or working standard solution into glass tubes. Subsequently add 0.1 mL of the internal standard solution and 0.7 mL of PBS (*see* **Note 6**) to all tubes. Mix the contents of the tubes by vortexing.
4. Load the diluted standards and samples onto the SPE cartridges. Use a clean pipet tip for each sample. Since an internal standard is used, transfer of the sample from the tube to the SPE cartridge does not need to be quantitative, i.e., rinsing of the tubes is not necessary.
5. Apply vacuum to pull the samples through the SPE columns (*see* **Note 7**).
6. Perform a first washing step with 1.0 mL of 100 m*M* HCl.
7. Perform a second washing step with 1.0 mL of methanol.
8. Remove the lid with the SPE cartridges from the vacuum chamber and replace the rack with the waste collection tubes by a rack with glass collection tubes.
9. Elute the basic amino acids with 1.0 mL of freshly prepared elution solvent (methanol/water/ammonia, 50/40/10 by vol).
10. Put the glass tubes with the samples in a heating block set at 40–60°C and dry the samples under a gentle stream of nitrogen gas (*see* **Notes 8** and **9**).

3.3. Derivatization

1. The OPA-MPA derivatization reagent stock solution is freshly prepared on the day of the analysis by dissolving 10 mg of OPA in 0.2 mL of methanol (*see* **Note 10**), followed by addition of 1.8 mL borate buffer (200 m*M* boric acid adjusted to pH 9.5 with potassium hydroxide [*see* **Note 11**]) and 10 μL of 3-mercaptopropionic acid. Just before derivatization, a working reagent solution is made by mixing 1 part of the stock solution with 4 parts of the borate buffer (*see* **Note 12**).
2. Add 0.1 mL of water to the tubes with the dried samples and put the tubes on a vortex mixer. Next, add 0.1 mL of derivatization working reagent and mix by vortexing. Let the samples stand for a few minutes and then vortex again (*see* **Note 13**).
3. Transfer the contents of the tubes to autosampler vials and cap the vials. Put the vials in the refrigerated sample compartment of the autosampler (*see* **Note 14**).

3.4. HPLC Analysis

1. Prepare buffer for mobile phase A (50 m*M* phosphate, pH 6.5) by dissolving 6.80 g potassium dihydrogen phosphate in 980 mL of water and adjusting the pH to 6.5 with potassium hydroxide. After filtration (0.45-μm filter), water is added to a final weight of 1000 g. Then add 74.3 g (95.3 mL) of acetonitrile to obtain a

Table 1
HPLC Gradient Conditions

Time (min)	Flow (mL/min)	Eluent A (%)	Eluent B (%)
0	1.1	100	0
18[a]	1.1	100	0
19	1.1	50	50
22	1.1	50	50
23	1.1	100	0
30[b]	1.1	100	0
35	1.1	100	0
36	1.1	0	100
50	1.1	0	100
51	0.0	0	100

[a]The gradient sequence between 18 and 23 min occurs after elution of the last analyte and serves as a strong solvent wash to elute strongly retained compounds.

[b]At 30 min a next injection occurs and the program is restarted; the remaining part of the gradient sequence is executed only after analysis of all samples.

final volume percentage of 8.7% (*see* **Note 15**). Mobile phase B is a mixture of water and acetonitrile (50/50).

2. Instrument settings
   a. Gradient conditions are shown in **Table 1** (*see* **Note 16**).
   b. Column oven temperature 30°C.
   c. Sample compartment temperature 4°C.
   d. Injection volume 20 µL.
   e. Analysis time 30 min.
   f. Fluorescence detector: excitation wavelength 340 nm; emission wavelength 455 nm; programmed sensitivity gain switch from 1 to 10 at approx 10 min (*see* **Note 17**).
3. After chromatography all chromatograms are inspected for adequate separation and absence of interfering peaks. Peak area is used to quantify components (*see* **Note 18**). The combined standard, run in duplicate, is used to construct calibration curves, by plotting peak area ratios of analyte over internal standard vs analyte concentration.

3.5. Results

Sample chromatograms of a standard and a plasma sample are shown in **Fig. 3**. Although the protocol as described above was designed for the analysis of plasma samples, it can also be used without modification for the determination of free ADMA in cerebrospinal fluid, tissue culture media, and urine. In the case of urine it may be necessary to dilute the samples, because concentrations of ADMA and SDMA in urine are an order of magnitude higher than in plasma. The method has also been applied for the determination of ADMA in proteins. In that case, protein-bound ADMA is first released by acid hydrolysis. A chromatogram of a hydrolyzed rat kidney homogenate is shown in **Fig. 4.**

4. Notes

1. The molecular mass of both ADMA and SDMA is 202.3 for the free base. The fact that the molecular masses of the salts are much higher (e.g., 758.8 for the di(p-hydroxyazobenzene-p'-sulfonate) salt of SDMA) should be taken into account in preparing standard solutions.
2. The gravimetric preparation of standards with high accuracy requires fairly large amounts of the pure compounds. For the inexpensive arginine this is not problematic. As ADMA and SDMA are rather expensive, it is more convenient to prepare stock solutions of these compounds with approximate concentrations and then determine the actual concentrations by HPLC, using the calibration curve for arginine. This procedure is based on the fact that under isocratic HPLC conditions, the OPA derivatives of ADMA, SDMA, and arginine have the same molar fluorescence response.
3. We use MMA as internal standard, as the endogenous amount of MMA in plasma is very low. For the analysis of other biological materials it is advised to check for the presence of endogenous MMA. The method can also be used for the analysis of MMA; in that case homoarginine can be used as internal standard.
4. We usually analyze series of 40 samples, consisting of the calibration standard and a quality control sample (both in duplicate) and 36 unknown samples. Since the capacity of the vacuum manifold is 20 samples, SPE is performed in two batches of 20 samples.
5. Both heparin and EDTA plasma can be used. If blood collection tubes with a fluid anticoagulant are used, appropriate corrections for sample dilution must be made. Serum can be used for the analysis of ADMA and SDMA, but is not suitable for the analysis of arginine, because arginine is released from platelets during coagulation.
6. The sensitivity of the method is sufficient to allow analysis of plasma volumes down to 0.05 mL. In that case the volume of PBS is increased to keep the final volume at 1 mL.
7. It is not necessary to precondition the SPE cartridges. Adjust the vacuum to achieve a flow rate of approx 1 mL/min during loading and elution steps. For the washing steps a higher flow rate can be used. It is no problem if the columns run dry during one of the steps. To start flow through the dry SPE cartridges it may be necessary to temporarily increase the vacuum.
8. Drying of the samples may take 30–60 min, because of the relatively high water content.
9. If it is not possible to start the HPLC analysis on the same day, the dried samples can be stored at room temperature.

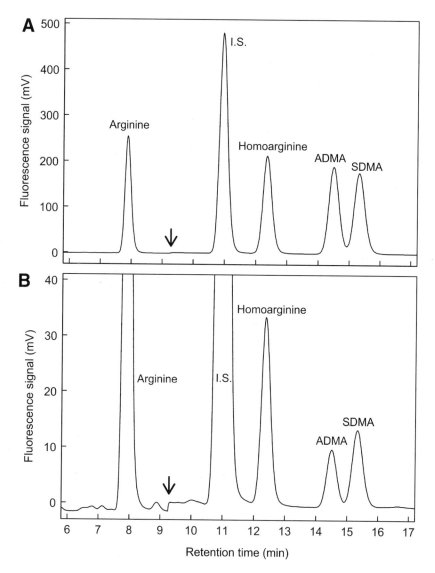

Fig. 3. Chromatograms of a combined standard solution (**A**) and a plasma sample (**B**). The arrow indicates a gain switch of the fluorescence detector (*see* **Note 17**). I.S., internal standard.

10. OPA should give a clear solution in methanol. If the batch of OPA is in use for a long time, it may be that the solution remains turbid. In that case it is time to use a fresh bottle of OPA.

11. Do not confuse boric acid (H_3BO_3) with borax (sodium tetraborate, $Na_2B_4O_7$).

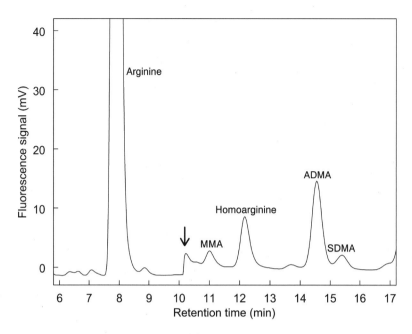

Fig. 4. Chromatogram of a hydrolysate of rat kidney. Renal tissue was homogenized in PBS and hydrolyzed in 6 *M* hydrochloric acid for 16 h at 110°C. The residue obtained after evaporation of the hydrochloric acid was dissolved in PBS and subjected to solid-phase extraction and derivatization as described under **Subheadings 3.2.** and **3.3.**, respectively. The arrow indicates a gain switch of the fluorescence detector (*see* **Note 17**). As no internal standard was added, the MMA peak represents endogenous MMA.

12. The final OPA concentration is sufficient for the analysis of plasma samples. For other sample types (i.e., protein hydrolysates) a higher concentration may be required, to ensure a complete derivatization. Completeness of the derivatization reaction can be assessed by inspection of the peak area of the internal standard (*see* **Note 18**). If a more concentrated working dilution is prepared, it is important to check that the final pH is above 8.0, because the stock solution is acidic due to the presence of mercaptopropionic acid. If complete derivatization cannot be achieved in this way, the amount of sample should be reduced or the volume of the derivatization reagent used in **step 2** should be increased.

13. The derivatization reaction proceeds almost instantaneously at room temperature. This sequence is followed to ensure that the analytes are fully dissolved from the tube's wall.

14. Cooling the samples increases stability of the OPA derivatives. During analysis of a series of 40 samples, peak areas of all components decrease approx 5 to 10%, but this loss of response is fully compensated for by the internal standard. It is possible to reanalyze the derivatized samples within a few days.

15. The retention time of the OPA derivatives depends very critically on the acetoni-

trile content of the mobile phase. Therefore preparation of mobile phase A is performed by weighing buffer and acetonitrile, which gives better accuracy and precision than can be obtained by using volumetric glassware.

16. Arginine, ADMA, and SDMA are eluted under isocratic conditions. The gradient starts after elution of SDMA and merely serves to elute strongly retained compounds from the column. If different HPLC equipment is used or if late-eluting peaks show up in subsequent chromatograms, it may be necessary to adapt the gradient, i.e., prolong the washing step or use a higher percentage of mobile phase B.

17. This programmed gain switch occurs between elution of arginine and the internal standard. For the analysis of plasma it is necessary, as the concentration of arginine is approximately 100–200-fold higher than the concentrations of ADMA and SDMA.

18. Peak area of the internal standard should approximately be the same for all samples. A low internal standard peak area may be indicative for several problems, e.g., pipetting errors, autosampler malfunctioning, or incomplete derivatization.

Acknowledgment

I thank Sigrid de Jong for her important role in fine-tuning of the method and for analyzing many hundreds of samples.

References

1. Andrew, P. J. and Mayer, B. (1999) Enzymatic function of nitric oxide synthases. *Cardiovasc. Res.* **43,** 521–531.
2. Vallance, P., Leone, A., Calver, A., Collier, J., and Moncada, S. (1992) Accumulation of an endogenous inhibitor of nitric oxide synthesis in chronic renal failure. *Lancet* **339,** 572–575.
3. Matsuoka, H., Itoh, S., Kimoto, M., et al. (1997) Asymmetrical dimethylarginine, an endogenous nitric oxide synthase inhibitor, in experimental hypertension. *Hypertension* **29,** 242–247.
4. Surdacki, A., Nowicki, M., Sandmann, J., et al. (1999) Reduced urinary excretion of nitric oxide metabolites and increased plasma levels of asymmetric dimethylarginine in men with essential hypertension. *J. Cardiovasc. Pharmacol.* **33,** 652–658.
5. Päivä, H., Laakso, J., Laine, H., Laaksonen, R., Knuuti, J., and Raitakari, O. T. (2002) Plasma asymmetric dimethylarginine and hyperemic myocardial blood flow in young subjects with borderline hypertension or familial hypercholesterolemia. *J. Am. Coll. Cardiol.* **40,** 1241–1247.
6. Kielstein, J. T., Bode-Böger, S. M., Frölich, J. C., Ritz, E., Haller, H., and Fliser, D. (2003) Asymmetric dimethylarginine, blood pressure, and renal perfusion in elderly subjects. *Circulation* **107,** 1891–1895.
7. Vallance, P. (2001) Importance of asymmetrical dimethylarginine in cardiovascular risk. *Lancet* **358,** 2096–2097.
8. Böger, R. H., Bode-Böger, S. M., Szuba, A., et al. (1998) Asymmetric

dimethylarginine (ADMA): a novel risk factor for endothelial dysfunction. Its role in hypercholesterolemia. *Circulation* **98**, 1842–1847.

9. Miyazaki, H., Matsuoka, H., Cooke, J. P., et al. (1999) Endogenous nitric oxide synthase inhibitor: a novel marker of atherosclerosis. *Circulation* **99**, 1141–1146.

10. Valkonen, V. P., Päivä, H., Salonen, J. T., et al. (2001) Risk of acute coronary events and serum concentration of asymmetrical dimethylarginine. *Lancet* **358**, 2127–2128.

11. Zoccali, C., Bode-Böger, S. M., Mallamaci, F., et al. (2001) Plasma concentration of asymmetrical dimethylarginine and mortality in patients with end-stage renal disease: a prospective study. *Lancet* **358**, 2113–2117.

12. Nijveldt, R. J., Teerlink, T., van der Hoven, B., et al. (2003) Asymmetrical dimethylarginine (ADMA) in critically ill patients: high plasma ADMA concentration is an independent risk factor of ICU mortality. *Clin. Nutr.* **22**, 23–30.

13. Gary, J. D. and Clarke, S. (1998) RNA and protein interactions modulated by protein arginine methylation. *Prog. Nucleic Acid Res. Mol. Biol.* **61**, 65–131.

14. Leiper, J. M., Santa Maria, J., Chubb, A., et al. (1999) Identification of two human dimethylarginine dimethylaminohydrolases with distinct tissue distributions and homology with microbial arginine deiminases. *Biochem. J.* **343**, 209–214.

15. Ogawa, T., Kimoto, M., and Sasaoka, K. (1989) Purification and properties of a new enzyme, N^G,N^G-dimethylarginine dimethylaminohydrolase, from rat kidney. *J. Biol. Chem.* **264**, 10205–10209.

16. Teerlink, T., Nijveldt, R. J., de Jong, S., and van Leeuwen, P. A. (2002) Determination of arginine, asymmetric dimethylarginine, and symmetric dimethylarginine in human plasma and other biological samples by high-performance liquid chromatography. *Anal. Biochem.* **303**, 131–137.

17. Mulder, C., Wahlund, L. O., Blomberg, M., et al. (2002) Alzheimer's disease is not associated with altered concentrations of the nitric oxide synthase inhibitor asymmetric dimethylarginine in cerebrospinal fluid. *J. Neural Transm.* **109**, 1203–1208.

18. Nijveldt, R. J., van Leeuwen, P. A., van Guldener, C., Stehouwer, C. D., Rauwerda, J. A., and Teerlink, T. (2002) Net renal extraction of asymmetrical (ADMA) and symmetrical (SDMA) dimethylarginine in fasting humans. *Nephrol. Dial. Transplant.* **17**, 1999–2002.

19. Teerlink, T., Neele, S. J., de Jong, S., Netelenbos, J. C., and Stehouwer, C. D. (2003) Oestrogen replacement therapy lowers plasma levels of asymmetrical dimethylarginine in healthy postmenopausal women. *Clin. Sci.* **105**, 67–71.

20. Post, M. S., Verhoeven, M. O., van der Mooren, M. J., Kenemans, P., Stehouwer, C. D. A., and Teerlink, T. (2003) Effect of hormone replacement therapy on plasma levels of the cardiovascular risk factor asymmetric dimethylarginine: a randomized, placebo-controlled 12-week study in healthy early postmenopausal women. *J. Clin. Endocrinol. Metab.* **88**, 4221–4226.

19

Proteomic Approaches in the Analysis of Hypertension

Soren Naaby-Hansen, Gayathri D. Warnasuriya, Claire Hastie, Piers Gallney, and Rainer Cramer

Summary

The completion of the genomic sequence and the definition of the genes provide a wealth of data to interpret cellular protein expression patterns and relate them to protein function. Proteomics is the large-scale study of proteins in the post-genomic era, aimed at identifying and characterizing protein expression, function, posttranslational modification, regulation, trafficking, interaction and structure, and their perturbation by disease and drug action. The multigenetic background and essentially unknown etiology of hypertension, makes this main killer a prime candidate for proteomic analysis. The classical proteomic approaches are based on two-dimensional gel electrophoretic protein separation and their subsequent identification and characterization by mass spectrometry analysis. However, expression level analysis may not reflect the functional state of proteins and is biased towards long-lived abundant proteins. This review describes a variety of techniques that can be used to identify low-abundance proteins that may be of more functional interest. The modification of classical two-dimensional electrophoresis in order to study post-translational modifications, e.g., phosphorylation, is also discussed.

Key Words: Proteomics; two-dimensional electrophoresis (2-DE); mass spectrometry; difference gel electrophoresis (DIGE); cell surface/metabolic labeling; phosphorylation; cell signalling.

1. Introduction

High-throughput DNA analysis has generated a wealth of information on predicted gene products and resulted in databases containing the complete genome sequences from several organisms. However, a comprehensive functional interpretation of this huge amount of nucleic acid sequence data remains. The major challenges of the postgenomic era are understanding gene function and the regulatory perturbations induced by disease.

Transcriptomics allows a global, quantitative analysis of gene expression by measuring the mRNA transcribed by the genome at a given time. An integrated view of the gene activation patterns at different cellular states can thus be

From: *Methods in Molecular Medicine, Vol. 108: Hypertension: Methods and Protocols*
Edited by: J. P. Fennell and A. H. Baker © Humana Press Inc., Totowa, NJ

achieved by comparative transcriptomic analysis. However, protein isoforms generated by posttranscriptional mRNA splicing or by posttranslational modifications of proteins cannot be predicted from a nucleic acid sequence or from mRNA transcript levels. Temporal differences between gene transcription and translation, as well as differential stability and turnover rates of mRNA and proteins, may also participate in the observed lack of correlation between mRNA transcript levels and protein expression levels *(1)*.

To achieve a correct annotation of gene functions, transcriptional profiling must be complemented by other approaches, which allows the expression and activity levels of the gene products, i.e., the proteins, to be profiled. Proteomics is the large-scale study of proteins, aimed at identifying and characterizing all proteins expressed by an organism or in a tissue. This can lead to elucidation of the complex patterns of regulatory networks that lead to activation of the genes and determine activation, interactions, and compartmentalization of their products. Proteomics originates from the term *proteome*, a linguistic analog to *genome*, defined as the entire protein complement expressed by a genome or by a cell or tissue type *(2)*.

Proteomics dates back to the late 1970s, when a small number of laboratories started to build databases of protein expression profiles, employing the newly developed technique of two-dimensional gel electrophoresis (2-DE). The key steps in classical proteomics are the separation of proteins in a sample by 2-DE and their subsequent quantitation and identification. However, a proteins expression level may not reflect its functional state, and protein profiling provides no data regarding a protein's subcellular site of action or its interaction partners, which is why the focus of modern proteomics has broadened considerably to include these basic aspects of cell biology. Blackstock and Weir recently suggested terms to discern two related but distinct forms of proteomics, namely, "expression proteomics" and "cell-map proteomics" *(3)*. Expression proteomics aims to generate quantitative maps of protein expression levels, akin to EST maps, whereas cell-map proteomics generates "physical maps" of the functional cellular machines, i.e., the protein complexes, by their systematic isolation, identification, characterization, and localization. Protein interaction studies may employ surface plasmon resonance (Biacore™) technology, two-hybrid screening *(4)*, or phage display *(5)* methods, whereas multiprotein complexes can be isolated by affinity purification utilizing gene tagging, fusion proteins, antibodies, peptides, DNA, RNA, or small targeting molecules as bait *(6)*. Whereas expression proteomic approaches have relied almost entirely on 2-DE-generated maps in the past, more sensitive methods for quantitative analysis of proteins in complex mixtures, which omit sample separation by gel electrophoresis, are currently under development in many laboratories. Chemical derivatization of specific amino acid residues in the samples proteins or peptides, before separation by multidimensional liquid chromatography (MDLC) and mass spectrometry (MS) analysis, is one such approach, which hold the promise of true global coverage of all the proteins in the sample.

By focusing on the functional products of the genome, proteomics provides an indispensable complement to genomics. The proteins are ultimately responsible for all processes that take place within a cell, and the mechanism of action of the vast majority of drugs are mediated through proteins. Only 2% of diseases are believed to be monogenic *(7)*, so the major challenge now is to understand how the regulatory networks of proteins are related and lead to the other 98% of diseases *(8)*. Proteomics holds great promise for the field of cardiovascular biology; benefits will include the identification of marker proteins, dissection of signaling pathways affected by the underlying perturbation, and drug-target identification and validation.

In this chapter we will focus on a few examples of how the powerful combination of two-dimensional gel electrophoresis (for a technical review, *see* **ref. 9**), bioinformatics, and mass spectrometry analysis can be applied in the study of hypertension.

1.1. Protein Expression Analysis

Protein expression-level comparison (differential display of expression) is the classical example of how 2-DE-based proteomics can be employed in the study of the pathophysiological effects of hypertension. Usually, extracts of normal and pathological tissues (biological fluids or tissue biopsies) are separated by 2-DE, visualized, and subjected to quantitative computer comparison. Differentially expressed proteins are subsequently cored from the gels and identified by MS analysis and database searches. Such 2-D gel-based approaches have been used extensively to study the expression of human heart proteins and their perturbations by disease *(10)*.

However, routine broad-pH-range 2-DE analysis of complex mixtures such as total cell or tissue extracts is biased toward long-lived, abundant proteins *(11)*. Low-abundance proteins (which could functionally be the most interesting) tend to be masked by housekeeping proteins present at several orders of magnitude higher abundance and become invisible due to sensitivity detection limits and spot overlapping. Differentially expressed cytoskeletal proteins will consequently dominate a comparison of morphologically distinct cell lines. Sample handling, separation, and detection methods must therefore be modified, to ensure biological relevance of "expression proteomic" analysis of cell lines.

Sample prefractionation techniques (sequential extraction, subcellular fractionation, or prefractionation based on different physiochemical properties) aim to reduce the diversity and complexity of protein mixtures, thus increasing the number and concentration of distinct subsets of proteins that can be resolved in a series of complementary narrow-pH-range 2-D gels. This approach increases the number of features that can be separated and should be combined with sensitive, MS-compatible detection methods such as silver staining, metal chelate stains, or fluorescence dye staining for optimal analysis of complex samples.

Fluorescent dyes offer a broader dynamic and linear quantitative range of detection than silver staining (*see* **ref. *12*** for review). Proteins can be covalently derivatized with fluorophores before separation or subjected to postelectrophoretic staining with fluorescence dyes. **Figure 1A** demonstrates prelabeling of free cysteine residues in nonreduced extracts of cultured prostate cells. Triton X-100 extracts of a tumor cell line derived from a primary adenocarcinoma and of a cell line generated from autologous benign epithelium *(13)* were labeled with 15 mM of an iodoacetamide derivate of Cy3, for 30 min at 30°C. Unreacted fluorophore was removed from the sample by centricon centrifugation (5000 daltons molecular cutoff weight). The proteins were subsequently dialysed against H_2O overnight, speed vacuum concentrated, and dissolved in reducing 2-DE lysis buffer before being separated by 2-D gel electrophoresis.

Difference gel electrophoresis (DIGE), in which two or three samples labeled with different fluorescence probes can be run in a single 2-DE gel, offers the opportunity of direct comparison of different samples, thus avoiding gel-to-gel variations inherent to comparative gel analysis *(14)*. The currently available commercial dyes for DIGE were first reported by John Minden and colleagues *(15)* and are built around the relatively photobleaching-resistant Cy3 and Cy5 dye cores. In our hands the original one-pot preparative procedures proved extremely unreliable, but pure samples of both dyes could be obtained with some modification of the conditions and, at each stage, separation from byproducts of the desired intermediates. The fluorophores of the Cy3 and Cy5 cores are very similar, but differ in the length of their central $(CH)_3$ and $(CH)_5$

Fig. 1. Comparison of protein expression levels in immortalized normal and adenocarcinoma cell lines derived from the same patient *(13)*. (**A**) Comparison of proteins levels following Cy3-labeling of free cysteine residues (A_1 and A_2). Proteins were separated by carrier ampholyte-based IEF/PAGE. The gels were stained with zinc *(9)* (A_3 and A_4), after the fluorescence-labeled proteins had been visualized by laser scanning. This procedure stains the gel but leaves the protein containing areas transparent and unstained, and the scanned gel image was reversed using Adobe Photoshop software. The horizontal arrow shows a protein labeled with the cysteine-reactive dye in normal but not in cancer cells. Interesting, this protein migrates as would be expected of the lipid phosphatase PTEN, which is frequently mutated or deleted in cancers. Phosphatases are among the expected targets for cysteine-directed affinity labels. Note

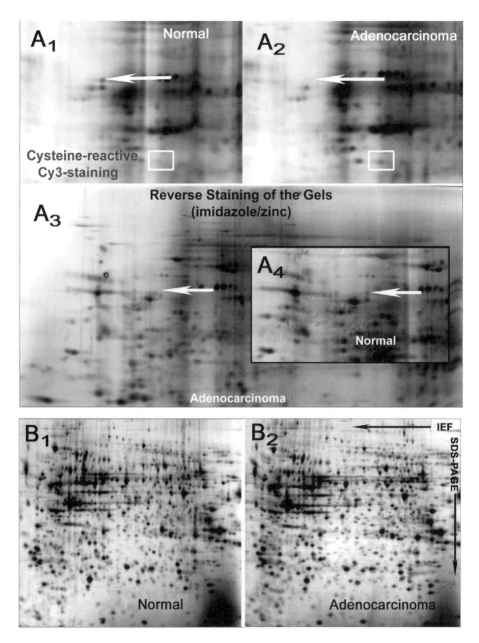

Fig. 1. (*continued*) that the differential labeled protein is also absent from the zinc-stained gel image, in accordance with it being downregulated or deleted in the tumor cells. (**B**) Comparison of the same two cell lines by postseparational fluorescence staining. Proteins were separated by immobilized pH gradient-based 2-DE, employing nonlinear broad-pH-range strips (pH 3.0–10.0). More than 1300 protein spots were matched on the two images using Melanie software.

poly-methine chains, respectively. This difference in size is compensated for by replacing a methyl in the Cy5 derivative with a propyl in the Cy3. Thus, these matched dyes are nearly the same size and proteins labeled with either have nearly identical electrophoretic mobilities.

Because some proteins that are likely to be of interest in hypertension have low cellular abundances, one would prefer to label all accessible reactive residues to maximize sensitivity. Saturation labeling of lysine, with an average occurrence of 5.8% among protein sequences, at first appears a reasonable choice, and the dyes of Minden et al. are N-hydroxysuccinimide esters, which react readily with primarily amines. However, such a large degree of labeling interferes with the physical properties of tagged proteins, as well as tryptic digestion, so that in practice minimal labeling is necessary, in which just one in six proteins is cross-linked to a single dye molecule. Apart from the loss in sensitivity, this has an additional disadvantage in that the detectable-labeled protein spot does not necessarily exactly coincide with the prevalent unlabeled protein. Consequently, a post-DIGE stain is still required to visualize the bulk of the protein before coring and subsequent MS analysis.

Saturation labeling of cystine residues, which have an occurrence of only 1.8%, might be expected to circumvent the difficulties inherent in saturation lysine labeling for DIGE. To this end, we have synthesized propyl-Cy3 and methyl-Cy5 dyes in which the carboxylate moities of the original lysine-reactive dyes have been replaced with a primary amine that may be readily converted to cystine-reactive iodoacetamides, or more selective maleimides. Initial experiments show much promise, with the expected gains in sensitivity. Additionally, cystine-reactive dyes target significantly different protein populations to lysine labeling and the populations sampled can be further selected depending on whether or not a reducing agent is included in the labeling protocol. However, saturation labeling amplifies small differences between Cy3- and Cy5-derivatized proteins so that a significant number, if still the minority, of paired spots do not exactly overlap, complicating the analysis.

Several dyes are available for noncovalent fluorescence staining of proteins following electrophoretic separation (12). **Figure 1B** demonstrates a classical expression-level comparison between total cell extracts from the same two cell lines as were used in **Fig. 1A**. More than 1300 proteins were visualized by post-separational staining with an analog of SYPRO dyes, which is intercalated into SDS micelles (14). This type of staining offers detection sensitivity competitive with silver staining and is compatible with downstream MS analysis. However, as some proteins may be detected by one procedure but not the other and vice versa, the most complete 2-D map is generally achieved by the computer-assisted assembly of images obtained from several staining and labeling techniques.

As mentioned earlier, difference gel electrophoresis offers the opportunity of direct comparison of different samples, thus avoiding gel-to-gel variations inherent to comparative gel analysis. However, as both carrier ampholyte-based isoelectric focusing gels and immobilized pH gradient gels (IPG strips) have practical thresholds for protein loads, above which loss of buffering capacity leads to spot fusion and comigration, the sensitivity of the DIGE technique becomes inferior to the one-sample, one-gel approach.

Non-gel separation techniques such as multidimensional liquid chromatography and the isotope-coded affinity tag (ICAT) method *(16)* are currently being optimized for large-scale proteomic application to circumvent the problems associated with gel electrophoresis. These techniques further increase the compatibility of the sample for mass spectrometry analysis, resulting in less discrimination of proteins, which are difficult to analyze on/from gels. Isotope labeling or chemical derivatization of peptides generated by enzymatic digestion of samples also enables quantification via mass spectrometry and can therefore be used for the proteins which are differentially expressed.

1.2. Cell Surface Labeling

The most desirable disease markers are present in easy accessible biological fluids and are expressed on the surface of the transformed cells. Several methods are available for more or less specific labeling of cell surface components.

Vectorial surface labeling can be achieved by chemical incorporation of radioisotopes (such as ^{125}I or ^{3}H) in the core of the protein or its carbohydrate or lipid side chain(s) *(17,18)*. A less hazardous and thus more desirable approach than performing vectorial radiolabeling is to derivatize surface proteins with fluorophores, biotin, or, even better, with compounds possessing properties for both peptide quantification and affinity purification, such as isotope-coded affinity tagging *(16)*. The latter method, which involves a deuterated biotin derivative, has been successfully combined with whole-cell trypsination, avidin-bead precipitation of the tagged peptides, and MS analysis.

Proteins expressed on the surface of the targeted cells can similarly be labeled with the water-soluble, cell-impermeable biotin analog sulfo-NHS-LC-biotin. Biotinylated proteins can then be visualized by blotting with enzyme-conjugated avidin or concentrated for further analysis via affinity chromatographic purification. Combined with final separation by SDS-PAGE or liquid chromatography (LC), the latter approach enables transmembrane surface proteins to be quantitated, identified, and their modifications characterized, and provides a valuable method to study their regulation by external signals (unpublished data). **Figure 2** shows the technique employed to demonstrate upregulated density of surface proteins in response to long-term interferon treatment. The number of surface-exposed proteins that can be labeled with biotin usually comprise less than 10% of the number of proteins that can be stained with silver or flourophobes. However, such interpretation based on spot numbers alone must be taken with caution, as only approx 60–70% of proteins readily stain with silver *(19)* and hydrophobic proteins are underrepresented in 2-D gels *(20)*. The latter tend to be aggregated when IPG strips are employed for first-dimensional separation, compared to gels in which the proteins were initially separated by carrier ampholyte-based isoelectric focusing in tube gels. The latter approach enables separation and detection of at least some integral membrane proteins on 2-D gels (unpublished data). Interpretation of the protein patterns are further complicated by the negative charge of the sulfo group in sulfo-NHS-LC-biotin. Multiple forms of a protein migrating at distinct horizontal positions can be generated by both posttranslational modifications (i.e., glycosylation or phosphorylation) and by biotin labelling. If a protein possesses multiple lysine groups accessible for NHS biotinylation, labeling will produce charge trains, in which each form represents a protein with a different number of sulfo-biotin molecules attached (suspected examples are enclosed in black in **Fig. 2**).

Nevertheless, by careful analysis and critical interpretations, 2-DE-based proteomics can be successfully employed to identify putative cell surface markers and to study the regulation of peripheral attached membrane proteins, including GPI-anchored proteins.

1.3. Metabolic Labeling

The effect of biological stimuli and/or drug action on the synthesis of proteins and their posttranslational modifications can be studied by metabolic radiolabeling strategies, employing isotope-labeled precursors (e.g., amino acid, monosaccharide, or lipid) or [$^{32/33}$P]-orthophosphate. In combination with 2-DE and quantitative computer analysis, such approaches can reveal important differences between the patterns of coordinate regulation in normal and diseased cells, and provide a valuable method for drug mode-of-action studies.

The effect of long-term interferon gamma (IFN-γ) stimulation on epithelial protein synthesis was studied (**Fig. 3**). Metabolic labeling with [^{35}S]-methionine/cysteine for various time periods in the presence or absence of IFN-γ was used to monitor protein synthesis. IFN-γ stimulation of the epithelial cell line resulted in changes in both the rate of protein synthesis (as judged by the amount of radioisotopes incorporated in the two samples) and posttranslational modifications of the newly synthesized proteins (examples are boxed in white in **Fig. 3**). The synthesis of a protein with molecular weight of 61 kDa and pI of 4.2 was increased by long-term stimulation with IFN-γ. The protein spot was cored from a fluorescence stained semi-preparative 2-D gel and identified as calreticulin by MS analysis (see below).

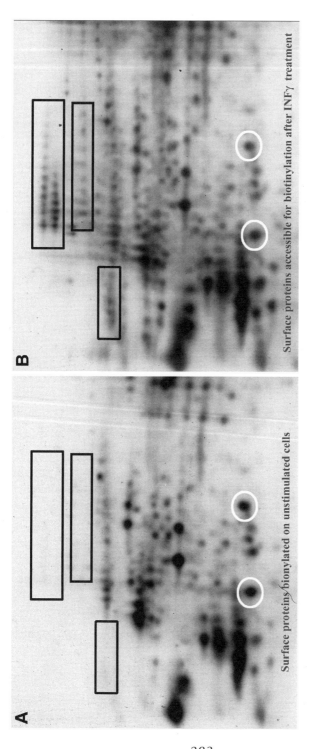

Surface proteins accessible for biotinylation after INFγ treatment

B

Surface proteins bionylated on unstimulated cells

A

Fig. 2. Biotinylated cell surface proteins detected by avidin blotting following 2-D gel electrophoresis. Exposure to INF-γ for 72 h leads to an increase in the density of several surface proteins (examples highlighted by black rectangles), while other proteins were downregulated (encircled in white). The charge trains seen in the black rectangles may be generated by posttranslational modifications of the proteins (e.g., glycosylation terminated by polysialic acids or multiple phosphorylation sites being activated) or may be artifactual due to polybiotinylation (*see* text for details).

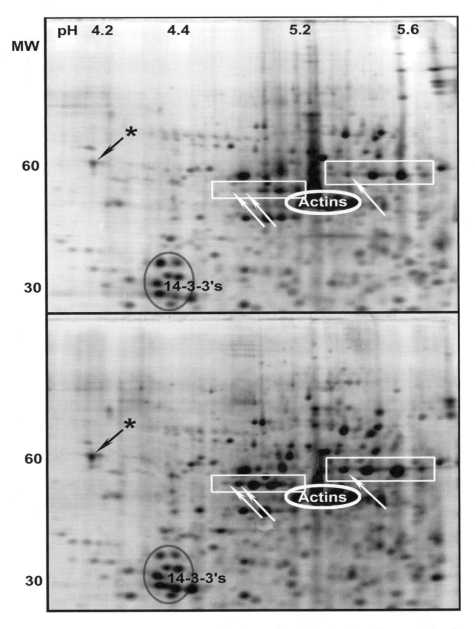

Fig. 3. Analysis of interferon-γ regulated protein synthesis. Proteins were visualized by 2D autoradiography following biosynthetic labeling with [^{35}S]-methionine/cysteine for 18 h, in the absence of stimuli (top) or during continuous stimulation with IFN-γ (500 U/mL) (bottom). The positions of actins and 14-3-3 proteins are circled. Note the increased synthesis rates of several 14-3-3 forms in response to INF-γ. The

Calreticulin is the major Ca^{2+}-binding/storage protein in the endoplasmic reticulum (ER) of a variety of non-muscle cell types, and like the closely related ER chaperone calnexin, calreticulin is a lectin that interacts specifically with partially trimmed, monoglucosylated, *N*-linked oligosaccharides via its P-domain *(21)*. The upregulation of a chaperone involved in ER processing of newly synthesized proteins is hardly surprising, as IFN-γ stimulation resulted in a general increase in protein synthesis in the cultured epithelial cells (compare **Fig. 3A,B**).

1.4. Analysis of Cell Signaling Pathways

The high resolution of 2-DE-based proteomic analysis offers unique opportunities for dissection of the signaling pathways in, for example, myocardial, endothelial, or kidney cells, and for studies of their perturbations by disease and drug actions. Epidermal growth factor-induced changes of the phosphoprotein population can thus be visualized by [$^{32/33}$P]orthophosphate labeling (**Fig. 4A**), by blotting with mAbs to specific phosphoresidues (**Fig. 4B**), or by the changes in migration patterns, which are induced by phosphatase treatment of the samples. Phosphorylation results in a more acidic migration pattern, which can easily be demonstrated by immunoblotting with antibodies to the modified protein (**Fig. 4C**). Computer-assisted analysis of changes in the global phosphosignaling activity, visualized by orthophosphate labeling and immunoblotting with phosphoresidue-specific antibodies, also provides a highly efficient method for detailed mode-of-action analysis of therapeutic compounds.

1.5. Protein Identification by Mass Spectrometry

Although 2-DE separates proteins with high resolution, it is practically impossible to identify proteins from 2-DE gel spots just by their position on the gel. Protein modification and degradation can lead to substantial gel spot shifts in both dimensions. Another practical limitation is the physical size of gels and gel spots. On a standard 2-DE gel, less than 12,000 spots can theoretically be resolved (gel size of 180 mm × 200 mm and an average spot size of 2 mm diameter). However, there are about 30,000 predicted human genes, plus two

---

Fig. 3. (*continued*) protein indicated by an oblique black arrow and asterisk was excised and subjected to mass spectrometry analysis (*see* **Fig. 5**). White oblique arrows indicate examples of acidic isoforms generated by IFN-γ-induced phosphorylation of the newly synthesized proteins. The unaltered protein forms migrate at the right end of the charge trains enclosed by white rectangles.

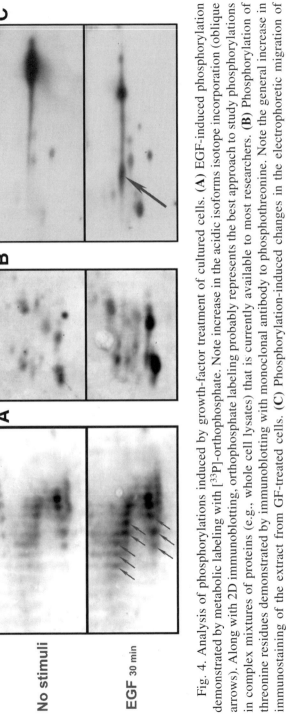

Fig. 4. Analysis of phosphorylations induced by growth-factor treatment of cultured cells. (**A**) EGF-induced phosphorylation demonstrated by metabolic labeling with [^{33}P]-orthophosphate. Note increase in the acidic isoforms isotope incorporation (oblique arrows). Along with 2D immunoblotting, orthophosphate labeling probably represents the best approach to study phosphorylations in complex mixtures of proteins (e.g., whole cell lysates) that is currently available to most researchers. (**B**) Phosphorylation of threonine residues demonstrated by immunoblotting with monoclonal antibody to phosphothreonine. Note the general increase in immunostaining of the extract from GF-treated cells. (**C**) Phosphorylation-induced changes in the electrophoretic migration of ERK1 demonstrated by 2D immunoblotting. Note the shift toward the acidic end of the gel in response to EGF-regulated phosphoactivation of the kinase (arrow).

No stimuli

EGF 30 min

286

to four times as many splice variants. Including their posttranslational modifications and degradation products, it becomes quite obvious that subsequent analyses have to be carried out to identify 2-DE-separated human proteins. The technique widely recognized to be best for this task is mass spectrometry *(6,11,22,23)*.

Mass spectrometric analysis can be extremely accurate, sensitive, and fast. In a time-of-flight (TOF) mass spectrometer the primary analysis time is less than 1 ms for even large macromolecules (> 100,000 kDa). High analytical sensitivity has been demonstrated on zeptomole amounts of sample *(24,25)*, although for 2-DE gel spot analysis realistic sensitivity limits are around the low femtomole level *(26)*. It has recently been reported that mass spectrometric sensitivity exceeds the analytical sensitivity of silver staining *(27)*. Equally important to sensitivity is its mass measurement accuracy *(11,28)* of usually 5–200 ppm for low-mass (< 5-kDa) analysis, leading to an extremely high confidence in protein identification by techniques such as peptide mass mapping (PMM) using peptide mass fingerprints from MS experiments and peptide sequencing using peptide fragmentation mass spectra from tandem mass spectrometry (MS/MS) experiments *(6,11)*.

In proteomics, mass spectrometric analysis is dominated by two ionization techniques: matrix-assisted laser desorption/ionization (MALDI) MS *(29)* and electrospray ionization (ESI) MS *(30,31)*. Because of their distinct sample desorption/ionization mechanisms these two ionization techniques are usually interfaced to rather different sample introduction systems and mass analyzers. For high-throughput protein identification from 2-DE gel spots, PMM by MALDI TOF MS is unchallenged, because of its speed and simplicity. However, higher confidence in protein identification can be achieved by employing MS/MS to obtain sequence information by peptide-ion fragmentation. The fragmentation method usually employed is low-energy collision-induced dissociation (CID), and coupled with ESI this method has been most widely established for MS/MS peptide sequencing.

The vast majority of identification strategies by MS are based on the analysis of proteolytic peptides, because the direct analysis of proteins by mass spectrometry is generally unfavorable due to severe limitation in several key areas such as detection, resolution, and fragmentation. Protein heterogeneity due to modifications and degradation further complicates identification by direct protein analysis. MS analysis of proteolytic products, on the other hand, can be undertaken with higher mass spectrometric performance but without significantly losing information necessary for high-confidence identification.

The strategy used to identify the 2-DE gel spot, which is marked by an asterisk in **Fig. 3**, comprises tryptic in-gel digestion and PMM. For PMM, a MALDI

TOF mass spectrum of the tryptic peptide mixture was acquired (**Fig. 5A**). From this spectrum a peptide ion mass list was compiled and submitted to a database search program (MS-Fit, ProteinProspector, UCSF, http://prospector.ucsf.edu) searching the SWISS-PROT protein database. The in-gel digestion protocol can be found under **Subheading 3.2.1.**, and the search parameters can be obtained from **Fig. 5B**. In this case the masses of 16 peptides of the human protein calreticulin (SWISS-PROT accession number P27797) match peptide-ion masses measured by MALDI TOF MS. These peptides cover 40% of the amino acid sequence. Although 197 entries have been selected by the search shown in **Fig. 4B**, only matches for human calreticulin and its homologs in other species have more than 20% sequence coverage. Together with the number of matching peptide-ion masses, protein identification can be achieved with extremely high confidence. In addition, information obtained from the gel, such as approximate values for molecular weight and pI of the protein, can dramatically increase the accuracy of the search. In the case presented, limiting the molecular-weight range in accordance with a gel molecular-weight measurement accuracy of ±25% results in the selection of the five calreticulin entries only.

In our institute, the majority of all identifications of the main protein in a 2-DE gel spot are obtained with PPM by MALDI TOF MS. The remaining identifications are achieved by ESI MS/MS employing CID and a directly coupled nano-HPLC to the ion source for online sample purification and concentration. Usually, 0.5 µL of the tryptic in-gel digest mixture is used for MALDI TOF MS, leaving 4.5 µL for further analysis such as ESI MS/MS. The routine sensitivity for protein identification lies in the low femtomole range of sample loaded on a 2-DE gel.

1.6. Summary

Currently, two-dimensional gel electrophoresis is the only well-established technique that can deliver fast, qualitative, and quantitative analysis of com-

---

Fig. 5. (*opposite page*) Protein identification by peptide mass mapping of the gel spot sample marked by a star in **Fig. 3**. (**A**) MALDI MS tryptic peptide mass fingerprint from the in-gel digest. (**B**) Database search results using the 55 monoisotopic masses of the most intense unknown isotope-resolved-ion signals in (A). Tryptic peptide-ion signals matching peptide masses of human calreticulin (SWISS-PROT accession number P27797) are marked with a circle. Trypsin autolysis product ion signals are marked with T. The spectrum is internally calibrated using the two protonated trypsin autolysis products at the monoisotopic m/z 842.5100 and 2211.1046. The search engine MS-FIT (ProteinProspector, UCSF, http://prospector.ucsf.edu) was used for database searching.

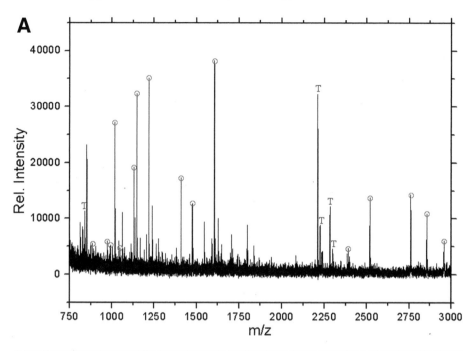

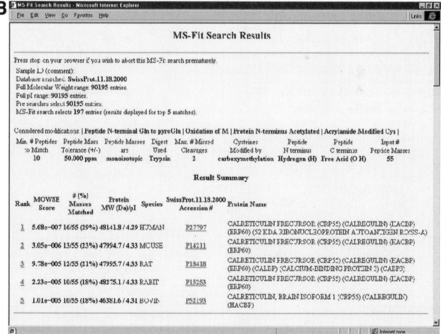

plex protein distributions in combination with parallel protein purification. However, 2-DE is not only applicable to study steady-state expression level differences, but can be employed in studies of dynamic cellular events to gain full potential of the technique.

The use of 2-DE in combination with specific labeling techniques and subcellular fractionation enables detailed studies of spatio-temporal cellular changes such as signal transduction pathways and translocation processes as well as their perturbations by disease and drug treatment.

In proteomics, particularly in global proteome mapping, mass spectrometry is so far the only technique that is sensitive, accurate, and fast enough to cope with the future challenges for large-scale protein identification. In addition, mass spectrometry can also provide structural information for further characterization of proteins and their modifications such as phosphorylation and glycosylation. Bioinformatic integration of data from such versatile, conditional studies combined with data obtained by cell-map proteomics and by transcriptomic analysis will hopefully lead to a more comprehensive understanding of the etiology and to new approaches in diagnosis, prevention, and treatment of hypertension.

2. Materials

2.1. Metabolic Labeling Protocols

2.1.1. Long-Term Biosynthetic Labeling of Methionine- and Cysteine-Containing Proteins

1. Labeling medium: 90% methionine/cysteine-free Dulbecco's modified Eagle's medium (DMEM), 10% DMEM with 0.2 mCi/mL Promix (Amersham).
2. Lyses buffer: 8 M urea, 2 M thiourea, 4% CHAPS, 65 mM dithiothreitol (DTT), protease inhibitors (e.g., Cocktail tablets from Boehringer Mannheim) and phosphate inhibitors (1 µM Okadaic acid, Fenvalerate, and bpVphen).

2.1.2. Labeling of Phosphoproteins

1. Sodium phosphate-free DMEM.
2. Fatty acid-free bovine serum albumin (BSA).
3. ^{33}P-orthophosphate (NEN).
4. Recombinant growth factor (EGF).
5. Phosphate-buffered saline (PBS).
6. Fetal calf serum (FCS).

2.1.3. Biotinylation of Surface Proteins on Cultured Cells Grown in Monolayer

1. Dulbecco's PBS.
2. Sulfo-HNS-LC-biotin (Pierce).
3. NH$_4$Cl.

2.2. Protein Identification by Mass Spectrometry

2.2.1. In-Gel Digestion

All solvents are HPLC-grade from Rathburn, Walkerburn, UK.
1. DTT from Pierce, Rockford, IL.
2. Iodoacetic acid (IAA) from Sigma, Poole, UK.
3. Modified trypsin (Promega, Southampton, UK).
4. SlickSeal tube (hydrophobic tubes, Bioquote Ltd, York, UK).
5. Prepare the following solutions:
    a. 25 m*M* Ammonium bicarbonate (ABC)/50% acetonitrile (ACN) in water.
    b. 10 m*M* DTT/25 m*M* ABC in water.
    c. 50 m*M* IAA/25 m*M* ABC in water.
    d. 25 m*M* ABC in water.
    e. 50% ACN/5% trifluoroacetic acid (TFA).

2.2.2. MALDI Sample Preparation and Analysis

1. HPLC-grade water (Rathburn, Walkerburn, UK).
2. 2,5-Dihydroxybenzoic acid (DHB) from Aldrich, Gillingham, UK.

3. Methods

All procedures should be optimized according to cell line/tissue and experimental design. You may benefit from extensive piloting with one-dimensional gels, especially in time-course studies and pulse-chase experiments.

3.1. Metabolic Labeling Protocols

3.1.1. Long-Term Biosynthetic Labeling of Methionine- and Cysteine-Containing Proteins

The protocol employed for biosynthetic labelling of proteins is essentially identical to the classical long-term ^{35}S-labeling procedure, published by numerous authors, including Patterson and Garrels *(32)*.

1. Remove culture medium by aspiration and wash twice in methionine/cysteine-free DMEM, leave cells in this medium for 15 min at 37°C in a 5% CO_2 incubator.
2. Aspirate the medium off and incubate in labeling medium for 18 hr with or without cytokines. Use 4 mL of medium per 10-cm dish and 7.5 mL per 15-cm dish.
3. Remove the medium and wash twice with plain PBS. Remove washing medium thoroughly by aspiration.
4. Add lysis buffer (minimum 400 µL for 10-cm dish and 600 µL for 15-cm dish) and scrape cells (you may perform this and the following steps cold [on ice]).
5. Pass the mixture through a 25-gage needle several times and then centrifuge at 20,000*g* for 10 min to pellet nonsolubilized material.
6. Remove aliquot for determination of protein concentration (e.g., by Bradford) and snap-freeze sample.

3.1.2. Labeling of Phosphoproteins

1. Synchronize cells by serum starvation overnight (if possible). Use the same confluency throughout experimental series, as this influences signaling in most cell types grown in monolayer.
2. Wash cells twice in sodium phosphate-free DMEM plus 0.1% FCS and incubate for 30 min in this buffer.
3. Initiate labeling by adding ^{33}P-orthophosphate (100 μCi/mL) to the sodium phosphate-free medium for 1–6 h (optimize according to cell line and experimental design).
4. Stimulate (or sham-stimulate) cells with growth factor (optimal concentration should be determined experimentally for each cell line) for variable periods at 37°C (e.g., start with 5, 10, 20, 30, and 60 min).
5. Remove medium by aspiration.
6. Lyse cells on ice as described under **Subheading 3.1.1.** Leave sample on ice and perform quick Bradford analysis.
7. Phosphoproteins should be separated immediately following determination of protein concentration (to avoid loss of labile sites). We find separation by carrier ampholyte IEF to be superior to immobilized pH gradients for this type of analysis.

Radioisotope incorporation can be determined following TCA precipitation of the sample as described by Link and Bizios *(33)*, and absolute quantitation of 2D gel protein spots following biosynthetic radiolabeling can be performed as described by Gygi and Aebersold *(34)*.

3.1.3. Biotinylation of Surface Proteins on Cultured Cells Grown in Monolayer

1. Remove medium by aspiration and wash cells twice with chilled PBS.
2. Add fresh solution of sulfo-HNS-LC-biotin (1.7 m*M* [1 mg/mL] in PBS).
3. Remove solution carefully after 5 min.
4. Quench reaction by adding 50 m*M* NH$_4$Cl in PBS. Incubate for 10 min at 4°C.
5. Remove solution and wash cells three times with PBS.
6. Lyse cells as described under **Subheading 3.1.1.**

The given biotin concentration is optimized for an epithelial cell line and optimal concentration could, depending on cell line/tissue, be as high as 5 m*M*. Aim for as short labeling time as possible, as the probe will be internalized (i.e., endocytosed) over time, despite the sulfo group.

3.2. Protein Identification by Mass Spectrometry

3.2.1. In-Gel Digestion

The purer the materials used, the lower the sample contamination will be. This can prevent potential problems for the mass spectrometric analysis. A clean environment and careful sample handling is mandatory in order to avoid sample contamination, particularly by keratins from skin and hair.

1. Excise gel pieces. Choose a piece size that represents a good compromise between maximal protein recovery and minimal interference of gel-associated contaminants. Bigger gel pieces should be cut into smaller pieces to increase the surface-to-volume ratio for higher protein accessibility.
2. Wash the gel pieces twice with 25 mM ABC/50% ACN for approx 5 min. Use a volume sufficient to cover the gel pieces. After each wash, remove the supernatant and discard the gel-loading pipet tips (*see* **Note 1**).
3. Dry gel pieces in a speed vacuum drier.
4. Rehydrate gel pieces with 20 μL of a 10 mM DTT/25 mM ABC solution.
5. Incubate the sample at 50°C for 45 min.
6. Remove supernatant.
7. Add 20 μL of a 50 mM IAA/25 mM ABC solution.
8. Incubate the sample in the dark at room temperature for 1 h.
9. Remove supernatant.
10. Wash gel pieces twice with 25 mM ABC/50% ACN as in **step 1**.
11. Dry gel pieces in a speed vacuum drier.
12. Prepare a 25-mM ABC solution containing modified trypsin with a trypsin concentration of 10 ng/μL.
13. Rehydrate the gel pieces with 3-6 μL of the trypsin containing 25 mM ABC solution. (Note: For 2-DE gel spots with a diameter of 2 mm, a total amount of 30 ng modified trypsin usually ensures moderate detection of trypsin autolysis products, which can then be used for internal mass calibration. This may vary depending on the protein amount.)
14. Add 15 μL of 25 mM ABC solution to immerse the gel piece sufficiently.
15. Incubate the sample at 37°C overnight.
16. Add 20 μL of 50% ACN/5% TFA.
17. Extract and store the supernatant in a second SlickSeal tube. Undertake an additional extraction of the digest mixture with 20 μL of 50% ACN/5% TFA and add the second extraction to the first.
18. Concentrate the recovered digest mixture by drying in a speed vacuum drier (*see* **Note 2**).
19. Resuspend the dried digest mixture in 5 μL of water.
20. Store samples in refrigerator for subsequent mass spectrometric analysis.

3.2.2. MALDI Sample Preparation and Analysis

1. Prepare a saturated aqueous 2,5-dihydroxybenzoic acid (DHB) solution (*see* **Note 3**).
2. Spot 0.5 μL of the peptide digest mixture on the MALDI target plate.
3. Add 1 μL from the supernatant of the DHB solution to the sample droplet.
4. Dry the sample droplet with a warm stream of air.
5. MALDI analysis. Because of the variety of MALDI mass spectrometers and

possible parameter settings, these aspects of the MALDI analysis will not be discussed. For protein identification of MALDI results, *see* **Note 4** and **Fig. 5**.

4. Notes

1. **Step 2** destains coomassie-stained gel pieces. Any other staining techniques might require further destaining steps. However, this protocol can also be used for silver-stained gel pieces, if superficial silver staining has been performed using a protocol published by Shevchenko et al. *(35)*.

2. **Steps 18–20** can be omitted in order to avoid any sample loss due to peptide adhesion to the tube walls during these steps, particularly the drying step.

3. After the preparation of the saturated DHB solution it is advisable to produce a clear supernatant for further usage. The solution should therefore be microcentrifuged, and undissolved DHB, found mainly on the surface, should be removed. Sample crystallization is very important in MALDI MS. Sometimes the sample might not crystallize completely, and a thin gel-like sample film is obtained. In these cases, diluting the initial peptide digest mixture with water often improves crystallization and the MALDI process. Another important issue seems to be the purity of DHB. Commercially available DHB varies dramatically in its effective use as MALDI matrix. Recrystallization of DHB can then improve its quality. DHB as well as other matrices can also be bought as a ready-to-use matrix solution (Hewlett Packard, Böblingen, Germany). One alternative is α-cyano-hydroxycinnamic acid. This matrix compound is probably used in many more MS laboratories because of its ease of use. However, DHB is substantially more tolerant to contaminants and is better suited for labile analyte molecules because of its "colder" ionization character. This can ultimately result in higher sensitivity, because additional sample cleaning and preparation steps such ZipTip™ clean-ups can be omitted. Although MALDI sample preparation with DHB is the simplest, even for relatively contaminated samples, the MALDI data acquisition is complicated as a result of the necessity to find a "sweet spot" for analyte-ion production. Samples with DHB as matrix typically crystallize with bigger, often needle-like crystals forming a rim and a more amorphous crystalline area inside. Best MALDI MS results can usually be obtained from the rim area and big crystals. Spectra obtained from the inside area are generally inferior, with lower analyte-ion signal and a higher degree of cation-adduct formation. It seems that DHB as matrix provides on-target inherent sample purification as a result of its crystallization.

4. The following web pages provide programs for database searching of MS and MS/MS data: http://prospector.ucsf.edu; http://prowl.rockefeller. edu/cgi-bin/ProFound; www.matrixscience.com. At these sites further links to database search engines and mass spectrometry sites can be found.

References

1. Gygi, S. P., Rochon, Y., Franza, B. R., and Aebersold, R. (1999) Correlation between Protein and mRNA abundance in yeast. *Mol. Cell. Biol.* **19**, 1720–1730.

2. Wasinger, V. C., Cordwell, S. J., Cerpa-Poljak, A., et al. (1995) Progress with gene-product mapping of the Mollicutes: *Mycoplasma genitalium*. *Electrophoresis* **16,** 1090–1094.

3. Blackstock, W. P. and Weir, M. P. (1999) Proteomics: Quantitative and physical mapping of cellular proteins. *TIBTECH* **17,** 121–127.

4. Uetz, P., Giot, L., Cagney, G., et al. (2000) A comprehensive analysis of protein-protein interactions in Saccharomyces cerevisiae. *Nature* **403,** 623–627.

5. Zozulya, S., Lioubin, M., Hill, R. J., Abram, C., and Gishizky, M. L. (1999) Mapping signal transduction pathways by phage display. *Nat. Biotechnol.* **17,** 1193–1198.

6. Pandey, A. and Mann, M. (2000) Proteomics to study genes and genomes. *Nature* **405,** 837–846.

7. Strohman, R. (1994) Epigenesis: the missing beat in biotechnology? *Biotechnology* **12,** 156–164.

8. Wang, J. H. and Hewick, R. M. (1999) Proteomics in drug discovery. *DDT* **4,** 129–133.

9. Link, T. L., ed. (1999) *2-D Proteome Analysis Protocol*. Humana, Totowa, NJ.

10. Jager, D., Jungblut, P. R., and Muller-Werdan, U. (2002) Separation and identification of human heart proteins. *J. Chromatogr. B* **771,** 131–153.

11. Naaby-Hansen, S., Waterfield, M. D., and Cramer, R. (2001) Proteomics—postgenomic cartography to understand cell function. *TIPS* **22,** 376–384.

12. Patton, W. F. (2000) A thousand points of light: the application of fluorescence detection technologies to two-dimensional gel electrophoresis and proteomics. *Electrophoresis* **21,** 1123–1144.

13. Bright, R. K., Vocke, C. D., Emmert-Buck, M. R., et al. (1997) Generation and genetic characterization of immortal human prostate epithelial cell lines derived from primary cancer specimens. *Cancer Res.* **57,** 995–1002.

14. Page, M. J., Amess, B., Townsend, R. R., et al. (1999) Proteomic definition of normal human luminal and myoepithelial breast cells purified from reduction mammoplasties. *Proc. Natl. Acad. Sci. USA* **96,** 12589–12594.

15. Unlu, M., Morgan, M. E., Minden, J. S., et al. (1997) Difference gel electrophoresis: a single gel method for detecting changes in protein extracts. *Electrophoresis* **18,** 2071–2077.

16. Gygi, S. P., Rist, B., Gerber, S A., Turecek, F., Gelb, M. H., and Aebersold, R. (1999) Quantitative analysis of complex protein mixtures using isotope-coded affinity tags. *Nat. Biotechnol.* **17,** 994–999.

17. Naaby-Hansen, S., Flickinger, C. J., and Herr, J. C. (1997) Two-dimensional gel electrophoretic analysis of vectorially labeled surface proteins of human spermatozoa. *Biol. Reprod.* **56,** 771–787.

18. Naaby-Hansen, S. (1990) Electrophoretic map of acidic and neutral human spermatozoal proteins. *J. Reprod. Immunol.* **17,** 167–185.

19. Patton, W. F., Pluskal, M. G., Skea, W. M., et al. (1990) Development of a dedicated two-dimensional gel electrophoresis system that provides optimal pattern reproducibility and polypeptide resolution. *Biotechniques* **8,** 518–527.

20. Chevallet, M., Santoni, V., Poinas, A., et al. (1998) New zwitterionic detergents improve the analysis of membrane proteins by 2-D electrophoresis. *Electrophoresis* **19**, 1901–1909.
21. Krause, K.-H. and Michalak, M. (1997) Calreticulin. *Cell* **88**, 439–443.
22. Jungblut, P. and Thiede, B. (1997) Protein identification from 2-DE gels by MALDI mass spectrometry. *Mass Spectrom. Rev.* **16**, 145–162.
23. Yates, J. R. III. (1998) Mass spectrometry and the age of the proteome *J. Mass Spectrom.* **33**, 1–19.
24. Guetens, G., Van Cauwenberghe, K., De Boeck, G., et al. (2000) Nanotechnology in bio/clinical analysis. *J. Chromatogr.* B **739**, 139–150.
25. Belov, M. E., Gorshkov, M. V., Udseth, H. R., Gordon, A. A., and Smith, R. D. (2000) Zeptomole-sensitivity electrospray ionization-fourier transform ion cyclotron resonance mass spectrometry of proteins *Anal. Chem.* **72**, 2271–2279.
26. Wilm, M., Shevchenko, A., Houthaeve, T., et al. (1996) Femtomole sequencing of proteins from polyacrylamide gels by nano-electrospray mass spectrometry. *Nature* **379**, 466–469.
27. Eckerskorn, C., Strupat, K., Schleuder, D., et al. (1997) Analysis of proteins by direct-scanning infrared-MALDI mass spectrometry after 2D-PAGE separation and electroblotting. *Anal. Chem.* **69**, 2888–2892.
28. Clauser, K., Baker, P., and Burlingame, A. L. (1999) Role of accurate mass measurement (±10 ppm) in protein identification strategies employing MS or MS/MS and database searching. *Anal. Chem.* **71**, 2871–2882.
29. Gross, J. and Strupat, K. (1998) Matrix-assisted laser desorption/ionisation-mass spectrometry applied to biological macromolecules. *TrAC* **17**, 470–484.
30. Kebarle, P. (2000) A brief overview of the present status of the mechanisms involved in electrospray mass spectrometry. *J. Mass Spectrom.* **35**, 804–817.
31. Cole, R. B. (2000) Some tenets pertaining to electrospray ionization mass spectrometry. *J. Mass Spectrom.* **35**, 763–772.
32. Patterson, S. D. and Garrels, J. I. (1994) Two-dimensional gel analysis of posttranslational modifications. In *Cell Biology, a Laboratory Handbook* (Celis, J., ed.), Academic.
33. Link, A. J. and Bizios, N. (1999) Measuring the radioactivity of 2-D protein extracts. In *2-D Proteome Analysis Protocols* (Link, A. J., ed.), Humana, Totowa, NJ.
34. Gygi, S. P. and Aebersold R. (1999) Absolute quantitation of 2-D protein spots. In *2-D Proteome Analysis Protocols* (Link, A. J., ed.), Humana, Totowa, NJ.
35. Shevchenko, A., Wilm, M., Vorm, O., and Mann, M. (1996) Mass spectrometric sequencing of proteins from silver-stained polyacrylamide gels. *Anal. Chem.* **68**, 850–858.

V

GENE TRANSFER

20

Gene Transfer in Endothelial Dysfunction and Hypertension

Sabyasachi Sen, Padraig M. Strappe, and Timothy O'Brien

Summary

Gene transfer represents a method for treatment of several cardiovascular disorders, including endothelial dysfunction and hypertension. For effective and safe gene therapy in vascular disease, a suitable therapeutic gene needs to be identified and delivered to the vasculature by appropriate delivery devices. In this chapter, we review the different vectors used, both viral and nonviral, suitable genes identified, and associated delivery devices. Several genes have been identified with a view to improve endothelial dysfunction, and we have elaborated the advantages and disadvantages of these approaches. Strategies to treat hypertension, both systemic and pulmonary, have also been described. The optimal vector has not yet been discovered although a wide variety of choices is available, each with properties that may render it suitable for specific applications. The individual characteristics of these vectors are described in relation to the proposed therapeutic paradigm. Although there are several unanswered questions in this arena, the future application of gene transfer technology to diseases of the vasculature holds significant promise.

Key Words: Gene transfer; endothelial dysfunction; hypertension; pulmonary hypertension; viral and nonviral vectors; nitric oxide synthase.

1. Introduction

Since the first demonstration of gene transfer to the vasculature in 1990 (*1*), the field of vascular gene therapy has grown considerably. The application of several different types of viral vectors to vascular gene delivery and the combination of viral vector or naked DNA with implant devices have led to improvements in specific targeting of vascular cells and increased transgene expression. The majority of cardiovascular gene therapy regimens involve the transduction of myocardium or the vessel wall. Depending on the methodology used, the endothelium, smooth muscle cells, or the adventitia may be targeted. This can

From: *Methods in Molecular Medicine, Vol. 108: Hypertension: Methods and Protocols*
Edited by: J. P. Fennell and A. H. Baker © Humana Press Inc., Totowa, NJ

be achieved through local gene delivery by direct injection of the vector to the target cell/blood vessel or through systemic administration of the vector. The former is the most common method employed. Gene transfer represents an opportunity to treat many cardiovascular disorders by replacement of a defective gene, overexpression of a therapeutic gene, or inhibition of toxic gene expression. For effective gene therapy in vascular disease, a therapeutic gene must first be identified, then delivered to the vasculature in a safe and efficient manner. The means of gene delivery to the blood vessel wall is the main obstacle to the translation of this technology to the clinic and will be reviewed here. Preclinical studies in suitable animal models must also be performed to evaluate the efficacy and safety of the gene and vector in question.

2. Vectors for Gene Delivery

One of the main barriers to the translation of vascular gene transfer to the clinical area is the need for a safe and efficient vector. Vector systems, both viral and nonviral, have been applied to vascular diseases.

2.1. Nonviral Vectors

The ability to achieve efficient therapeutic gene expression with nonviral vectors would have immense benefit to clinical studies, in which biosafety and toxicity issues are paramount. An early study with DNA complexed with liposomes demonstrated transfection of endothelial and vascular smooth muscle cells of the arterial wall in an animal model *(1)*. Within a decade, the field of DNA delivery by nonviral methods resulted in several clinical trials aimed at promoting angiogenesis in ischemic peripheral vascular beds and in diseased myocardial tissue *(2)*. Delivery mechanisms to the vasculature have included complexing naked DNA with liposomes *(3)*, or other cationic polymers such as polyethylenimines (PEIs) *(4)*, or a PEI/Liposome combination *(5)*. Whereas nonviral methods of DNA delivery demonstrate limited immune or inflammatory reactions, their major limitations include a low transfection efficiency of target cells and a limited duration of transgene expression. Novel approaches to improve DNA transfection efficiency in vitro and in vivo have included incorporation of the SV40 nuclear localizing signal for increased nuclear uptake *(6)* and the inclusion of integrin targeting peptides *(7)* for specific transfection of endothelial cells. A combination of plasmid DNA complexed with PEI and an artificial retroviral envelope expressing an RGD peptide to target integrin-receptors on tumor endothelial cells *(8)* could also provide increased and specific gene transfer to the endothelium.

New experimental methods of DNA delivery to the vasculature have included the use of high-intensity focused ultrasound *(9)*, which increased gene expression without vessel damage when contrast was excluded. Electroporation of DNA to the intact vasculature has also been reported to increase gene expression without tissue damage or ischemia *(2)*. Complexing DNA to a cationic nanoparticle coupled to an integrin-targeting ligand has been used to deliver genes specifically to the endothelium, resulting in targeted gene delivery to the neovasculature of tumor-bearing mice *(10)*.

2.2. Viral Vectors

2.2.1. Retroviruses

Retroviruses are double-stranded RNA viruses that convert their RNA genome to a cDNA copy by reverse transcription following entry into a cell. The cDNA stably integrates into the host chromosome as a provirus, which can lead to long-term transgene expression. Retroviral vectors have limited utility for vascular gene transfer owing to the requirement for cell division for successful transduction of the target. However, ex vivo approaches have been performed with transplantation of transduced cells into the vasculature. In these experiments vascular wall cells are harvested and transduced ex vivo with retroviral vectors. This is feasible because the cells are replicative in culture. The transduced cells are then delivered to the animal. This method has been shown to result in long-term transgene expression in the blood vessel wall *(11)*. In that study smooth muscle cells were transduced ex vivo with a marker gene and seeded into balloon-injured carotid arteries. Transgene expression was detected 1 yr later. The same group later demonstrated that eNOS delivered to the arterial wall in the same fashion inhibited intimal hyperplasia *(12)*. Retroviral vectors have also been used to transduce endothelial progenitor cells ex vivo with plasminogen activator (t-PA) and hirudin followed by local infusion into freshly balloon-injured rabbit carotid *(13)*. The need to isolate autologous cells before transduction is obviously a significant drawback to this method of gene delivery. In addition, random integration of the vector into the host genome is also a concern. Random insertional mutagenesis has been implicated in the development of a lymphoproliferative disorder in two children in a recent human gene therapy trial, in which hematopoietic stem cells were transduced ex vivo by a retroviral vector expressing the γc-chain of the interleukin receptor *(14)*.

2.2.2. Lentiviruses

Lentiviruses are complex retroviruses that offer major advantages over other retroviral vectors, as they do not depend on the proliferation of target cells for stable transduction *(15)*. Lentiviral vectors based predominantly on human immunodeficiency virus type 1 (HIV-1) have demonstrated stable transgene expression in a variety of nondividing cells. However, concerns have been raised that lentivirus-mediated prolonged transgene expression *(16)*, and random integration with host gene *(17)* may lead to vascular tumors at the site of implantation *(18)*.

Lentiviral vectors are often pseudo-typed with a heterologous envelope such as the G-protein of vesicular stomatitis virus (VSV-G). They have been derived from primate lentiviruses such as human immunodeficiency virus types 1 and 2 (HIV-1, HIV-2) and simian immunodeficiency virus (SIV) and other nonprimate lentiviruses such as feline immunodeficiency virus (FIV) and equine infectious anemia virus. Vectors that are based on HIV retain less than 5% of the parental genome, and less than 25% of the genome is incorporated into packaging constructs, which minimizes the possibility of the generation of replication-competent HIV. Safety has been further increased by the development of self-inactivating vectors that contain deletions of the regulatory elements in the downstream long terminal repeat (LTR) sequence, eliminating the transcription of the packaging signal that is required for vector mobilization. Reverse transcription of the retroviral RNA genome occurs in the cytoplasm and, unlike C-type retroviruses, the lentiviral cDNA is complexed with other viral proteins, to form a preinitiation complex (PIC), which translocates across the nuclear membrane allowing transduction of nondividing cells. Lentiviral vectors are produced by cotransfection of 293T cells with separate DNA constructs that include the gene transfer plasmid containing the viral LTRs, the packaging signal linked to a heterologous promoter expressing the transgene of interest, a gag-pol expression plasmid providing the viral structural and enzymatic proteins, and a heterologous envelope. There have been a limited number of studies using lentiviral vectors in the vasculature. Recently, Dishart et al. *(19)* demonstrated increased transduction efficiency of endothelial and smooth muscle cells with a lentiviral vector compared to adeno-associated virus, serotype 2 (AAV-2), and lentiviral vectors expressing a noncatalytic domain of matrix metalloproteinase 2 have been used to transduce human endothelial cells, resulting in inhibition of tumor-induced angiogenesis in a nude mouse model *(20)*. However, much work needs to be done in examining the use of this vector system for vascular gene delivery.

2.2.3. Adenoviruses

Viral vectors based on adenoviruses are the preferred gene delivery vehicle for modification of the vasculature at the current time. Adenoviruses are well characterized, with more than 50 serotypes having been identified to date. First-generation, replication-defective adenoviral vectors are generated simply by deletion of the E1 region and grown in 293 helper cells *(21,22)*. Importantly, adenoviral vectors can transduce both dividing and nondividing vascular cells with high efficiency. However, adenoviral vectors do not integrate into the host genome, remaining as an episome, providing transient overexpression of delivered genes that may be sufficient for certain acute cardiovascular disorders such as early vein graft failure or restenosis following balloon angioplasty *(23)*. In addition, adenoviruses are highly immunogenic *(24)* and are cleared rapidly from the vessel wall. It has been suggested that many of these complications may be avoided using second-generation vectors, but a recent study has demonstrated that using second-generation adenoviruses alone does not reduce the immune response after vascular gene delivery *(25)*. Deletion of viral genes from the vector backbone, leading to generation of high-capacity third-generation adenovirus vectors may increase the longevity of gene expression through a reduction in the immune response to virally transduced cells *(26)*.

Adenoviral vectors have not been linked to any human malignancies and have been used in a number of human trials. Although the overall safety record of adenoviral vectors has been reasonable, they have resulted in inflammatory reactions, formation of antibodies to the virus, transient fever, and increases in liver transaminases. However, these side effects appear to be dose-related. In spite of the adverse effects, the safety profile of adenoviruses is well established, and the US Food and Drug Administration and other regulatory authorities have approved their use in clinical trials.

2.2.4. Adeno-Associated Virus

Adeno-associated virus (AAV) is a small dependovirus of the single-stranded DNA parvovirus family. Vectors based on AAV have a packaging capacity of approx 4.7 kb following removal of the viral rep and cap genes. Its principal host cell-binding receptor is heparan sulfate proteoglycan (HSPG), and co-receptors include the αV-$\beta 5$ integrin receptor and the FGF1 receptor. Cellular transduction by AAV vectors results in stable transgene expression, limited toxicity, and efficient gene transfer in vivo *(27)*. These properties have been demonstrated in liver, skeletal muscle, and nervous system. Wild-type AAV integrates into the host chromosome at a specific and non-oncogenic site on chromosome 19 through the action of the rep protein, leading to long-term persistence in the genome *(28)*. AAV may be an ideal vector when persistent gene expression is required, and vectors based on AAV have been considered for gene-based therapy of genetic diseases through gene replacement strategies in conditions such as cystic fibrosis and muscular dystrophy *(29,30)*. However, rep-deficient recombinant AAVs do not have the site-specific integration capacity and may therefore integrate in a random manner through the genome. However, recent evidence suggests that cells transduced by AAV retain the genome in a nonintegrated, episomal manner in the long term *(31,32)*.

Disadvantages of AAV include lack of site-specific integration in rep-negative rAAV, limited transgene size of 4.7 kb, and lack of efficient large-scale production systems. In addition, AAV vectors have a limited range of target cells, particularly those lacking its principal receptor HSPG or co-receptors, and inefficient conversion from single- to double-stranded DNA after cellular transduction. The latter may result in a delayed onset of transgene expression.

Several different serotypes (1–8) of AAV are known to exist *(33)*, of which AAV-2 has been the most extensively used and tested. The eight serotypes of AAV have a varied cell tropism due to a preference for different receptors. Using different AAV serotypes, Gao et al. have shown improved liver cell transduction using serotype 7 and 8 compared to AAV serotype 2 *(33)*, and Walters et al. have shown that AAV5 uses a different principal receptor, 2,3-sialic acid, and transduces airway epithelial cells more efficiently *(34)*.

In addition to different serotypes having specific cell tropisms, targeting AAV2 to specific cell types such as endothelial cells may be possible by genetic modification of the capsid. Girod et al. *(35)* reported that genetic incorporation of RGD-containing sequences into the AAV2 capsid protein expanded tropism to previously nonpermissive cell types. Shi et al. *(36)* have shown that an RGD capsid insertion mutant of an AAV vector displayed a significantly improved gene transfer profile, with cellular transduction independent of the HSPG receptor and dependent on an RGD–integrin interaction.

While long-lived transgene expression is obtained with AAV, regulated transgene expression would be advantageous and improve the biosafety profile of this vector. AAV vectors have been developed that are responsive to the tetracycline analog, doxycycline, using a tetracycline-responsive promoter *(37)*. Regulated transgene expression from an AAV vector has also been demonstrated using an analog of rapamycin as a heterodimerizer of a DNA-binding domain and a transactivation domain *(38)*.

There are a limited number of reports of AAV-mediated gene delivery to the vasculature *(39–42)*. Although results have been inconsistent and comparison between studies difficult due to the variety of animal models and vector doses used, the following pattern is emerging. AAV2 appears to be less efficient than adenoviral vectors at transducing vascular cells. Indeed, AAV serotype 2 appears to be incapable of transducing endothelial cells. In contrast, AAV2 can transduce the media even in the presence of an intact endothelium. In this setting, adenoviral-mediated gene delivery is limited to the endothelium. Finally, as expected, the duration of expression is longer and does not appear to be associated with blood vessel wall inflammation. Our group has recently shown that AAV serotype 1 and 5 can transduce endothelial cells, but much work remains to be done on the characteristics of AAV serotypes for vascular gene delivery *(43)*. See **Table 1**, describing the characteristics of different vectors used in gene transfer.

Table 1
Common Vectors Used in Vascular Gene Transfer

Vectors	Advantages	Disadvantages
Naked DNA	Nonimmunogenic, useful for IM injection and vaccine	Poor transduction efficiency, rapid clearance, poor specificity
Cationic lipids	Safe and easy to produce	Poor efficiency
Retrovirus	Integration to host DNA long-term expression	Transduction efficiency to nondividing cells is poor, possible insertional mutagenesis
Lentivirus	Stable transduction, both dividing and nondividing cells, low immune response	Chance of insertional and mutagenesis, ethical safety issues in vivo
Adenovirus	High transduction efficiency in dividing and nondividing cells; produced in high titers	Immune response, lack of cell specificity of viral transduction
Adeno-associated virus	Less immunogenic, longer transgene expression, Nonpathogenic to humans, infects proliferative and quiescent cells	Limited packaging capacity, slow to show expression, difficult to produce in large quantities

3. Therapeutic Applications of Vascular Gene Transfer

Vascular gene transfer has numerous potential therapeutic applications including but not limited to the following:

1. Improving endothelial function
2. Hypertension
3. Atherosclerosis
4. Therapeutic angiogenesis
5. Anti-restenosis strategies
6. Ischemia reperfusion
7. Inhibition of thrombosis

We will now review the data examining gene therapy approaches to the first two of these disorders.

3.1. Gene Therapy Approaches to Improve Endothelial Function

Endothelial dysfunction characterized by abnormal endothelium-dependent vasorelaxation is found in a wide variety of disorders, including diabetes mellitus, hypertension, hypercholesterolemia, atherosclerosis, pulmonary hypertension, and subarachnoid hemorrhage-induced vasospasm. These conditions are associated with reduced nitric oxide bioavailability in the blood vessel wall. The pathophysiology of this defect is complex but may include decreased L-arginine availability, increased concentrations of asymmetric dimethylarginine, decreased tetrahydrobiopterin levels, alterations of NOS isoforms expression, or increased levels of oxygen free radicals *(44)*. Thus, in terms of gene therapy approaches to reversing endothelial dysfunction, there are many gene targets. In addition to the choice of gene, the optimal vector type for gene delivery based on the characteristics outlined above needs to be considered. For example, short-lived transgene expression such as that provided by an adenoviral vector would suffice in conditions such as subarachnoid hemorrhage-induced vasospasm, assuming the toxicity profile is acceptable. In contrast, conditions such as systemic or pulmonary hypertension would require more prolonged transgene expression, and AAV or lentivirus may be more suitable.

There have been a large number of studies focusing on the reversal of endothelial dysfunction via overexpression of NOS isoforms. Our group has shown that adenoviral-mediated gene transfer of eNOS results in improved endothelial function in hypercholesterolemia, hypertension, diabetes mellitus, atherosclerosis, vein bypass grafts, and subarachnoid hemorrhage-induced vasospasm *(45–50)*. Other groups have confirmed these results and extended them to the neuronal NOS isoform *(51)*. In contrast, iNOS over expression resulted in deterioration in endothelial function in a hypercholesterolemic rabbit model *(52)*. Thus, individual NOS isoforms may have unique characteristics when used for vascular gene modification.

An alternative gene therapy approach to vascular dysfunction would aim to increase the antioxidative capacity of the blood vessel wall by overexpressing genes such as superoxide dismutase (SOD). We and others have shown that endothelial dysfunction associated with hypercholesterolemia and diabetes mellitus can be reversed by such a strategy *(53,54)*. Endothelial dysfunction, in a hypertensive rat model, has also been shown to improve with adenovirus-mediated expression of human extracellular SOD (ECSOD) *(55)*.

Tetrahydrobiopterin (BH4) is an essential cofactor for endothelial nitric oxide synthase that protects against superoxide (O_2^-)-induced endothelial damage. An additional gene therapy approach to improving endothelial dysfunction may attempt to augment vascular wall levels of tetrahydrobiopterin. A recent study has shown that gene transfer of human guanosine 5'-triphosphate (GTP) cyclohydrolase (GTPCH I), the first and rate-limiting enzyme for BH4 biosynthesis, reverses BH4 deficiency and improves endothelial function *(56)*.

3.2. Gene Therapy for the Treatment of Hypertension

Systemic and pulmonary hypertension are polygenic diseases in which certain key mediators may have significant roles that could be modified by gene transfer. Although all of the genes implicated in hypertension have not been elucidated, certain gene targets have recently been validated. Similar to the situation with the reversal of endothelial dysfunction, both the therapeutic gene and the optimal vector system need to be considered. Gene therapy may allow chronic hypertension control, obviating life-long daily drug therapy. This would require long-lived transgene expression or the ability to readminister the chosen vector periodically. Gene therapy approaches to hypertension may involve overexpression of vasodilator molecules or inhibition of vasoconstrictor molecules via antisense strategies. In the latter case the antisense is delivered using a vector.

Intravenous delivery of plasmid DNA encoding vasodilator proteins has been tested. Delivery of the atrial natriuretic peptide gene led to reduction in blood pressure after 1 wk; the effect lasted up to 7 wk *(57)*. Similarly, decrease in blood pressure was obtained by intravenous delivery of a plasmid encoding eNOS *(58)*. In addition, systemic hypertension has been reversed in adult rats by overexpressing atrial natriuretic peptide, kallikrein, or adrenomedullin *(59–61)*.

In addition to modulating the NO system, attempts to increase the scavenging of oxygen free radicals may have beneficial effects in hypertension. Increased levels of reactive oxygen species, particularly O_2^-, have been demonstrated in blood vessels and in several tissues in experimental models of hypertension, including spontaneously hypertensive rats (SHR), Dahl salt-sensitive rats, hypertension induced by angiotensin II, and hypertension associated with obesity *(62)*. Increased O_2^- may contribute to hypertension by inactivation of vascular NO and by formation of the deleterious free radical peroxynitrite. Thus, reduction of O_2^- levels might be expected to attenuate hypertension. In some but not all studies, antioxidants appear to attenuate hypertension. The explanation for variability in the effects of antioxidants on blood pressure is not clear, but this variability may be due to several factors, including differences in cellular binding and/or cell permeability of the antioxidants. For example, copper/zinc superoxide dismutase (CuZnSOD) protein given intravenously, which does not bind to cells and is not cell-permeable, does not reduce blood pressure in SHR, in angiotensin II-induced hypertensive rats, or in patients with essential hypertension. In contrast, CuZnSOD protein, with fusion of a heparin-binding domain (HBD), which is able to bind to cells, reduced blood pressure in experimental animals with hypertension *(63)*. ECSOD is the only isoform of SOD that is expressed extracellularly and binds to tissues. A study to examine the effects of ECSOD on arterial pressure in experimental hypertension showed beneficial effects of ECSOD gene transfer on arterial pressure *(64)*.

Engelhardt, Chen et al. have reported that angiotensin (Ang) II induces the expression of vascular cellular adhesion molecule-1 (VCAM-1), a key early marker in the development of atherosclerotic lesions in Ang II-induced hypertensive rats *(65)*. Indeed, O_2^- has been shown to stimulate VCAM-1 expression through activation of redox-sensitive transcription factor nuclear factor (NF)-κB *(66)*. It has been demonstrated that enhanced arterial VCAM-1 expression is suppressed by gene transfer of manganese superoxide dismutase (Mn-SOD), suggesting that O_2^- plays an important role in mediating VCAM-1 expression and that overexpression of this gene may be beneficial in the hypertensive vasculature *(67)*.

Another potential gene target for treatment of hypertension is heme oxygenase. Overexpression of the human heme oxygenase (HO) gene by targeted gene transfer has become a powerful tool for studying the role of this human enzyme. Successful and functional HO gene transfer has been shown using a variety of viral vectors *(68)*. HO gene delivery must be site and organ-specific. Site-specific delivery of HO-1 to renal structures in SHR, specifically mTAL, using Na^+-K^+ Cl^- cotransporter (NKCC2 promoter), has been shown to normalize blood pressure and provide protection to mTAL against oxidative injury, respectively. Human HO-1 gene transfer into endothelial cells has been shown to attenuate angiopoietin II-, TNF-, and heme-mediated DNA damage. Furthermore, delivery of human HO-1 into SHR has been shown to enhance somatic body growth and endothelial cell proliferation *(68)*. The ability to transfect human HO gene and to demonstrate its expression may offer a new therapeutic strategy for treating systemic hypertension.

An alternative approach to the treatment of hypertension would be to knock down the expression of genes involved in the renin angiotensin system. The renin–angiotensin system (RAS) is probably the most significant regulator of hypertension and delivery of antisense gene to the angiotensin II type 1 receptor (AT1R) successfully prevented blood pressure elevation, alterations in calcium homeostasis, and cardiovascular ultrastructure changes in spontaneously hypertensive rats (SHR) for 18 mo *(69)*. In that report, a single intracardiac injection to 5-d-old spontaneously hypertensive rats of a retroviral vector encoding antisense to the AT1 receptor resulted in attenuation of hypertension for 210 d. This demonstrates the long-lived efficacy of retroviral-based gene delivery as discussed above. In addition, intravenous delivery of liposomes carrying antisense to the β1 receptor decreased blood pressure in the SHR *(70)*.

3.3. Gene Therapy for the Treatment of Pulmonary Hypertension

Gene therapy approaches may also be used to treat pulmonary hypertension. The expression of eNOS in the pulmonary vasculature of patients with primary pulmonary hypertension is markedly diminished *(71)*; increasing eNOS activity in these patients may be life-saving. Evidence for the efficacy of modulating NO in the pulmonary vasculature as a therapeutic approach to pulmonary hypertension is provided by the observation that inhaled NO is used in the management of this disorder and aerosolized type V phosphodiesterase inhibitors selectively reduce pulmonary arterial pressure by increasing cGMP levels in the lung *(72)*. Gene transfer to the pulmonary vascular bed has been used to deliver adenoviral vectors to the pulmonary artery and pulmonary airway epithelium and alters pulmonary vascular function *(72,73)*. In addition, adenovirus-mediated transfer of the gene coding for prepro-calcitonin gene-related peptide (CGRP) has been shown to have a beneficial effect in chronic hypoxia-induced pulmonary hypertension in the mouse *(73)*. Adenoviral transfer of the eNOS gene to the lung of the mouse and rat may reduce hypoxic pulmonary vasoconstriction and transfer of the eNOS gene to the lung may correct pulmonary hypertension in eNOS-deficient mice *(72)*. Monocyte/macrophage chemoattractant protein-1 (MCP-1), a potent chemoattractant chemokine and an activator for mononuclear cells, may play a role in the initiation and/or progression of pulmonary hypertension (PH). Blockade of a systemic MCP-1 signal pathway in vivo has been shown to prevent PH, by intramuscular transduction using a naked plasmid encoding a 7-NH_2 terminus-deleted dominant negative inhibitor of the MCP-1 (7ND MCP-1) gene in monocrotaline-induced PH *(74)*. Several other genes such as angiopoietin-1 and kallikrein have been used to improve pulmonary hypertension in hypertensive rat models using different vector systems, showing satisfactory and sustained effect *(75,76)*.

4. Future Directions

Although many advances have been made in vascular gene delivery, translation of preclinical research to the clinic has been slower than expected. The key barriers to the translation of this research are suitable vectors and adequate delivery devices.

The optimal vector should be safe, target-specific, regulatable, and result in a suitable temporal pattern of therapeutic transgene expression. Currently available vectors meet a number of criteria for specific interventions such as improving endothelial function and treating hypertension, but significant advances are still required.

References

1. Nabel, E. G., Plautz, G., Nabel, G. J., et al (1990) Site-specific gene expression in vivo by direct gene transfer into the arterial wall. *Science* **249**, 1285–1288.
2. Yla-Herttuala, S. and Martin, J. F. (2000) Cardiovascular gene therapy. *Lancet* **355**, 213–222.
3. Takeshita, S., Losordo, D. W., Isner, J. M., et al. (1994) Time course of recombinant protein secretion after liposome-mediated gene transfer in a rabbit arterial organ culture model. *Lab. Invest.* **71**, 387–391.
4. Turunen, M. P., Urtti, A., Yla-Herttuala, S., et al. (1999) Efficient adventitial gene delivery to rabbit carotid artery with cationic polymer-plasmid complexes. *Gene Ther.* **6**, 6–11.
5. Lampela, P., Yla-Herttuala, S., Raasmaja, A., et al. (2002) The use of low-molecular-weight PEIs as gene carriers in the monkey fibroblastoma and rabbit smooth muscle cell cultures. *J. Gene Med.* **4**, 205–214.
6. Young, J. L., Benoit, J. N., Dean, D. A., et al. (2003) Effect of a DNA nuclear targeting sequence on gene transfer and expression of plasmids in the intact vasculature. *Gene Ther.* **10**, 1465–1470.
7. Hart, S. L., and Coutelle, C. (1995) Gene delivery and expression mediated by an integrin-binding peptide. *Gene Ther.* **2**, 552–554.
8. Harbottle, R. P., Miller, A. D., Coutelle, C., et al (1998) An RGD-oligolysine peptide: a prototype construct for integrin-mediated gene delivery. Hum. Gene Ther. 9(7), 1037–1047.
9. Huber, P. E., Dzau, V. J., Hynynen, K., et al. (2003) Focused ultrasound (HIFU) induces localized enhancement of reporter gene expression in rabbit carotid artery. *Gene Ther.* **10**, 1600–1607.
10. Hood, J. D. and Cheresh, D. A. (2002) Targeted delivery of mutant Raf-kinase to new vessels causes tumour regression. *Cold Spring Harb. Symp. Quant. Biol.* **67**, 285–291.
11. Clowes, M. M., Lynch C. M., Clowes, A. W., et al. (1994) Long-term biological response of injured rat carotid artery seeded with smooth muscle cells expressing retrovirally introduced human genes. *J. Clin. Invest.* **93**, 644–651.
12. Chen, L., Walter, U., Clowes, A. W., et al. (1998) Over expression of human endothelial nitric oxide synthase in rat vascular smooth muscle cells and in balloon-injured carotid artery. *Circ. Res.* **82**, 862–870.
13. Griese, D. P., Weil, J., Riegger, G. A., et al. (2003) Vascular gene delivery of anticoagulants by transplantation of retrovirally-transduced endothelial progenitor cells. *Cardiovasc. Res.* **58**, 469–477.
14. Marshall, E. (2003) Gene therapy. Second child in French trial is found to have leukaemia. *Science* **299**, 320.

15. Naldini, L., Trono, D., Verma, I. M., et al. (1996) Efficient transfer, integration, and sustained long-term expression of the transgene in adult rat brains injected with a lentiviral vector. *Proc. Natl. Acad. Sci. USA* **93**, 11382–11388.

16. Kay, M. A., Glorioso, J. C., Naldini, L., et al (2001) Viral vectors for gene therapy: the art of turning infectious agents into vehicles of therapeutics. *Nat. Med.* **7**, 33–40.

17. George and Baker (2002) Gene transfer to the vasculature. *Mol. Biotechnol.* **22**, 153–164.

18. Lee, R. J., Springer, M. L., Blanco-Bose, W. E., et al. (2000) VEGF gene delivery to myocardium: deleterious effects of unregulated expression. *Circulation* **102**, 898–901.

19. Dishart, K. L., Denby, L., Baker, A. H., et al. (2003) Third-generation lentivirus vectors efficiently transduce and phenotypically modify vascular cells: implications for gene therapy. *J. Mol. Cell. Cardiol.* **35**, 739–748.

20. Pfeifer, A., Cheresh, D. A., Verma, I. M., et al. (2000) Suppression of angiogenesis by lentiviral delivery of PEX, a noncatalytic fragment of matrix metalloproteinase 2. *Proc. Natl. Acad. Sci. USA* **97**, 12227–12232.

21. Graham, F. L. and Prevec, L. (1992) Adenovirus based expression vectors and recombinant vaccine. In *Vaccines: New Approaches to Immunological Problems.* (Ellis, R. W., ed.), Butterworth-Heinemann, Boston, 363–390.

22. Bett, A. J., Haddara, W., Prevec, L., et al. (1994) An efficient and flexible system for construction of adenovirus vectors with insertions or deletions in early regions 1 and 3. *Proc. Natl. Acad. Sci. USA* **91**, 8802–8806.

23. Hedman, M. and Yla-Herttuala, S. (2000) Gene therapy for treatment of peripheral vascular disease and coronary artery disease. *Drugs Today* **36**, 609–617.

24. Newman, K. D., Dunn, P. F., Owens, J. W., et al. (1995) Adenovirus-mediated gene transfer into normal rabbit arteries results in prolonged vascular cell activation, inflammation, and neointimal hyperplasia. *J. Clin. Invest.* **96**, 2955–2965.

25. Wen, S., Schneider, D. B., Dichek, D. A., et al. (2000) Second generation adenoviral vectors do not prevent rapid loss of transgene expression and vector DNA from the arterial wall. *Arterio Thromb. Vasc. Biol.* **20**, 1452–1458.

26. Wilson, J. M. (1996) Adenoviruses as gene-delivery vehicles. *N. Engl. J. Med.* **334**, 1185–1187.

27. Monahan, P. E. and Samulski, R. J. (2000) Adeno-associated virus vectors for gene therapy: more pros than cons? *Mol. Med. Today* **6**, 433–440.

28. Surosky, R. T., Urabe, M., Godwin, S. G., et al. (1997); Adeno-associated virus Rep proteins target DNA sequences to a unique locus in the human genome. *J. Virol.* **71**, 7951–7959.

29. Wagner, J. A., Messner, A. H., Moran, M. L., et al. (1999) Safety and biological efficacy of an adenoassociated virus vector-cystic fibrosis transmembrane regulator (AAV-CFTR) in the cystic fibrosis maxillary sinus. *Laryngoscope* **109**, 266–274.

30. Stedman, H., Wilson, J. M., Mendell, J., et al. Phase I clinical trial utilizing gene therapy for limb girdle muscular dystrophy: a-, b-, g, or f-sarcoglycan gene delivered with intramuscular instillations of adeno-associated vectors. *Hum. Gene Ther.* **11**, 777–790.

31. Rabinowitz, J. and Samulski, R. J. (1998) Adeno-associated virus expression systems for gene transfer. *Curr. Opin. Biotechnol.* **9,** 470–475.

32. Huttner, N. A., Girod, A., Hallek, M., et al. (2003) Analysis of site-specific transgene integration following cotransduction with recombinant AAV and a rep encoding plasmid. *J. Gene Med.* **5,** 120–129.

33. Gao, G. P., Alvira, M. R., Wilson, J., et al. (2002) Novel adeno-associated viruses from rhesus monkeys as vectors for human gene therapy. *Proc. Natl. Acad. Sci. USA* **99,** 11854–11859.

34. Walters, R. W., Chiorini, J. A., Zabner J., et al. (2001) Binding of adeno-associated virus type 5 to 2, 3-linked sialic acid is required for gene transfer. *J. Biol. Chem.* **276,** 20610–20616.

35. Girod, A. (1999) Genetic capsid modifications allow efficient re-targeting of adeno-associated virus type 2, (published erratum appears in *Nat. Med.* **5,** 1438). *Nat. Med.* **5,** 1052–1056.

36. Shi, W. and Bartlett, J. S. (2003) RGD Inclusion in VP3 provides adeno-associated virus type 2 (AAV2)-based vectors with a heparan sulfate-independent cell entry mechanism. *Mol. Ther.* **7,** 515–525.

37. Folliot, S., Briot, D., Rolling, F., et al. (2003) Sustained tetracycline-regulated transgene expression in vivo in rat retinal ganglion cells using a single type 2 adeno-associated viral vector. *J. Gene Med.* **5,** 493–501.

38. Rivera, V. M., Wilson, J., Gilman, M., et al. (1999) Long-term regulated expression of growth hormone in mice after intramuscular gene transfer. *Proc. Natl. Acad. Sci. USA* **96,** 8657–8662.

39. Lynch, C. M., Hara, P. S., Geary, R. L., et al, (1997) AAV vectors for vascular gene delivery. Circulat. Res. **80,** 497–505.

40. Maeda, Y., Ikeda, U., Ozawa, K., et al. (1997) Gene transfer into vascular cells using AAV vectors. *Cardiovasc. Res.* **35,** 514–521.

41. Pajusola, K., Seppo, Y., Beuler, H., et al. (2002) Cell-type-specific characteristics modulate the transduction efficiency of AAV type 2 and restrain infection of endothelial cells. *J. Virol.* **76,** 11530–11540.

42. Richter, M., Halbert, C. L., Allen, M. D., et al. (2000). Adeno-associated virus vector transduction of vascular smooth muscle cells in vivo. *Physiol. Genom.* **2,** 117–127.

43. Sen, S., Bartlett, J. S., O'Brien, T., et al. (2003) Effect of adeno-associated virus (AAV) serotype on vascular gene delivery in-vivo. *Circulation* **108,** Suppl. 4.

44. Sen, S. and O'Brien, T. (2003) Improving endothelial function. *Irish Med. News* May(2), 40–42.

45. Cable, D. G., O'Brien, T., Pompili, V. J., et al. (1997) Recombinant endothelial nitric oxide synthase-transduced human saphenous veins: gene therapy to augment nitric oxide production in bypass conduits. *Circulation* **96** (Suppl.), II-173–II-178.

46. Mozes, G., Katusic, Z. S., O'Brien, T., et al. (1998) Ex vivo gene transfer of endothelial nitric oxide synthase to atherosclerotic rabbit aortic rings improves relaxations to acetylcholine. *Atherosclerosis* **141,** 265–271.

47. Alexander, M. Y., O'Brien, T., Dominiczak, A. F., et al. (1999) Gene transfer of endothelial nitric oxide synthase improves nitric-oxide dependent endothelial function in a hypertensive rat model. *Cardiovasc. Res.* **43**, 798–807.

48. Zanetti, M., Katusic, Z., O'Brien, T., et al. (2000) Gene transfer of endothelial nitric oxide synthase improves endothelium-dependent relaxations in aorta from diabetic rabbits. *Diabetologia* **43**, 340–347.

49. Sato, J., Katusic, Z. S., O'Brien, T. et al. (2000) In vivo gene transfer of endothelial nitric oxide synthase to carotid arteries from hypercholesterolemic rabbits enhances endothelium-dependent relaxations. *Stroke* **31**, 968–975.

50. Khurana, V. G., O'Brien, T., Katusic, Z. S., et al. (2002) Protective vasomotor effects of in vivo recombinant endothelial nitric oxide synthase gene expression in a canine model of cerebral vasospasm. *Stroke* **33**, 782–789.

51. Channon, K. M., Qian, H., Neplioueva, V., et al. (1998) In vivo gene transfer of nitric oxide synthase enhances vasomotor function in carotid arteries from normal and cholesterol fed rabbits. *Circulation* **98**, 1905–1911.

52. Kullo, I. J., Simari, R. D.,Schwartz, R. S., et al. (1999) Vascular gene transfer. From bench to bedside. *Arterioscler. Thromb. Vasc. Biol.* **19**, 196–207.

53. Zanetti, M., Katusic, Z. S., O'Brien, T., et al. (2001) Gene transfer of superoxide dismutase isoforms reverses endothelial dysfunction in diabetic rabbit aorta. *Am. J. Physiol. Heart Circ. Physiol.* **280**, H2516–H2523.

54. Zanetti, M., Katusic, Z. S., O'Brien, T., et al. (2001) Gene transfer of manganese superoxide dismutase reverses vascular dysfunction in the absence but not in the presence of atherosclerotic plaque. *Hum. Gene Ther.* **12**, 1407–1416.

55. Fennell, J. P., Heistad, D., Baker, A. H., et al. (2002) Adenovirus-mediated overexpression of extracellular superoxide dismutase improves endothelial dysfunction in a rat model of hypertension. *Gene Ther.* **9**, 110–117.

56. Zheng, J. S., Kovesdi, I., Chen, A. F., et al. (2003) Gene transfer of human guanosine 5' triphosphate cyclohydrolase I restores vascular tetrahydrobiopterin level and endothelial function in low renin hypertension. *Circulation* **108**, 1238–1245.

57. Lin, K. F., Chao, J., and Chao, L. (1995) Human atrial natriuretic peptide gene delivery reduces blood pressure in hypertensive rats. *Hypertension* **26**, 847–853.

58. Lin, K. F., Chao, L., and Chao, J. (1997) Prolonged reduction of high blood pressure with human nitric oxide synthase gene delivery. *Hypertension* **30**(3 Pt 1), 307–313.

59. Chao, J., Jin, L., Chao L., et al. (1997) Adrenomedullin gene delivery reduces blood pressure in spontaneously hypertensive rats. *Hypertens. Res.* **20**, 269–277. Errata: *Hypertens. Res.* **22**, 229 (1999); *Hypertens. Res.* **24**, 611 (2001).

60. Lin, K. F., Chao, L., and Chao, J. (1998) Atrial natriuretic peptide gene delivery attenuates hypertension, cardiac hypertrophy, and renal injury in salt-sensitive rats. *Hum. Gene Ther.* **9**, 1429–1438. Errata: *Hum. Gene Ther.* **12**, 2034 (2001).

61. Dobrzynski, E., Chao, J., Chao, L., et al. (1999) Adenovirus-mediated Kallikrein gene delivery attenuates hypertension and protects against renal injury in deoxycorticosterone-salt rats. *Immuno-Phamacology* **44**, 57–65.

62. Gardon, M. L., Katovich, M. J., Raizada, M. K., et al. (1999) The potential use of gene therapy in the control of hypertension. *Drugs Today* **35**, 925–930.

63. Nakazono, K., Watanabe, N., Matsuno, K., Sasaki, J., Sato, T., Inoue, M. (1991) Does superoxide underlie the pathogenesis of hypertension? *Proc. Natl. Acad. Sci. USA* **88**, 10045–10048.

64. Chu, Y., Iida, S., Heistad, D. D., et al. (2003) Gene transfer of extracellular superoxide dismutase reduces arterial pressure in spontaneously hypertensive rats: role of heparin-binding domain. *Circ. Res.* **92**, 461–468.

65. Engelhardt, J. F., Heistad, D. D., Chen, A. F., et al. (2003) Endothelin-1 stimulates arterial VCAM-1 expression via NADPH oxidase-derived superoxide in mineralocorticoid hypertension. *Hypertension* **42**, 997–1003.

66. Tummala, P. E., Chen, X. L., Sundell, C. L., et al. (1999) Angiotensin II induces vascular cell adhesion molecule-1 expression in rat vasculature: a potential link between the renin-angiotensin system and atherosclerosis. *Circulation* **100**, 1223–1229.

67. Li, L., Crockett, E., Wang, D. H., Galligan, J. J., Fink, G. D., and Chen, A. F. (2002) Gene transfer of endothelial NO synthase and manganese superoxide dismutase on arterial vascular cell adhesion molecule-1 expression and superoxide production in deoxycorticosterone acetate-salt hypertension. *Arterioscler. Thromb. Vasc. Biol.* **22**, 249–255.

68. Abraham, N. G. (2003) Therapeutic applications of human heme oxygenase gene transfer and gene therapy. *Curr. Pharm. Des.* **9**, 2513–2524.

69. Reaves, P. Y., Katovich, M. J., Raizada, M. K., et al (1999) Permanent cardiovascular protection from hypertension by the AT(1) receptor antisense gene therapy in hypertensive rat offspring. *Circ. Res.* **85**, e44–e50.

70. Zhang, Y. C., Shen, L., Phillips, M. I., et al. (2000) Antisense inhibition of β_1-adrenergic receptor mRNA in a single dose produces a profound and prolonged reduction in high blood pressure in spontaneously hypertensive rats. *Circulation* **101**, 682–688.

71. Giaid, A. and Saleh, D. (1995) Reduced expression of endothelial nitric oxide synthase in the lungs of patients with pulmonary hypertension. *N. Engl. J. Med.* **333**, 214–221.

72. Champion, H. C., Bivalacqua, T. J., Kadowitz, P. J., et al. (2002) Adenoviral gene transfer of endothelial nitric-oxide synthase (eNOS) partially restores normal pulmonary arterial pressure in eNOS-deficient mice. *PNAS* **99**, 13248–13253.

73. Champion, H. C., Heistad D. T. J., Kadowitz, P. J., et al. (2000) In vivo gene transfer of prepro-calcitonin gene-related peptide to the lung attenuates chronic hypoxia-induced pulmonary hypertension in mouse. *Circulation* **101**, 923–930.

74. Ikeda, Y., Yonemitsu, Y., Sueishi, K., et al. (2002) Anti-monocyte chemoattractant protein-1 gene therapy attenuates pulmonary hypertension in rats. *Am. J. Physiol. Heart Circ. Physiol.* **283**, H2021–H2028.

75. Zhao, Y. D., Ng, D., Stewart, D. J., et al. (2003) Protective role of angiopoietin-1 in experimental pulmonary hypertension. *Circ. Res.* **92**, 984–991.

76. Bledsoe, G., Chao, L., and Chao, J. (2003) Kallikrein gene delivery attenuates cardiac remodeling and promotes neovascularization in spontaneously hypertensive rats. *Am. J. Physiol. Heart Circ. Physiol.* **285**, H1479–H1488.

21

Nonviral Gene Delivery Methods in Cardiovascular Diseases

Marika Ruponen, Zanna Hyvönen, Arto Urtti, and Seppo Ylä-Herttuala

Summary

Nonviral gene delivery methods with naked plasmids and various plasmid carrier complexes have been used for intravascular, intramuscular and periadventitial gene delivery to cardiovascular system. Efficacy, homogenity and quality of the nonviral gene delivery complexes can be significantly affected by the way they are produced. This chapter presents basic methods to produce nonviral gene delivery complexes and describes common models to test their properties in cardiovascular applications in vivo.

Key Words: Nonviral vectors; cardiovascular diseases; plasmids; liposomes.

1. Introduction

Gene therapy has become an alternative method for the treatment of cardiovascular diseases. Both viral and nonviral methods have been used in experimental animal studies and in human trials. Treatment targets have been therapeutic vascular growth, restenosis, vascular graft failure, and transplant atherosclerosis. Also, some forms of hyperlipidemias and myocardial diseases have been targeted with gene therapy. Methods for nonviral gene delivery have been significantly improved over the last decade. Even though nonviral vectors are still less efficient than adenoviruses, they seem to have a more favorable safety profile and the risk of virus-associated immunological and inflammatory responses is less apparent. Also, manufacturing of clinical-grade nonviral vectors is relatively easy, and formulation of nonviral gene medicines is easier to accomplish than with viral vectors.

1.1. General Considerations

Delivery of transcriptionally active DNA into the cell nucleus is required for successful transduction (*1*). Since plasmid DNA is a large and negatively

From: *Methods in Molecular Medicine, Vol. 108: Hypertension: Methods and Protocols*
Edited by: J. P. Fennell and A. H. Baker © Humana Press Inc., Totowa, NJ

charged macromolecule, its delivery is difficult and often inefficient. In order to improve the efficacy of the DNA transfer, several nonviral delivery systems have been developed. Most commonly used systems are based on positively charged polymers (dendrimers, polyethyleneimines), liposomes (DOTAP, DOGS, DOTMA, DOPE), or peptides (poly-L-lysine). Cationic lipids, polymers, and peptides form complexes spontaneously when they are mixed in aqueous solutions with the polyanionic DNA. Upon complexation, DNA is condensed and its cellular uptake is facilitated by the positive charge of the complexes. The preparation of the complexes is easy, but the activity of the complexes depends on various practical factors: DNA complexing agent, concentration, charge ratio (carrier/DNA), medium, cell type, and storage conditions.

Many transfection reagents are available as kits (e.g., Lipofectin, Superfect, Transfectam, FuGene, Lipofectamine). These kits contain ready-to-use delivery systems that are mixed with DNA. Transfection kits are easy to use, but they are usually very expensive. Several useful nonviral DNA delivery reagents (e.g., polyethyleneimines, poly-L-lysines, DOTAP; *see* **Subheading 2.**) are available as raw materials. These carriers are relatively easy to use in the transfections, and the price is much lower than the cost of the commercial transfection kits.

The purpose of this chapter is to describe some basic aspects of the preparation of nonviral plasmid-based gene delivery systems and their testing in vitro and in vivo.

2. Materials

1. Poly-L-lysine (PLL; mol wt of the monomer unit is 128 g/mol) (Sigma or Aldrich): Prepare stock solution in water at appropriate concentrations and store stock solution at +4°C. Stock solution can be used for several months.
2. Polyethyleneimines (PEI; Sigma and Aldrich): Prepare 10 mM stock solution in water.
3. (N-[1-(2,3-dioleoyloxy)propyl]-N,N,N-trimethyl ammonium methylsulfate (DOTAP; a monovalent lipid [mol wt 698.55 g/mol]) (Avanti Polar Lipids, Alabaster, AL, USA): Prepare stock solution of lipid in chloroform (10 mg/mL) and store at –20°C under nitrogen or argon.
4. 1,2-dioleyl-3-phosphatidylethanolamine (DOPE; a neutral fusogenic lipid [mol wt 744 g/mol]) (Avanti Polar Lipids, Alabaster, AL, USA): Prepare stock solution of lipid in chloroform (10 mg/mL) and store at –20°C under nitrogen or argon.
5. 2-[N-morpholino] ethanesulfonic acid hydrate-N-[2-hydroxyethyl] piperazine-N'-(2-ethanesulfonic acid) (MES-HEPES) buffer: 150 mM NaCl or 50 mM MES, 50 mM HEPES, 75 mM NaCl, pH adjusted to 7.2.
6. Dulbecco's modified Eagle's medium (DMEM; Invitrogen; Scotland).

7. 5% glucose: 5 w/v glucose solution in water.
8. 5X loading buffer: 30% glycerol, 0.25% sodium dodecylsulfate (SDS), 50 mM Tris-HCl (pH 8.0), 50 mM NaCl, 20 mM EDTA (pH 8.0), 0.1% bromphenol blue. Prepare stock solution in water and store aliquots at 4°C.
9. 1X TBE buffer: 8.9 mM Tris-borate, 2 mM EDTA, pH 8.0.
10. RAASMC cells growth medium: DMEM supplemented with 10% inactivated (56°C, 30 min) fetal bovine serum (FBS), penicillin (100 U/mL), streptomycin (100 µg/mL).
11. 2% Triton X-100: Prepare 10% (m/v) Triton stock solution by dissolving Triton X-100 in water. Dissolve appropriate amount of stock solution five times in 250 mM Tris-HCl (pH 8.0) to obtain 2% Triton X-100.
12. *o*-Nitrophenylgalacto-pyranoside (ONPG; [Sigma] used as a substrate for β-galactosidase): Dissolve ONPG (2 mg/mL) in 60 mM phosphate buffer, pH 8.0, containing 1 mM MgSO$_4$, 10 mM KCl, and 50 mM β-mercaptoethanol. Add β-mercaptoethanol to the buffer and dissolve ONPG just before use.
13. β-Galactosidase (Sigma): Prepare stock solution in 0.1 M NaH$_2$PO$_4$/0.1 M Na$_2$HPO$_4$ buffer, pH 7.3. Store aliquots (2 U/20 µL) at –70°C.
14. Dissolve ethidium monoazide (EMA) (Molecular Probes) in dimethyl sulfoxide (DMSO) (1 mg/mL) and store stock-solution aliquots at –20°C.
15. Cesium chloride (CsCl)-saturated isopropanol: Prepare CsCl-saturated water by adding the CsCl to water until part of CsCl remains undissolved. Prepare CsCl saturated isopropanol by adding an equal volume of CsCl-saturated water to isopropanol.
16. Tris-EDTA buffer: 10 mM Tris, 1 mM EDTA, pH 8.0.
17. Trypsin-EDTA: 0.5% trypsin, 5.3 mM EDTA · 4Na (Euroclone Ltd, UK).
18. 1% Paraformaldehyde (PFA): Prepare 8% (m/V) stock solution by dissolving PFA in 1X PBS. Place solution on magnetic stirrer and heat to 70°C until solution becomes clear. Cool stock solution to room temperature, make aliquots and store at –20°C. Dissolve the stock solution to 1% in 1X PBS just before use. Once thawed, aliquot should be used within 1 wk. PFA is toxic; handle solutions with gloves and under the hood.
19. Phosphate-buffered saline (PBS), pH 7.2.
20. 1% (m/v) Agarose gel. For small gel: 1 g agarose (Sigma) in 100 mL 1X TBE buffer, heat and cool to 60°C. Place solution into a gel-casting platform with inserted appropriate comb and allow to harden.
21. 10 mg/mL ethidium bromide (EtBr) (Molecular Probes): Gel staining solution: 20 µL in 0.5 L water. Prepare fresh solution every time (*see* **Note 1**).

3. Methods

3.1. Nonviral Gene Delivery Systems

Poly-L-lysines (PLL) and polyethyleneimines (PEI) are polymers with high cationic charge density. PLL contains primary amino groups, while PEI contains primary, secondary, and tertiary amino groups. Both polymers are commercially available at different mean molecular weights ranging from 1000 to 1 million. Synthetic polymers are not monodisperse, therefore the molecular weights are mean values in polydisperse mixtures. In general, higher transfection efficiencies are obtained with PEI than with PLL. In most cell types, 25-kDa PEI has higher transfection activity than higher-molecular-weight forms (700 or 800 kDa), while the low-molecular-weight PEI works only in combination with cationic lipids. High-molecular-weight (200-kDa) PLL is preferred over lower molecular weights (4 kDa or 20 kDa).

3.1.1. Preparation of PEI Solution (2)

1. Dissolve 50% (w/v) commercial PEI in water to a concentration of 0.9 mg/10 mL.
2. Adjust the pH of the solution to neutral with 0.2 M HCl.
3. Sterilize the solution by filtering.
4. PEI stock solution is stored at 4°C and can be used for several months.

3.1.2. Preparation of Cationic Liposomes (DOTAP or DOTAP/DOPE at Molar Ratio 1:1)

1. Evaporate the chloroform solution of lipids under nitrogen stream for 2 h.
2. Remove traces of chloroform under vacuum for 3 h.
3. Add water to get lipid concentration of 3.2 mM and incubate for 1 h to hydrate the thin film.
4. Sonicate liposomes until clear liposomal solution is obtained.
5. Always sonicate the liposomes before complex preparation.
6. The liposomes preserve maximally for 3 mo at 4°C under nitrogen or argon.

3.1.3. Calculating ± Charge Ratios

The amount of DNA and carrier in complexes is expressed as ± charge ratio or nitrogen/phosphorus (N/P) ratio. At a charge ratio of ± 1 the positive charges of carrier equals the negative charges of DNA. When the charge ratio is over ±1 there are more positive charges (i.e., carrier) than negative charges (i.e., DNA). The basic principle in calculating ± charge ratios is that the moles of positive groups of carrier, such as amino groups, and moles of negative groups of DNA (phosphates), are compared. The amount of phosphates in 1 μg of DNA is 3 nmol, and to obtain, for example, PEI complexes at an N/P ratio of 1, the amount of amine nitrogen should also be 3 nmol (1 μL of PEI stock solution contains 10 nmol of amine nitrogen). To obtain PEI complexes at charge ratio N/P = 2 the amount of amine nitrogen should be 6 nmol, i.e., twice as much as the amount of phosphates of DNA. The optimal ± charge ratio varies among carriers and cell lines. Therefore, the preliminary transfections with new cell lines and carriers should be done at various ± charge ratios. For carriers that contain fully protonated primary (e.g., PLL) or quaternary amino groups (e.g., DOTAP), ratios based on N/P and ± are calculated similarly. Since PEI also contains secondary and tertiary amino groups, which may be only partly protonated, calculation of N/P ratio is preferable.

3.1.4. Complexation

DNA/carrier complexes are not stable, and therefore complexes must always be prepared just before transfection. The complexes can be prepared in various kinds of media such as water, buffers (such as MES-HEPES), 5% glucose, or cell growth media (DMEM). The choice of medium is important because the medium affects the size of the complexes, as discussed later. First, DNA and carrier are diluted separately in medium. Here we use an example:

1. Dilute DNA (0.6–2 μg) in 75 μL medium (*see* **Note 2**).
2. Then add carrier solution (75 μL; the amount of carrier depends on the ± charge ratio) by mixing gently.
3. Incubate at room temperature for 15 min.
4. Complexes are ready for transfection.

3.2. Testing of Carrier/DNA Complexes In Vitro

3.2.1. DNA Binding

Binding of carrier to DNA is necessary for successful gene transfer. Ability of carrier to bind DNA can be examined by measuring the changes in DNA migration during agarose gel electrophoresis. DNA that is associated with the cationic carrier does not migrate into the gel during electrophoresis as free DNA does. For example, the electrophoresis of PEI/DNA complexes shows that PEI effectively binds DNA (Fig. 1). At charge ratios of ± 1 and higher, plasmid DNA does not migrate into the gel (**Fig. 1**).

3.2.1.1. GEL ELECTROPHORESIS PROCEDURE

1. Prepare 1% agarose gel and place it into the electrophoresis tank containing 1X TBE buffer to cover the gel about 2 mm.
2. Prepare the carrier/DNA complexes at different ± charge ratios in desired complexation medium as described above.
3. Add an appropriate amount (usually 8% w/v) of 5X loading buffer to each complex.
4. Load the complexes on the gel with a pipet. Include free DNA as control or appropriate DNA molecular-weight marker.
5. Apply a voltage of 60 V (59 mA) to the electrophoresis system for 2 h.
6. Remove the gel and stain with EtBr (5 μg/mL) for 10–15 min. Visualize DNA bands on a UV transilluminator and photograph using Video Documentation System (Biometra, BioDoc II/NT) or with a Polaroid camera.

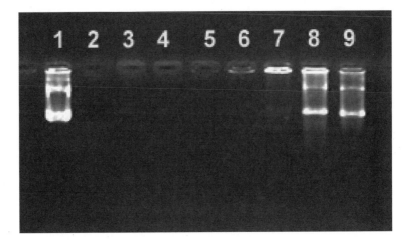

Fig. 1. Gel electrophoresis of PEI/DNA complexes: (lane 1) plasmid DNA alone (0.6 μg) (positive control); (lane 2) PEI (2 μ*M*) alone (negative control); (lanes 3–9) PEI/DNA complexes at charge ratios ±: 16, 8, 4, 2, 1, 0.5, 0.25, respectively.

3.2.2. Size and Zeta Potential

The sizes and zeta-potentials of the carrier/DNA complexes are determined by NICOMP™ 380 ZLS (Particle Sizing Systems, Santa Barbara, CA, USA) quasi-elastic light-scattering apparatus with a 5-mW He–Ne laser at 632.8 nm. Complexes are prepared in the desired solution by the addition of plasmid DNA to liposomes at different ± charge ratios as described above. 6 × 50 mm borosilicate glass culture tubes are used for particle size determination and 10 × 10 × 45 mm polystyrene cuvets are used for zeta-potential determination. The following parameters are used: particle suspension temperature 23°C, the viscosity of medium 0.933 cP, medium refraction index 1.333, and dielectric constant 78.5. Sizes of the complexes were measured in deionized water, 5% (w/v) glucose solution or MES-HEPES buffer. Zeta potentials are measured in de-ionised water or mild buffer (less than 10 m*M*) to avoid shielding effects by the ions at high ionic strengths.

Charge ratio between the carrier and DNA defines various properties of the complexes: size disribution, zeta-potential, colloidal stability, and transfection activity. The complexes with excess of cationic charges (± ratios ≥ 4) exhibit fairly homogeneous size distribution and small mean diameters. The complexes prepared at the charge ratio close to neutrality are more heterogeneous and tend to aggregate. This is due to the lack of electrostatic repulsive forces between the complexes. Accordingly, the sizes of the complexes at charge ratios ±2 and ±1 are significantly increased (**Fig. 2**). The complexes that are

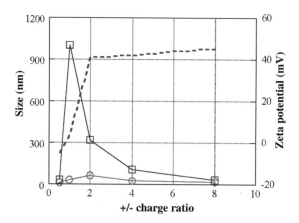

Fig. 2. Mean diameters of the DOTAP/DNA complexes. Different ± charge ratios were prepared in deionized water (○) and MES-HEPES buffer, pH 7.2 (□); zeta-potential of the complexes prepared in deionized water (dashed line). Complexes were incubated for 20 min before the measurements. Size distributions are assessed on the bases of NICOMP number-weighted analysis.

prepared in solutions with low ionic strength (water or glucose) are much smaller than complexes in high ionic strength (buffer, DMEM).

Zeta potentials (the surface charge of the complexes and the solvent layer that moves with the complexes) of the complexes at the excess of the cationic carrier are positive, significantly decreased at charge ratio of ±1, and shifted to negative values at charge ratio below ±1 (**Fig. 2**).

3.2.3. Transfection Assays

Transfections can be monitored with several marker genes. The properties of different marker genes are listed in **Table 1** (*see* **Note 3**).

1. Culture the cells and seed them on 96-well plates (Nunclon) in 100 µL growth medium.
2. After 24 h, change medium to medium without serum (150 µL/well). At the time of transfection, the cells should be about 80% confluent.
3. Prepare the carrier/DNA complexes in MES-HEPES buffer at desired ± charge ratios as described above (0.6 µg DNA per well; pCMV-β-galactosidase plasmid is used).
4. Add the complexes to the cells (50 µL/well) and transfer the plates to the incubator for 5 h.
5. Remove the medium with the complexes, wash the cells with 1X PBS (150 µL/well), and add the growth medium (150 µL/well). Incubate the cells for an additional 45 h.

Table 1
Commonly Used Marker Genes for Testing Nonviral Gene Delivery Systems

Gene	Localization of product	Analysis/end point	Sensitivity	Reference
β-Galactosidase	Intracellular	X-gal staining/no. of transfected cells	Medium	*16,17*
β-Galactosidase	Intracellular	ONPG assay/total expression	Low	*18*
Luciferase	Intracellular	Luminometer/total expression	High	*18–20*
CAT[a]	Intracellular	Radiochemical/total expression	High	*18*
SEAP[b]	Secreted	Luminesence/total expression	High	*21*
GFP[c]	Intracellular	Fluorescence microscopy/number of cells transfected	Low	*22*

[a]Chloramphenicol acetyltransferase.
[b]Secreted alkaline phosphatase.
[c]Green fluorescent protein.

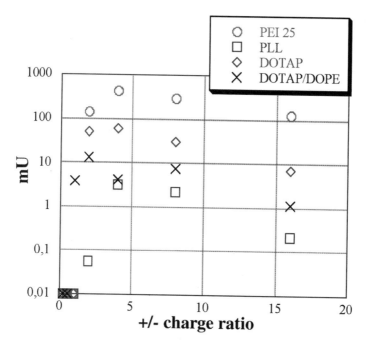

Fig. 3. In vitro transfection. Aortic smooth muscle (RAASMC) cells were transfected with pCMV-βGal complexed with cationic carriers at different ± charge ratios. β-Galactosidase activity was determined as described in the text. Note the logarithmic scale of gene expression.

6. Remove the medium and add 2% Triton X-100 (50 μL/well).
7. Subject the plates to two cycles of freezing and thawing.
8. Add 0.5% (v/v) FBS in PBS (50 μL/well).
9. Add ONPG solution (150 μL/well).
10. Determine β-galactosidase activity in each well spectrophotometrically with an Elx 800 automated microplate reader (Bio-Tek Instruments, Winooski, VT, USA) by monitoring of the hydrolysis of ONPG at 405 nm. Purified β-galactosidase from *Escherichia coli* is used to construct a standard curve for calculation of the β-galactosidase activity in the transfected cells *(10)*.

Transfection efficacy is dependent on ± ratio of carrier/DNA complexes (**Fig. 3**). At low ± values the interactions between the complexes and the anionic cell surfaces are weak and transfection levels are low. At higher ± ratios the complexes are taken into cells more easily, but at too high carrier concentrations (e.g., ±16), toxicity hampers the transfections. Although this kind of profile (transfection vs charge ratio) is very typical, the exact values of optimal charge ratios depend on the carrier and cell type.

3.2.4. Cellular Uptake of DNA

3.2.4.1. EMA-Labeling of Plasmid DNA *(3,4)*

1. Add EMA in water (5 µg/500 µL) to plasmid DNA in water (200 µg/500 µL).
2. Incubate EMA/DNA solution for 10 min at room temperature.
3. Expose the mixture to UV light (312 nm) for 2 min. During this time EMA binds covalently to the bases of DNA.
4. Remove free EMA label by gel filtration on NAP-10 columns (Amersham Pharmacia Biotech).
5. Add CsCl to eluted EMA-DNA solution (1.5 mL) at the concentration of 1.1 g/mL.
6. Remove intercalated EMA by extractions (four times) with equal volume of CsCl-saturated isopropanol (1.5 mL).
7. Remove CsCl by overnight dialysis against Tris-EDTA buffer. Change the dialysis buffer at least four times during dialysis.
8. Recover covalently labeled EMA-DNA by ethanol precipitation.
9. Store EMA-DNA at 4°C. Stock solution should be used within 1 mo.

3.2.4.2. Cellular Uptake of EMA-DNA

1. Seed cells onto 6-well plates at 80% confluency the day before transfection.
2. Next day, replace the medium (2 mL) with serum-free medium (1.5 mL).
3. Add freshly prepared complexes to the cells.
4. Remove EMA-labeled complexes after 5 h exposure to cells.
5. Wash cells twice with 2 mL PBS and once with 1 mL of 1 M NaCl to remove the attached complexes from the cell surface.
6. Detach cells with 1 mL of trypsin-EDTA and fix with 1 mL of 1% PFA in PBS.
7. After 10 min incubation, wash cells twice with 1% PFA.
8. The samples can be stored for 1 wk at 4°C before analysis by flow cytometry.
9. Wash GFP plasmid complexes after 5 h exposure time.
10. Analyze levels of GFP expression at 24 h (*see* **Note 4**).

Figure 4 shows the cellular uptake of EMA-labeled plasmid DNA into RAASMC cells and the fraction of transfected cells by GFP-plasmid. Transfections by PLL (200 kDa), PEI (25 kDa), DOTAP, and DOTAP/DOPE complexes demonstrate that the cellular uptake of DNA is much higher than the levels of transfection. This is due to intracellular factors that limit the access of the transgene into the cell nucleus. Futhermore, the cellular DNA uptake and transfection do not always correlate. For example, PLL/DNA complexes show high levels of uptake, but the transfections are clearly lower than in the case of DOTAP/DNA complexes.

3.3. Potential In Vivo Applications

Here we assess and discuss the potential modes of delivery for such complexes for in vivo gene delivery.

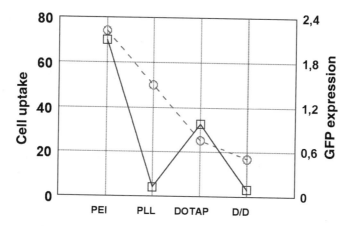

Fig. 4. GFP expression analysis. The cells were treated with EMA-labeled pCMV-β-galactosidase plasmid or with GFP plasmid complexed with various carriers. Percentage of cells with EMA-DNA (○) or GFP expression (□) was analyzed with flow cytometry as described in the text.

3.3.1. Local Intravascular Gene Delivery

Intravascular gene transfer is easily performed either using iv injections or during intravascular manipulations *(5)*. Limitations for the intravascular gene transfer include the presence of anatomical barriers, such as the internal elastic lamina and atherosclerotic lesions and the blood complement system, which efficiently inactivates many gene transfer vectors *(1)*. After iv injection, most gene delivery vectors end up in the liver or lungs *(6)*. Several catheters are commercially available that can be used for gene delivery. A double balloon catheter is made of two latex balloons that, when inflated in a target arterial segment, isolate a transfection chamber of varying length, into which a gene transfer solution can be infused. The major limitations of this catheter type are seized blood flow and leakage through arterial side branches. The Dispatch™ catheter is an infusion-perfusion balloon catheter that forms a separate compartment adjacent to the target vessel wall when the catheter is inflated. Prolonged gene transfer vector infusion can be performed, because blood flows through a central channel of the catheter. This system has been used successfully to achieve substantial gene delivery into the endothelium and other superficial layers of animal and human arteries *(7)*. Porous and microporous catheters have also been used for arterial delivery of marker genes. The channeled balloon catheter has 24 longitudinal channels, each containing 100-μm pores *(8)*. Iontophoretic catheters are catheters that use electroporation technique in combination with balloon catheter. New catheters are continuously being developed for intravascular injections.

3.3.2. Perivascular Gene Delivery

When gene transfer vector is administered on the adventitial surface of the vessel wall, it can stay in close contact with arterial cells for a long time. Adventitial gene transfer can be used for the delivery of therapeutic genes into the arterial wall during bypass operations, prosthesis and anastomosis surgery, and endarterectomies *(1)*. Adventitial gene delivery can be performed with silastic or biodegradable collar, biodegradable gel, or direct injection into the adventitia. The limitation of this technique is that surgical operation is needed for the gene transfer *(9)*.

3.3.3. Intramuscular Delivery

Intramuscular injection of nonviral vectors seems to provide an efficient means of transgene expression for longer periods of time than in most other tested tissues *(10)*. Typically, several injections are given intramuscularly along the muscles in the lower extremities. Muscle can be used for the production of systemically secreted factors. Also, local relief to conditions such as ischemia have been achieved in experimental animal models. For reasons that are still somewhat unknown, nonviral vectors can persist in muscles for several weeks.

3.3.4. Systemic Gene Delivery

Systemically administered gene transfer vectors usually transfect liver cells *(6)*. Therefore, diseases in which the liver is the target organ could be treated by systemic gene transfer. The inhibitory effect of blood components for many gene transfer vectors currently limits the use of systemic gene transfer. This has been tried to overcome by using so-called stealth technology. If vector is administered systemically it should, because of safety aspects, either have specificity to target cells or bear a specific promoter that is expressed only in certain cell types or diseased tissue *(11)*. Current peptide libraries may provide new targeting possibilities for future gene transfer vectors *(12)*. Hydrodynamic pressure-mediated delivery may improve gene transfer efficiency, at least in small-animal models *(13)*. New electroporation systems are also potential alternatives for cardiovascular gene delivery of plasmids and oligonucleotides *(14)*. Physical methods such as ultrasound *(15)* have also been used successfully for cardiovascular gene delivery.

4. Notes

1. Ethidium bromide is a potential carcinogen. Wear gloves when handling.
2. The concentration of DNA should not be too high, because it may cause aggregation of the complexes and precipitation. The complexes may aggregate especially

if a medium with high ionic strength is used (e.g., buffers, cell culture medium). If higher amounts of DNA must be used, then the complexes should be made in higher solution volume.

3. Usually, strong viral promoters, such as cytomegalovirus (CMV) or Rous sarcoma virus (RSV), are inserted into the plasmid to provide high levels of expression.

4. The analysis of the samples is performed by flow cytometry (FACScan, Becton Dickinson) using an argon-ion laser (488 nm) as the excitation source. For each sample, 10,000 events are collected. Fluorescence of EMA is collected at 670 nm and GFP at 525 nm. Living cells are defined by gating the major population of the cells from forward-angle light-scatter (FSC) vs 90° light-scatter (SSC) display. The number of EMA- or GFP-positive cells can be analyzed either from histograms or from dot plots. The gate of positive events for each carrier is adjusted according to a negative control. It is especially important to have negative controls for each carrier/DNA composition (nonlabeled DNA complexed by the carrier), to avoid any misinterpretations due to auto-fluorescence. The percentage of positive cells is defined by dividing the number of positive cells in the analysis gate by the total amount of cells in the live gate.

Acknowledgments

This work has been supported by Tekes, Finnish Academy and Sigrid Juselius Foundation. Authors thank Ms. Marja Poikolainen for preparing the manuscript.

References

1. Ylä-Herttuala, S. and Martin, J. F (2000) Cardiovascular gene therapy. *Lancet* **355**, 213–222.
2. Boussif, O., Lezoualch, F., Zanta, M. F., et al. (1995) A versatile vector for gene and oligonucleotide transfer into cells in culture and in vivo: polyethylenimine. *Proc. Natl. Acad. Sci. USA* **92**, 7297–7301.
3. Zabner, J., Fasbender, A. J., Moninger, K., Poellinger, K., and Welsh, M. J. (1995) Cellular and molecular barriers to gene transfer by a cationic lipid. *J. Biol. Chem.* **270**, 18997–19007.
4. Ruponen, M., Rönkkö, S., Honkakoski, P., Pelkonen, J., Tammi, M., and Urtti, A. (2001) Extracellular glycosaminoglycans modify cellular trafficking of lipoplexes and polyplexes. *J. Biol. Chem.* **276**, 33,875–33,880.
5. Hiltunen, M., Turunen, M., and Ylä-Herttuala, S. (2001) Gene therapy methods in cardiovascular diseases. *Meth. Enzymol.* **346**, 311–320.
6. Hiltunen, M. O., Turunen, M. P., Turunen, A-M., et al. (2000) Biodistribution of adenoviral vector to nontarget tissues after in vivo gene transfer to arterial wall using intravascular and periadventitial gene delivery methods. *FASEB J.* **14**, 2230–2236.
7. Laitinen, M., Mäkinen, K., Manninen, H., et al. (1998) Adenovirus-mediated gene transfer to lower limb artery of patients with chronic critical leg ischemia. *Hum. Gene Ther.* **9**, 1481–1486.

8. Mäkinen, K., Manninen, H., Hedman, M., et al. (2002) Increased vascularity detected by digital subtraction angiography after VEGF gene transfer to human lower limb artery. A randomized, placebo-controlled, double-blinded Phase II study. *Mol. Ther.* **6**, 127–133.

9. Turunen, M.P., Hiltunen, M.O., Ruponen, M., et al. (1999) Efficient adventitial gene delivery to rabbit carotid artery with cationic polymer-plasmid complexes. *Gene Ther.* **6**, 6–11.

10. Aihara, H. and Miyazaki, J. (1998) Gene transfer into muscle by electroporation in vivo. *Nat. Biotechnol.* **16**, 867–870.

11. Ylä-Herttuala, S. and Alitalo, K. (2003) Gene transfer as a tool to induce therapeutic vascular growth. *Nat. Med.* **9**, 694–701.

12. Koivunen, E., Arap, W., Valtanen, H., et al. (1999) Tumor targeting with a selective gelatinase inhibitor. *Nat. Biotechnol.* **17**, 768–774.

13. Budker, V., Zhang, G., Danko, I., Williams, P., and Wolff, J. (1998) The efficient expression of intravascularly delivered DNA in rat muscle. *Gene Ther.* **5**, 272–276.

14. Vicat, J. M., Boisseau, S., Jourdes, P., et al. (2000) Muscle transfection by electroporation with high-voltage and short-pulse currents provides high-level and long-lasting gene expression. *Hum. Gene Ther.* **11**, 909–916.

15. Lawrie, A., Brisken, A. F., Francis, S. E., et al. (1999) Ultrasound enhances reporter gene expression after transfection of vascular cells in vitro. *Circulation* **99**, 2617–2620.

16. Lin, W. C., Pretlow, T. P., Pretlow 2nd, T. G., and Culp, L. A. (1990) Bacterial lacZ gene as a highly sensitive marker to detect micrometastasis formation during tumor progression. *Cancer Res.* **50**, 2808–2817.

17. Weiss, D. J., Liggitt, D., and Clark, J. G. (1997) In situ histochemical detection of beta-galactosidase activity in lung assessment of X-Gal reagent in distinguishing lacZ gene expression and endogenous beta-galactosidase activity. *Hum. Gene Ther.* **8**, 1545–1554.

18. Sambrook, J. and Russell, D. W. (2001) *Molecular Cloning: A Laboratory Manual*, 3rd ed., Cold Spring Harbor Laboratory Press, Cold Spring Harbor, NY, 17.33–17.51.

19. Seliger, H. H. and McElroy, W. D. (1960) Spectral emission and quantum yield of firefly bioluminescence. *Arch. Biochem. Biophys.* **88**, 136–141.

20. de Wet, J. R., Wood, K. V., Helinski, D. R., and DeLuca, M. (1985) Cloning of firefly luciferase cDNA and the expression of active luciferase in *Escherichia coli. Proc. Natl. Acad. Sci. USA* **82**, 7870–7873.

21. Berger, J., Hauber, J., Hauber, R., Geiger, R., and Cullen, B. R. (1988) Secreted placental alkaline phosphatase: a powerful new qualitative indicator of gene expression in eukaryotic cells. *Gene* **66**, 1–10.

22. Chalfie, M., Tu, Y., Euskrirchen, G., Ward, W. W., and Prasher, D. C. (1994) Green fluorescent protein as a marker for gene expression. *Science* **263**, 802–805.

22

Construction and Characterization of Helper-Dependent Adenoviral Vectors for Sustained In Vivo Gene Therapy

Kazuhiro Oka and Lawrence Chan

Summary

A helper-dependent adenoviral (HDAd) vector is the most recently developed adenoviral vector. It does not contain any viral coding sequences except the inverted terminal repeat for replication origin and the packaging signal. Its safety profile and duration of transgene expression in vivo have improved substantially compared to early generation adenoviruses. Despite its usefulness for experimental gene therapy, technical difficulties in producing the HDAd vector have hampered its wide application. This chapter illustrates important considerations in vector design, unique features of this system, and an overview of vector production, which is followed by a step-by-step protocol for vector production. Vector characterization and troubleshooting are also provided at appropriate steps.

Key words: Helper-dependent adenoviral vector; helper virus; packaging cell line; Cre-*lox*P system; quantitative PCR; vector purification.

1. Introduction

A safe and effective gene delivery vehicle is central to all in vivo gene therapy protocols. Of the currently available viral gene delivery systems, adenovirus (Ad) has attracted wide attention because of its efficient transduction of a wide range of cell types in vitro and in vivo, independent of cell cycle. Although first- and second-generation Ads are useful in DNA vaccination or cancer gene therapy, the use of such Ad vectors for genetic diseases or for long-term treatment is limited by their substantial acute and chronic toxicity and the short-lived nature of transgene expression *(1)*. Leaky viral gene expression, even in the absence of the E1 gene, induces an immune response against transduced cells. In an attempt to reduce toxicity associated with early generation Ads, a novel Ad vector lacking all viral protein coding sequences has been developed *(2,3)* (for review, *see* **ref. 4**). This vector has been referred

From: *Methods in Molecular Medicine, Vol. 108: Hypertension: Methods and Protocols*
Edited by: J. P. Fennell and A. H. Baker © Humana Press Inc., Totowa, NJ

to as "helper-dependent," "high-capacity," "gutless," or "gutted" Ad. The only *cis* elements needed for Ad packaging are the inverted terminal repeat (ITR) and the packaging signal. Other factors can be supplied in *trans* by a helper virus. The term "helper-dependent" reflects the most popular production strategy currently in use, and we will refer to this Ad vector as a HDAd. Significant contamination of helper virus, a first-generation E1-deleted Ad, annuls the potential advantages of HDAd vectors; hence, removal of helper virus from HDAd vectors is critical in HDAd production. This problem has been resolved in part by taking advantage of the Cre-*lox*P system to remove the packaging signal of helper virus during vector production *(5)*. HDAd vectors have become the vector of choice for Ad vector-mediated experimental gene therapy because of their low toxicity and long-term transgene expression. Although HDAd vectors may exhibit superior performance over early-generation Ads in many applications, they have proven most useful in liver-directed gene transfer in vivo in experimental animals *(6–9)*. However, the large-scale production of HDAd free from helper virus contamination is still a challenge. In this chapter, we describe the HDAd production protocol based on our experience over the last several years. The following is a basic protocol that can be tried and modified according to the specific needs of individual laboratories.

1.1. Vector Design

The genome size of HDAds must be between 27 and 38 kb for efficient packaging. Smaller genome sizes can be packaged as head-to-tail and tail-to-tail concatamers within the size limit *(10)*. In order to bring the vector genome size within the packagable range, one can insert stuffer DNA into the vector construct (**Fig. 1**). The nature of stuffer DNA influences the efficiency of transgene expression. Fully characterized DNA of mammalian origin that does not contain any genes or repetitive sequences should be used as stuffer DNA in order to avoid rearrangement during serial passages *(11)* as well as to eliminate its effects on transgene expression. The presence of the matrix attachment site in the HDAd vector has been reported by some to enhance transgene expression *(12)*, but not by others *(13)*. Because the HDAd vector contains no viral coding sequence, transgene expression is independent of the orientation and only marginally influenced by the location of the transgene cassette within the vector genome *(12)*. HDAd vectors containing natural genes appear to have more sustained transgene expression than those containing cDNAs driven by heterologous promoters *(6–9,13,14)*. However, large genes exceeding the packaging limit or genes containing no endogenous tissue-specific promoter for target tissues must depend on the use of heterologous promoters. We have reported in abstract form that LDL receptor driven by the phosphoenolpyruvate carboxykinase promoter produces prolonged LDLR expression in the liver

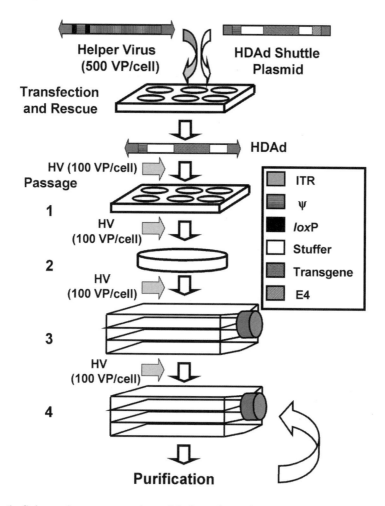

Fig. 1. Schematic representation of helper-dependent adenoviral vector (HDAd) production using Cre-*lox*P system. Typical structures of HDAd shuttle vector and helper virus. ITR, inverted terminal repeat; ψ, packaging signal; E4, the 400-bp fragment containing the E4 promoter. The 293 Cre66 cells are transfected with a HDAd shuttle vector (pC4HSU containing a transgene cassette) and infected with a helper virus (AdLC8cluc) at 500 vector particles (VP)/cell. Since the packaging signal of a helper virus is flanked by *lox*P sequences, it is excised in 293Cre66 cells, leaving a helper virus unpackagable. Only HDAd vector is packaged. The titer of HDAd vector is increased by serial passages. The 293Cre66 cells in a 6-well plate are co-infected with HDAd vector and a helper virus (100 VP/cell) in passage 1. Co-infection is repeated in a 10-cm dish for passage 2, a triple flask (TF) for passage 3, and 8X TF for passage 4. After passage 4, HDAd vector is purified by CsCl density centrifugation. The typical yield of HDAd vector is $1–2 \times 10^{12}$ VP. The purified HDAd vector is used as a seed stock to produce more vectors.

of LDL receptor-deficient mice for over a year *(15)*. Therefore, even for cDNAs
driven by heterologous promoters, long-term transgene expression is possible
and factors that determine duration of expression are complex and poorly
understood in individual vectors. Target tissue-specific promoters are preferable to ubiquitous promoters for sustained transgene expression, and the use of
promoters active in antigen-presenting cells should be avoided to minimize the
generation of neutralizing antibodies against transgene products. The inclusion of the first 400 bp from the right end containing the E4 promoter without
any coding sequence into a HDAd vector has been reported to increase vector
production, by enhancing either replication or packaging of the vector DNA
(11). Although we have inconsistent results using this element, its presence
does not negatively impact viral production and we include it in the standard
vector design (**Fig. 1**). The woodchuck hepatitis virus posttranscriptional
regulatory element (WPRE) is a cis-acting element that increases the amount
of unspliced RNA in both the nuclear and cytoplasmic compartments *(16)*. The
insertion of WPRE in the 3'-untranslated region upstream to the polyadenylation signal is a useful strategy to increase transgene expression without
affecting promoter specificity *(17)*.

1.2. Other Features of Helper-Dependent Adenoviral Vectors

Despite the long-term transgene expression mediated by HDAd *(6,8)*, it is
poorly integrated in the host chromosome *(18,19)*. Vector DNA is eventually
eliminated from the tissues by cell division or cell turnover. Therefore, to maintain a therapeutic level of transgene expression, one needs to readminister the
HDAd. The generation of neutralizing antibodies by the host animal against
Ad precludes repeated Ad administration. However, as neutralizing antibodies
are serotype-specific, one can circumvent the immune response by retreatment
using a HDAd produced with a helper virus of an alternate serotype *(8,20)*.
Importantly, the current HDAd vector production strategy allows HDAd vectors with various serotypes to be produced readily by co-infection of the same
vector backbone and a helper virus of the second serotype during large-scale
production (serotype switching). Another approach to overcome the essentially
transient transgene expression is to incorporate elements that permit stable
integration of the vector into the host chromosome. This approach takes
advantage of the cloning and transduction efficiency of Ad vectors and the
capability of DNA integration of other systems such as adeno-associated virus
(AAV) *(21,22)*, retrovirus *(23)*, lentivirus *(24)*, or transposon *(25,26)*. In most
of the hybrid HDAd vectors, the transgene is integrated at random sites except
for Ad/AAV hybrid viruses expressing Rep78 gene *(21)*. Site-specific integration mediated by AAV vectors has been confirmed in humans and in the African green monkey *(27–29)*, but not in rodents. Another hybrid system that could

effect site-specific integration is produced by the incorporation of phage φC31 integrase *(30)* in the vector. The utility of such hybrid HDAd vector systems remains to be tested in animals.

The cellular tropism of HDAd vectors is no different from that of a first-generation Ad. It is determined by the presence of surface Coxsackie and aden-ovirus receptor as primary attachment sites for the fiber. The integrin molecules $\alpha_V\beta_3$ and $\alpha_V\beta_5$ serve as secondary internalization receptors for the penton base protein *(31)*. Cell-surface heparan sulfate glycosaminoglycans have also been reported to be involved in the initial binding *(32)*. Despite the wide spectrum of Ad infection, several cell types are poorly transduced by Ad because of poor expression of these receptors. Much effort has been directed toward targeting first-generation Ad vectors to these cell types. The knowledge from these stud-ies can be applied to generate targeting helper viruses *(33)*. Because the helper virus determines the targeting specificity of HDAds, one can easily produce HDAds targeting specific cells and tissues using a library of helper viruses with such targeting capabilities.

One other major advantage of HDAd vector is its large cloning capacity. Genes containing endogenous promoters and regulatory elements up to 37 kb can be inserted into the vector. There are many polygenic diseases for which a multiple-gene treatment is considered. A single HDAd vector expressing mul-tiple genes may be a useful feature for gene therapy in the future.

1.3. Overview of the Production Protocol of Helper-Dependent Adenoviral Vectors

The current HDAd production system depends on the inhibition of helper virus packaging without interfering with its ability to provide necessary helper function to propagate HDAd virions. The most common strategies utilize Cre-*lox*P *(5,33,34)*, or FLP-*frt* *(35,36)* systems. The packaging signal of a helper virus is flanked by *lox*P or *frt* sites. Following infection of E1 complementing cells expressing either recombinase, the packaging signal is excised from the helper virus by site-specific recombination. Consequently, the helper virus genome cannot be packaged into virions, whereas the HDAd vector is nor-mally packaged (**Fig. 1**). Replication of helper virus is not impaired and con-tinues to supply helper function for HDAd. The titer of the HDAd vector is increased by serial propagation until it reaches an appropriate level. However, the excision of the packaging signal is not always complete. The remaining helper virus in the final HDAd vector preparation is removed by CsCl density-gradient ultracentrifugation.

The possibility exists for the generation of replication competent Ad as a consequence of homologous recombination between the helper virus and the overlapping sequence present in E1 complementing cell lines. To eliminate such a possibility, it is necessary to use PERC6-Cre- *(34)* or N52.E6-derived cells *(37)*, in which the truncated E1 gene does not have the overlapping sequence with the current Ad vectors. Because of the ease of handling, suspension culture is preferred for the large-scale vector production. Although Sakhuja et al. have reported the adaptation of PERC6-Cre cells for suspension cell culture, helper virus contamination appears to be a practical problem *(34)*. Shiedner et al. have adapted 293Cre66 cells for suspension, which produce HDAd vectors at similar levels with similar helper virus contamination as those produced with adherent cells (Schiedner et al., manuscript in preparation). Palmar and Ng have recently reported improved HDAd vector production using 293 suspension cells expressing Cre protein *(38)*. These encouraging developments will likely be incorporated into future routine large-scale HDAd vector production protocols.

2. Materials

2.1. E1-Complementing Cells Expressing Site-Specific Recombinase and Helper Virus

One of the following cells and compatible helper virus:

1. E1 function complementing cell lines (for amplification of helper virus) such as 293, PERC6 *(39)*, or N52.E6 *(37)*.
2. The E1 function complementing cell lines expressing Cre or FLP recombinase such as 293Cre4 *(5)*, 293Cre66 (Schiedner et al., manuscript in preparation), C7-Cre *(40)*, PERC6-Cre *(34)*, 293FLP *(36)*, or 293-FLPe6 *(35)*.
3. Helper virus with the packaging signal flanked by *lox*P sites or *frt* sites: AdLC8cluc *(5)*, H14 *(11)*, Av1nBgflx *(34)*, Av1S4BflxFE3 *(34)*, AdCBfrt3 *(36)*, or FL helper virus *(35)*.

Early passages of 293, 293 N3S (suspension cell), and 293Cre4 cells, as well as helper virus H14 and pC4HSU shuttle vector, are available through Microbix (www.microbix.com) (*see* **Note 1**).

2.2. Cell Culture

The following reagents are based on 293Cre66 cells in combination with AdLC8cluc as a helper virus.

1. Minimum essential medium alpha (α-MEM, Invitrogen, cat. no. 12571-063).
2. Geneticin (G418; Invitrogen, cat. no. 10131-027).
3. 0.25% Trypsin-EDTA (Invitrogen, cat. no. 25200-056).
4. Antibiotic-antimycotic (100X, Invitrogen, cat. no. 15240-062).
5. PBS^{++} (Invitrogen, cat. no. 14040-133).
6. Growth medium: α-MEM supplemented with 10% fetal bovine serum (FBS; heat-inactivated at 56°C for 30 min), 1X antibiotic-antimycotic and 0.4 mg/mL of G418.

7. Complete medium: α-MEM supplemented with 10% FBS (heat inactivated) and 1X antibiotic-antimycotic.
8. Maintenance medium (used after infection): α-MEM supplemented with 5% horse serum (heat-inactivated) and 1X antibiotic-antimycotic.
9. 40% sucrose (tissue-culture grade, Sigma, cat. no. S1888): autoclave, filter through 0.22-μm filter (Corning, cat. no. 431097), and store at room temperature.

2.3. Transfection

One of the following transfection reagents.

1. Calcium phosphate transfection kit (Promega, cat. no. E1200). Calcium phosphate transfection reagents can be prepared as described *(41,42)*.
2. SuperFect transfection reagent (Qiagen, cat. no. 301305).

2.4. Characterization of HDAd Vector DNA

1. Phenol/choloroform/isoamyl alcohol (25/24/1, v/v; Invitrogen, cat. no. 15593-031).
2. 1 M Tris-HCl, pH 8.0 (Invitrogen, cat. no. 15568-025).
3. 10% Sodium dodecyl sulfate (SDS) (Invitrogen, cat. no. 15553-035).
4. 0.5 M EDTA, pH 8.0 (Invitrogen, cat. no. 15575-038).
5. Agarose gel electrophoresis system.
6. Slot-blot apparatus (Bio-Rad, cat. no. 170-6542).
7. TE: 10 mM Tris-HCl, pH 8.0, 0.1 mM EDTA.
8. Proteinase K reaction mixture (freshly prepare, 176 μL of H_2O, 20 μL of 10% SDS, 4 μL of Proteinase K stock solution [10 mg/mL in H_2O, stored in small aliquots at –20°C]).
9. 3 M Sodium acetate buffer, pH 5.2: Dissolve 40.8 g sodium acetate·$3H_2O$, adjust pH to 5.2 with 3 M acetic acid, add H_2O to 100 mL. Sterilize by autoclave.
10. 6X Gel loading buffer (1X TAE, 0.25% bromophenol blue, 0.25% xylene cyanol, 30% glycerol; Invotrogen, cat. no. 750005).
11. 50X TAE buffer: 242 g Tris base, 57.1 mL glacial acetic acid, 37.2 g $Na_2EDTA.2H_2O$, H_2O to 1 L (Invitrogen, cat. no. 750001).
12. 20X SSC: 175 g NaCl, 88 g Na_3-citrate·$2H_2O$, adjust pH to 7.0 with 1 M HCl and H_2O to 1 L (Invitrogen, cat. no. 750020).
13. 10X citric-saline (1.35 M KCl, 0.15 M sodium citrate, autoclave and store at 4°C).
14. Radioactive or nonradioactive random priming DNA labeling kit. For nonradioactive method, we use DIG DNA labeling kit/wash and block buffer kit (Roche, cat. no. 1-585-614 and 1-585-761).
15. QIAamp DNA kit (Qiagen, cat. no. 52304).
16. SYBR Green QPCR master mix (Stratagene, cat. no. 600548, or MJ Research, cat. no. F-400L).
17. Phosphoimager.
18. Real-time QPCR platform.

2.5. HDAd Vector Purification

1. CsCl (Invitrogen, cat. no. 15507-023).
2. Dialysis cassette (Pierce, cat. no. 66332).
3. 1 M MgCl$_2$.
4. 10X Tris density buffer (TD). Dissolve 80.0 g NaCl, 3.8 g KCl, 30.0 g Tris base, and 1.87 g Na$_2$HPO$_4$·7H$_2$O, adjust pH to 7.4–7.5 with 5 M NaOH, and make the final volume to 1 L with double-distilled H$_2$O.
5. CsCl density solutions (d = 1.25, 1.35, and 1.41 g/mL). Pour 350 mL of 1X TD into a beaker. Add 135 g CsCl for d = 1.25 (for d = 1.33 add 160 g CsCl, and for d = 1.41 add 180 g CsCl) and mix with a stir bar, then let come to room temperature. Weigh out 1 mL of the CsCl solution on the small weigh boat using a 1-mL pipet (calibrated 1 mL of H$_2$O–1.00 g), and add more 1X TD or CsCl powder until exact density concentration is reached (add each weighing back into beaker). Sterilize by a 0.22-μm filter (Corning, cat. no. 431097) and store at room temperature.
6. Dialysis buffer (DB): 10 mM Tris-HCl, pH 8.0, 2 mM MgCl$_2$, 4% sucrose.

3. Methods

The following basic protocol is based on the use of 293Cre66 cells, AdLC8cluc helper virus and pC4HSU shuttle vector, though it is generally applicable to other cell lines with appropriate modifications.

3.1. Cell Culture

293Cre66 cells are maintained in T162 culture flask, or a TripleFlask (Nunc, cat. no. 132867) using a growth medium containing G418 (0.4 mg/mL). In general, approx 90% confluent cells are split 1:4 twice a week (the doubling time of 293Cre66 is about 2 d). The following is the TripleFlask (TF) version.

1. Remove the medium from flasks.
2. Add 10 mL trypsin and incubate at room temperature for 3–5 min. 293Cre66 cells should not be rinsed with PBS before adding trypsin, because this cell line is loosely attached to the flask and tends to become detached by doing so.
3. Cells will begin to detach from the flask. Tap the side of the flask, if necessary, to detach any remaining cells.
4. Add 20 mL of growth medium.
5. Pour cell suspension into an appropriate container, mix well, and distribute into new plates, dishes, or flasks.

3.2. Rescue and Serial Amplification of Helper-Dependent Adenoviral Vector

1. Prepare the shuttle vector plasmid DNA using a commercial kit. An ample amount of plasmid DNA is provided by 100 mL of LB culture.
2. Linearize the shuttle vector DNA with an appropriate restriction enzyme (*Pme* I for pΔ21[8]-, pΔ28[7]-, or pC4HSU[11]-based shuttle vector).

3. Extract with phenol/chloroform/isoamyl alcohol, precipitate with ethanol, and resuspend in nuclease-free H_2O under sterile conditions.

3.2.1. Transfection and Rescue HDAd Vector

The 293Cre66 cells can be transfected by one of two methods: calcium phosphate precipitation or liposome-mediated transfection. The calcium phosphate precipitation method is slightly more effective than liposome-mediated transfection; however, the latter method requires less DNA and appears to be more reproducible. The two methods are described below. It is recommended that a shuttle vector containing a reporter gene included for the first time to easily monitor vector amplification and to ensure a properly functioning system.

3.2.1.1. CALCIUM PHOSPHATE TRANSFECTION METHOD USING A KIT (PROMEGA)

Seed 293Cre66 cells with complete medium into a 6-well plate or 3.5-cm dish to reach 70–90% confluency at the day of transfection.

1. Add 5 µg linearized shuttle vector and 18.5 µL of 2 M $CaCl_2$ solution in a 1.5-mL tube to make a final volume of 150 µL with H_2O.
2. Add the DNA solution to a 15-mL polystyrene tube containing 150 µL of HEPES-buffered saline dropwise while gently vortexing the tube. The solution becomes slightly opalescent due to the formation of fine particles.
3. Incubate the solution at room temperature for 30 min under the hood.
4. Vortex the DNA solution, and apply it dropwise on top of cells without removing medium.
5. Incubate cells overnight in a CO_2 incubator.

3.2.1.2. LIPOSOME-MEDIATED TRANSFECTION METHOD

1. Dissolve 2.5 µg of linearized shuttle vector in 75 µL of α-MEM (no FBS or antibiotic-antimycotic).
2. Add 12.5 µL of SuperFect reagent to DNA solution, mix gently by pipetting up and down several times.
3. Incubate for 5–10 min at room temperature.
4. During incubation, wash the cells once with 2 mL of α-MEM prewarmed to 37°C.
5. Add 0.25 mL of α-MEM to DNA solution, mix by pipetting up and down.
6. Overlay DNA–liposome complex on top of cells (medium must be removed before DNA–liposome solution is overlayed).
7. Incubate cells for 2–3 h in a CO_2 incubator. Swirl every 30 min. Add 1 mL of complete medium.

Next day, wash the cells once with 2 mL of a-MEM (the rest of the protocol is common for both transfection methods).

1. Remove medium and infect with 0.25 mL of α-MEM containing 5×10^8 vector particles (VP) of helper virus (500 VP/cell) (*see* **Note 2**).

2. Incubate cells for 1 h in a CO_2 incubator. Swirl every 10–15 min.
3. Add 1 mL of maintenance medium.
4. Cells are incubated until >90% cells show cytopathic effect (CPE; cells are rounded and detached from the plate). This should occur between 48 and 72 h postinfection.
5. Transfer cell and medium (crude viral lysate, CVL) to a cryotube.
6. Add 0.1 vol of 40% sucrose for storage at –80°C.

3.2.2. Passage 1

All infections are carried out on cells 80–90% confluent.

1. Seed 293Cre66 cells in a 6-well plate.
2. On the day of infection, thaw the CVL in a 37°C water bath.
3. Remove medium and incubate cells with 0.5 mL of CVL together with helper virus at 100 VP/cell (1×10^8 VP).
4. Continue infection for 1 h as described under **Subheading 3.2.1.**
5. Add 1 mL of maintenance medium.
6. Incubate until >90% cells show CPE. If cells do not show CPE after 72 h, helper virus is not sufficient. Thus, more helper virus must be added.
7. Transfer CVL to a cryotube.
8. Add 0.1 vol of 40% sucrose to the CVL for storage at –80°C.

3.2.3. Passage 2

1. Seed 293Cre66 cells in a 10-cm dish.
2. Thaw CVL in a 37°C water bath.
3. Infect cells with 1 ml of CVL supplemented with 7×10^8 VP of helper virus.
4. Add 5 mL of maintenance medium after 1 h incubation.
5. Incubate until >90% cells show CPE (usually 2–3 d).
6. Aliquot 0.2 mL of CVL for vector DNA analysis.
7. Transfer the remaining CVL to a 15-mL tube.
8. Add 0.1 vol of 40% sucrose.
9. Store the CVL at –80°C (*see* **Note 3**).

3.2.4. Passage 3

1. Seed 293Cre66 cells in TF (or 3×15-cm dishes).
2. Thaw CVL in a 37°C water bath.
3. Dilute CVL with α-MEM to 10 mL.
4. Add 5×10^9 VP of helper virus to CVL and infect cells.
5. Add 20 mL of maintenance medium after 1 h incubation.
6. Incubate until CPE is nearly complete (2–3 d).
7. Transfer 0.2 mL of CVL to a 1.5-mL tube for DNA extraction.
8. Transfer the remaining CVL into a 50-mL tube.
9. Add 0.1 vol of 40% sucrose and store at –80°C.

Before proceeding to passage 4, vector DNA should be analyzed for vector amplification as described below, because appropriate vector titer is necessary for a large-scale infection. By plating cells at the appropriate density, the vector can be passaged at least twice per week.

3.2.4.1. ANALYSIS OF VECTOR DNA

1. Thaw the 0.2 mL of CVL collected from serial passages in a 37°C water bath.
2. Add 0.2 mL of proteinase K reaction mixture.
3. Incubate at 56°C for at least 2 h.
4. Add 400 μL of phenol/chloroform/isoamyl alcohol and vortex vigorously.
5. Centrifuge at 13,000g for 2 min.
6. Transfer the supernatant to a new 1.5-mL tube.
7. Precipitate DNA by adding 40 μL of 3 *M* sodium acetate buffer, pH 5.2, and 880 μL of 100% ethanol. DNA clump should be visible soon after adding ethanol, due to the presence of chromosomal DNA.
8. Incubate at room temperature for 10–30 min to prevent salt precipitation.
9. Centrifuge at 13,000g for 3 min in a microcentrifuge.
10. Discard supernatant.
11. Rinse DNA pellet with 500 μL of 70% ethanol.
12. Briefly air-dry DNA pellet, and reconstitute in 30 μL of TE. It is important not to excessively dry DNA, because dried DNA is difficult to dissolve.
13. Digest 4 μL of vector DNA with an appropriate enzyme (we routinely use *Hin*d III) in a total volume of 20 μL. In separate tubes, digest 0.1 μg (corresponding to 2.58×10^9 VP) of helper virus and 0.1 μg of plasmid HDAd shuttle vector predigested with *Pme* I.
14. Incubate at 37°C for at least 2 h.
15. Add 4 μL of 6X loading buffer, vortex, spin down, and separate on a 1.2% agarose gel (24 μL/well). Use 4 μL of 1 kbPlus DNA marker (Invitrogen, cat. no. 10787-018, diluted to 50 ng/μL in 1X loading buffer) as a molecular size standard.
16. Follow the standard Southern blot analysis. The 400-bp fragment containing the left ITR plus the packaging signal is used as a probe because it differentiates the left and right arms of the HDAd vector (**Fig. 2**) (*see* **Note 4**).

3.2.4.2. DETERMINATION OF INFECTIOUS TITER USING HDAD VECTOR CONTAINING A REPORTER GENE

With HDAd vectors containing a reporter gene such as LacZ or green fluorescence protein (GFP), the infectious titer can be easily determined by infection of 293 cells. In the following example, we determine the infectious titer of serial passages of HDAd vector containing a βgeo cassette using the β-Gal staining kit (Invitrogen, cat. no. K1465-01). For this assay, an additional 0.2 mL CVL containing 4% sucrose must be aliquoted at each passage.

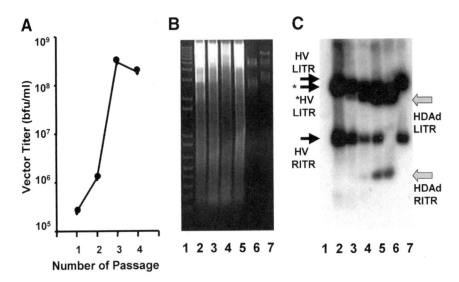

Fig. 2. HDAd vector amplification during serial passage using β-geo as a reporter gene. **(A)** Increase of infectious titer. The titer is expressed as blue-forming unit (bfu)/mL. **(B)** DNA stained by ethidium bromide. **(C)** Southern blot analysis. DNAs were digested with Hind III, and separated on a 1.2% agarose gel. The ^{32}P-labeled ITR + packaging signal was used as a probe. Lane 1, 1 KbPlus ladder; lane 2, DNA extracted from CVL collected at passage 1; lane 3, passage 2; lane 4, passage 3; lane 5, passage 4; lane 6, purified HDAd-βgeo vector; lane 7, 0.1 μg of helper virus (2.58 × 10^9 VP). HV-LITR: intact helper virus left inverted terminal repeat (3.3 kb); *HV-LITR: HV-LITR lacking the packaging signal (3.1 kb); HV-RITR: HV right ITR (1 kb), HDAd-LITR: HDAd-βgeo (pC4HSU backbone) left ITR (2.4 kb); HDAd-RITR: HDAd-βgeo right ITR (0.4 kb). The clear vector amplification is detected at passage 2 (lane 3), and the signal of HDAd vector is comparable to that of helper virus at passage 3 before to the large-scale vector production (lane 4).

1. Seed 293 cells in a 12-well plate 1 d before infection. Cells should be 80–90% confluent at the time of infection.
2. Remove the medium and incubate cells for 1 h in 0.2 mL of α-MEM containing various volumes of CVL from serial passages (10, 20, 40, and 80 μL).
3. Add 1 mL of maintenance medium and continue the incubation overnight.
4. Remove the medium, and fix cells with 0.5 mL of 1X fixative solution for 20 min at room temperature.
5. Rinse the wells twice with 1 mL of 1X PBS.
6. Add 0.2 mL of staining solution.
7. Incubate the plate at 37°C. Blue cells are visible after 15–30 min. Do not exceed 2 h.
8. Count the number of blue cells, and calculate the transducing unit as blue form-

ing unit (bfu)/mL of CVL. The titer should be about $0.5-1 \times 10^8$ bfu/ml prior to large-scale production (passage 4).

3.2.5. Large-Scale Adenovirus Production (Passage 4)

The first large-scale production of the HDAd vector is performed in 8X TF or 24X 15-cm dishes.

1. Seed 293Cre66 cells in 8X TF.
2. Thaw the CVL in a 37°C water bath.
3. Divide CVL evenly into two 50-mL tubes.
4. Bring volume to 40 ml with α-MEM in each 50-mL tube.
5. Add helper virus (5×10^9 VP × 4) for each 50-mL tube, and mix by inverting the tubes several times.
6. Remove the medium from the TF.
7. Add 10 mL of CVL containing helper virus to each TF.
8. Continue the infection for 1 h in a CO_2 incubator.
9. Add 20 mL of maintenance medium.
10. Check the cells every 12–24 h and collect CVL in 250-mL centrifuge tubes when CPE is nearly complete after 48–72 h.
11. Centrifuge at 800g for 10 min.
12. Discard the supernatant.
13. Resuspend cells in 9–10 mL of maintenance medium or α-MEM.
14. Aliquot 0.2 mL in a 1.5-mL tube for DNA extraction.
15. Transfer the remaining cell suspension into a 15-ml tube (Corning, cat. no. 430055).
16. Add 0.1 volumes of 40% sucrose, and store at –80°C.

3.2.5.1. PURIFICATION OF ADENOVIRUS

HDAd vectors are released from cells by freezing/thawing or disrupting cell membranes using sodium deoxycholate *(41,42)*. The yield of HDAd vectors by the deoxycholate method is about 10–20% higher than that of the freezing/ thawing method. Because cell suspensions are typically frozen prior to purification, we generally purify the vector from the supernatant after freeze/thaw. Ad vectors can be purified by various methods, including CsCl density centrifugation, ion exchange, or metal-chelating column chromatography *(41,43–45)*. The CsCl density gradient is the most popular method and will be included in this protocol.

1. Thaw frozen cells by incubation in a 37°C water bath.
2. Centrifuge the tube in the SS-34 rotor (Sorvall) at 5000g for 10 min.
3. Recover the clear supernatant.

3.2.5.2. First Ultracentrifugation

To purify the virus, sterilize NVT 65 tubes (Beckman, cat. no. 362181) either by autoclaving, irradiation under the UV light for several hours, or soaking in 100% ethanol followed by sterile water and air-dry in the hood (two tubes required for each viral preparation).

1. Place 3 mL of low-density (1.25-g/mL) CsCl in a centrifuge tube.
2. Underlay 3 mL of high density (1.41 g/mL) CsCl using a 2-mL pipet.
3. Carefully overlay 5 mL of clear supernatant collected under **Subheading 3.2.5.1., step 3**, using a 5-mL pipet.
4. Fill the tubes to the neck using a 2-mL or Pasteur pipet with either the clear supernatant or PBS^{++}, and cap the tubes (**Fig. 3A**). There is no need to weigh them.
5. Centrifuge for 30 min at 202,000g and 20°C (brake on) (*see* **Note 5**).
6. Remove caps from the tubes.
7. Collect the lower opalescent band (**Fig. 3B**) with a 1- or 3-mL syringe and 21G needle by side puncture. Clean the area for needle puncture with 70% ethanol before collection. It is useful to remove the empty capsid band (upper opalescent band) before collecting the infectious virus band, because they are physically close together and would be difficult to isolate one from the other.

3.2.5.3. Second Centrifugation

1. Place 8 mL of 1.35-g/mL CsCl in a new centrifuge tube.
2. Overlay the band recovered from the first centrifugation.
3. Fill in the tubes with 1.35-g/mL solution.
4. Centrifuge as above except for 3.5 h.
5. Recover the opalescent band with a syringe (**Fig. 3C**).
6. Transfer the virus into a dialysis cassette.
7. Dialyze against 3 L of DB without sucrose once for 1 h at 4°C, and then against 3 L of DB at 4°C overnight (*see* **Note 6**).

An alternative to dialysis is desalting with a PD10 disposable column (Amersham/Pharmacia, cat. no. 17-085-01).

1. Equilibrate the PD10 column with a total of 25 mL of DB in batches of 5 mL. The flow rate is about 0.25 mL/min. Therefore the column equilibration must be initiated after the second ultracentrifugation begins.
2. Load 2.5 mL of collected HDAd vector onto the column. If the volume is less than 2.5 mL, adjust the volume with DB.
3. Discard the effluent.
4. Elute the vector with 3.5 mL of DB into a 15-mL tube when the sample has run into the column.

3.3. Vector Characterization

The following are routine vector characterizations.

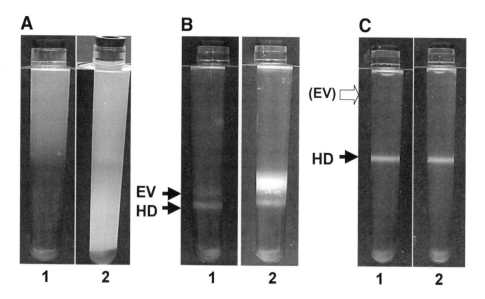

Fig. 3. Purification of HDAd vector by CsCl density centrifugation. (**A**) Prior to the first CsCl density centrifugation. (**B**) HDAd vector bands after the first CsCl centrifugation. (**C**) HDAd vector bands after the second CsCl centrifugation. 1, Freeze/thaw method; 2, sodium deoxycholate method. EV, empty virus (capsids); HD, HDAd vector. In lane 2 of (**B**), EV band overlaps with chromosomal DNA band. Open arrow in (**C**) indicates the position for EV, which is not visible in this preparation. The band corresponding to helper virus is not visible due to less than 0.1% contamination. It appears as a lower band relative to HDAd vector if helper virus contamination is significant.

3.3.1. Concentration of Vector Particles (VP) Using Optical Density

The most common method is based on optical density (*46*). OD_{260} titers are calculated using $\varepsilon = 9.09 \times 10^{-13}$ ml cm virion^{-1}, though the accuracy has been disputed (*43,47*).

1. Add 380 µL of TE/SDS solution (7.5 mL of TE + 80 µL of 10% SDS) to 20 µL of purified HDAd vector. For a blank, add 380 µL of TE/SDS solution to 20 µL of DB.
2. Incubate at 56°C for 20 min.
3. Measure OD at 260 nm. To check the purity, a ratio of 260 nm/280 nm is measured, which should be higher than 1.3.

The physical concentration (VP/ml) is calculated as follows: $OD_{260nm} \times$ Ddilution factor [400 (µL)/20 (µL)] $\times 1.1 \times 10^{12}$ VP/mL $\times$ size correction factor (36 kb/size of vector in kb)

3.3.2. Infectious Titer

The infectious titer of a first-generation Ad vector is determined by plaque assay, which relies on vector replication in E1-complementing cell lines. HDAd vectors do not contain any viral coding sequences, and therefore do not form plaques. Thus, it is necessary to perform an assay based on internalization of vector DNA as described by Kreppel et al. *(48)*. The assay is universal to all HDAd as well as early-generation Ad vectors.

1. Seed 293 cells in a 24-well plate with complete medium and wait until cells become 80–90% confluent.
2. Dilute HDAd vectors and reference HDAd vector containing a reporter gene such as βgeo or GFP (infectious titer should be known) to 5×10^9 VP/mL with α-MEM.
3. Remove medium and replace with 0.2 mL of α-MEM.
4. Add the following volume of diluted HDAd vector in duplicate. 0, 2, 4, 8, 16, and 32 μL.
5. Continue infection for 1 h.
6. Add 0.3 mL of maintenance medium, and incubate the plate overnight in a CO_2 incubator.
7. Wash the cells twice with 1 mL of PBS^{++}.
8. Add 0.2 mL of 1X citric saline.
9. Incubate at room temperature for about 20 min or until cells start to round up and detach from the well.
10. Transfer the cell suspension to a 1.5-mL tube by pipetting up and down.
11. Add 0.2 mL of 0.8 *M* NaOH, vortex vigorously, and incubate at room temperature for 15 min.
12. Assemble the slot-blot apparatus, and load 200 μL of the above cell suspension into each slot.
13. Proceed to hybridization. The ^{32}P-labeled ITR or packaging signal is used as a probe.
14. Quantify the radioactive bands by a phosphoimager. The infectious titer of HDAd vector is calculated from the standard curve obtained by HDAd containing the reporter gene (*see* **Note 7**).

3.3.3. Helper Virus Contamination

Helper virus contamination can be determined by semiquantitative Southern blot analysis as described under **Subheading 3.2.4.1.** using known amounts of helper virus DNA as a standard. The radioactive bands corresponding to the left arm are quantified by a phosphoimager and the amount of helper virus present in HDAd vector is calculated from the standard. However, real-time polymerase chain reaction (PCR) *(11)* is a more accurate way to quantify helper virus contamination. The following protocol is based on the use of SYBR Green I as a detection dye. For this analysis, DNA purified by a QIAamp DNA kit is preferable. The PCR primer sequences to detect helper virus or pC4HSU-based HDAd vector genomes are provided below.

Helper virus (AdLC8cluc): Primer 1, 5' – CCTACACCAACACAACAACTC – 3', and Primer 2, 5' – ATCCACCTCAAAAGTCATGTC – 3'

HDAd on pC4HSU backbone: Primer 3, 5' – AGTAGGGTGAAGGGATGGAG – 3', and Primer 4, 5' – TGTGGGAAGACAGAAAACAAAG – 3'.

1. Make serial dilutions of helper virus and *Pme* I linearized pC4HSU shuttle vector DNA by 10-fold increment dilutions starting at 0.1 ng/μL and ending at 10^{-7} ng/μL (seven dilutions) with H_2O.
2. Make serial dilution of HDAd vectors to be analyzed by 10-fold increments starting at 0.1 ng/μL and ending at 10^{-4} ng/μL (four dilutions).
3. Prepare PCR-primer mix for helper virus. For 24 wells, mix 25 × 26 μL (24 wells + 2 extra wells) of PCR master mix, 26 μL of Primer 1 (10 pmol/μL), 26 μL of Primer 2 (10 pmol/μL) and 13 × 26 μL of H_2O. Mix gently by pipetting up and down. Minimize exposure to light, because SYBR Green is light-sensitive.
4. Prepare PCR-primer mix for HDAd vector. Repeat above procedure with primers 3 and 4.
5. Dispense 40 μL of PCR-primer mix to each well in duplicate.
6. Add 10 μL of DNA solution to each well in duplicate. Include 10 μL of H_2O (no template control, NTC). Therefore, two rows include NTC, standards (seven dilutions) and HDAd vector to be assayed (four dilutions) in duplicate.
7. Follow the manufacture's instruction. The PCR cycle for the primers listed above is 95°C for 10 min, followed by 95°C for 20 s, 55°C for 20 s, and 72°C for 30 s for 40 cycles.

Helper virus contamination (%): (ng of helper virus/ng of HDAd vector)/ (ng of shuttle vector DNA/ng of HDAd vector) × 100 × size correction factor [31 (size of pC4HSU in kb)/35 (size of AdLC8cluc in kb)]

3.3.4. Assurance of Vector Structures/Quality Control

HDAd vectors are produced in serial passages by co-infection with helper virus. The existence of overlapping sequences between HDAd vector and helper virus potentially results in recombination between the two viruses *(11)*. Such vector recombination can be detected by Southern blot analysis, in which the vector containing recombination appears as extra bands of varying sizes other than HDAd vector or helper virus. However, we routinely compare the structures of HDAd vector and its plasmid shuttle vector by Southern blot analysis *(7,8)*. The probe for this analysis is the corresponding plasmid shuttle vector without plasmid backbone.

4. Notes

1. Helper virus should be plaque purified prior to large-scale production on 293 cells (*see* **ref. 41** for the production of a first generation Ad) and its structure verified. This is necessary because any variant (e.g., helper virus lost *lox*P or *frt* sequences) can outgrow HDAd vector during serial passages. Purified helper virus is stored at –80°C in small aliquots in 10 m*M* Tris-HCl, pH 8.0, 2 m*M* MgCl$_2$, 4% sucrose at concentrations of 1–3 × 10^{12} VP/mL. Higher concentrations may result in aggregation and precipitation of Ads.

2. The amount of helper virus is based on the ratio of infectious particles to vector particles being between 1:40 and 1:100. The exact amount of helper virus should be optimized for each helper virus preparation based on infectious titer. However, its amount described in the protocol is applicable in most cases without modification.

3. Collection of 0.2 mL of CVL for DNA extraction is omitted at the transfection/ rescue step and passage 1 because the vector titer is too low for detection at these stages. Some vectors (e.g., HDAd-βgeo) are efficiently amplified and passage 1 may be eliminated.

4. If no clear vector amplification is detected at passage 3, repeat one or two more serial passages in TF using the protocol described under **Subheading 3.2.3.** Passage 3, and analyze vector amplification by Southern blot analysis. With efficient vector amplification, the intensity of the band corresponding to the left arm of HDAd vector is comparable to that of helper virus lacking the packaging signal at passage 3 (**Fig. 2C**, lane 4). If no HDAd vector is detected after additional amplifications, it is likely due to inefficient transfection and repeating the transfection is recommended. We found that one or two more serial passages increase the titer without detectable vector rearrangement. However, unnecessary amplification should be avoided because it increases the chance of vector rearrangement. Vector DNA can be purified using QIAamp DNA kit (Qiagen cat. no. 52304). DNA is clean but diluted to 0.2 mL.

5. Any swinging rotors can be used, but require longer centrifugation time. Check for appropriate speed and centrifugation time at www.beckman.com/resource-center/labresources/centrifuges/rotorcalc.asp.

6. Efficient HDAd vector propagation at passage 4 results in less than 1% helper virus contamination in the supernatant after freeze/thaw. Defrost 0.2 mL of cell suspension in a 37°C water bath, centrifuge at 13,000*g* for 3 min, and extract DNA from the supernatant as described under **Subheading 3.2.4.1.** Analyze DNA by Southern blot analysis. This provides the approximate yield and helper virus contamination of HDAd vectors before CsCl purification. The typical yield of HDAd vector on pC4HSU backbone at passage 4 is 1–2 × 10^{12} VP with less than 0.1% helper virus contamination, and the ratio of infectious to vector particles is 1:20. For future vector amplification, the purified virus is used as a seed stock.

7. HeLa or A549 cells are preferred for this analysis. Although it is not ideal, a known amount of shuttle vector plasmid DNA or purified vector DNA can be added to cell suspensions recovered from uninfected cells for a standard. This

allows direct calculation of HDAd vector DNA taken up by cells. For 1 copy/cell of a 35-kb plasmid in 1×10^5 cells, add 3.85 pg of plasmid DNA.

Acknowledgments

We thank Dr. G. Schiedner and Dr. S. Kochanek for providing us the 293Cre66 cells and sharing unpublished data, and E. A. Nour and C. Dieker for their technical assistance. This work was supported by National Institutes of Health grant HL59314 and HL73144.

References

1. Oka, K. and Chan, L. (2002) Recent advances in liver-directed gene therapy for dyslipidemia. *Curr. Atheroscler. Rep.* **4**, 199–207.
2. Mitani, K., Graham, F. L., Caskey, C. T., and Kochanek, S. (1995) Rescue, propagation, and partial purification of a helper virus-dependent adenovirus vector. *Proc. Natl. Acad. Sci. USA* **92**, 3854–3858.
3. Kochanek, S., Clemens, P. R., Mitani, K., Chen, H. H., Chan, S., and Caskey, C. T. (1996) A new adenoviral vector: replacement of all viral coding sequences with 28 kb of DNA independently expressing both full-length dystrophin and beta-galactosidase. *Proc. Natl. Acad. Sci. USA* **93**, 5731–5736.
4. Kochanek, S. (1999) High-capacity adenoviral vectors for gene transfer and somatic gene therapy. *Hum. Gene Ther.* **10**, 2451–2459.
5. Parks, R. J., Chen, L., Anton, M., Sankar, U., Rudnicki, M. A., and Graham, F. L. (1996) A helper-dependent adenovirus vector system: removal of helper virus by Cre-mediated excision of the viral packaging signal. *Proc. Natl. Acad. Sci. USA* **93**, 13,565–13,570.
6. Morral, N., O'Neal, W., Rice, K., et al. (1999) Administration of helper-dependent adenoviral vectors and sequential delivery of different vector serotype for long-term liver-directed gene transfer in baboons. *Proc. Natl. Acad. Sci. USA* **96**, 12816–12821.
7. Oka, K., Pastore, L., Kim, I. H., et al. (2001) Long-term stable correction of low-density lipoprotein receptor-deficient mice with a helper-dependent adenoviral vector expressing the very low-density lipoprotein receptor. *Circulation* **103**, 1274–1281.
8. Kim, I. H., Jozkowicz, A., Piedra, P. A., Oka, K., and Chan, L. (2001) Lifetime correction of genetic deficiency in mice with a single injection of helper-dependent adenoviral vector. *Proc. Natl. Acad. Sci. USA* **98**, 13282–13287.
9. Belalcazar, L. M., Merched, A., Carr, B., et al. (2003) Long-term stable expression of human apolipoprotein A-I mediated by helper-dependent adenovirus gene transfer inhibits atherosclerosis progression and remodels atherosclerotic plaques in a mouse model of familial hypercholesterolemia. *Circulation* **107**, 2726–2732.
10. Parks, R. J. and Graham, F. L. (1997) A helper-dependent system for adenovirus vector production helps define a lower limit for efficient DNA packaging. *J. Virol.* **71**, 3293–3298.

11. Sandig, V., Youil, R., Bett, A. J., et al. (2000) Optimization of the helper-dependent adenovirus system for production and potency in vivo. *Proc. Natl. Acad. Sci. USA* **97**, 1002–1007.

12. Schiedner, G., Hertel, S., Johnston, M., Biermann, V., Dries, V., and Kochanek, S. (2002) Variables affecting in vivo performance of high-capacity adenovirus vectors. *J. Virol.* **76**, 1600–1609.

13. Ehrhardt, A. and Kay, M. A. (2002) A new adenoviral helper-dependent vector results in long-term therapeutic levels of human coagulation factor IX at low doses in vivo. *Blood* **99**, 3923–3930.

14. Schiedner, G., Morral, N., Parks, R. J., et al. (1998) Genomic DNA transfer with a high-capacity adenovirus vector results in improved in vivo gene expression and decreased toxicity. *Nat. Genet.* **18**, 180–183.

15. Nomura, S., Merched, A., Nour, E., Dieker, C., Oka, K., and Chan, L. (2004) Low density lipoprotein receptor gene therapy using helper-dependent adenovirus produces long-term protection against atherosclerosis in a mouse model of familial hypercholesterolemia. *Gene Ther.* advance online publication 22 July 2004; doi:10. 1038/sj.gt. 3302310.

16. Donello, J. E., Loeb, J. E., and Hope, T. J. (1998) Woodchuck hepatitis virus contains a tripartite posttranscriptional regulatory element. *J. Virol.* **72**, 5085–5092.

17. Loeb, J. E., Cordier, W. S., Harris, M. E., Weitzman, M. D., and Hope, T. J. (1999) Enhanced expression of transgenes from adeno-associated virus vectors with the woodchuck hepatitis virus posttranscriptional regulatory element: implications for gene therapy. *Hum. Gene Ther.* **10**, 2295–2305.

18. Harui, A., Suzuki, S., Kochanek, S., and Mitani, K. (1999). Frequency and stability of chromosomal integration of adenovirus vectors. *J. Virol.* **73**, 6141–6146.

19. Hillgenberg, M., Tonnies, H., and Strauss, M. (2001) Chromosomal integration pattern of a helper-dependent minimal adenovirus vector with a selectable marker inserted into a 27.4-kilobase genomic stuffer. *J. Virol.* **75**, 9896–9908.

20. Parks, R., Evelegh, C., and Graham, F. (1999) Use of helper-dependent adenoviral vectors of alternative serotypes permits repeat vector administration. *Gene Ther.* **6**, 1565–1573.

21. Recchia, A., Parks, R. J., Lamartina, S., et al. (1999) Site-specific integration mediated by a hybrid adenovirus/adeno-associated virus vector. *Proc. Natl. Acad. Sci. USA* **96**, 2615–2620.

22. Goncalves, M. A., Pau, M. G., de Vries, A. A., and Valerio, D. (2001) Generation of a high-capacity hybrid vector: packaging of recombinant adenoassociated virus replicative intermediates in adenovirus capsids overcomes the limited cloning capacity of adenoassociated virus vectors. *Virology* **288**, 236–246.

23. Soifer, H., Higo, C., Logg, C. R., et al. (2002) A novel, helper-dependent, adenovirus-retrovirus hybrid vector: stable transduction by a two-stage mechanism. *Mol. Ther.* **5**, 599–608.

24. Kubo, S. and Mitani, K. (2003) A new hybrid system capable of efficient lentiviral vector production and stable gene transfer mediated by a single helper-dependent adenoviral vector. *J. Virol.* **77,** 2964–2971.

25. Soifer, H., Higo, C., Kazazian, H. H., Jr., Moran, J. V., Mitani, K., and Kasahara, N. (2001) Stable integration of transgenes delivered by a retrotransposon-adenovirus hybrid vector. *Hum. Gene Ther.* **12,** 1417–1428.

26. Yant, S. R., Ehrhardt, A., Mikkelsen, J. G., Meuse, L., Pham, T., and Kay, M. A. (2002) Transposition from a gutless adeno-transposon vector stabilizes transgene expression in vivo. *Nat. Biotechnol.* **20,** 999–1005.

27. Kotin, R. M., Siniscalco, M., Samulski, R. J., et al. (1990). Site-specific integration by adeno-associated virus. *Proc. Natl. Acad. Sci. USA* **87,** 2211–2215.

28. Samulski, R. J., Zhu, X., Xiao, X., et al. (1991) Targeted integration of adeno-associated virus (AAV) into human chromosome 19. *EMBO J.* **10,** 3941–3950.

29. Amiss, T. J., McCarty, D. M., Skulimowski, A., and Samulski, R. J. (2003) Identification and characterization of an adeno-associated virus integration site in CV-1 cells from the African green monkey. *J. Virol.* **77,** 1904–1915.

30. Thyagarajan, B., Olivares, E. C., Hollis, R. P., Ginsburg, D. S., and Calos, M. P. (2001). Site-specific genomic integration in mammalian cells mediated by phage phiC31 integrase. *Mol. Cell Biol.* **21,** 3926–3934.

31. Nemerow, G. R. and Stewart, P. L. (1999) Role of alpha(v) integrins in adenovirus cell entry and gene delivery. *Microbiol. Mol. Biol. Rev.* **63,** 725–734.

32. Dechecchi, M. C., Melotti, P., Bonizzato, A., Santacatterina, M., Chilosi, M., and Cabrini, G. (2001) Heparan sulfate glycosaminoglycans are receptors sufficient to mediate the initial binding of adenovirus types 2 and 5. *J. Virol.* **75,** 8772–8780.

33. Biermann, V., Volpers, C., Hussmann, S., et al. (2001) Targeting of high-capacity adenoviral vectors. *Hum. Gene Ther.* **12,** 1757–1769.

34. Sakhuja, K., Reddy, P. S., Ganesh, S., et al. (2003) Optimization of the generation and propagation of gutless adenoviral vectors. *Hum. Gene Ther.* **14,** 243–254.

35. Umana, P., Gerdes, C. A., Stone, D., et al. (2001) Efficient FLPe recombinase enables scalable production of helper-dependent adenoviral vectors with negligible helper-virus contamination. *Nat. Biotechnol.* **19,** 582–585.

36. Ng, P., Beauchamp, C., Evelegh, C., Parks, R., and Graham, F. L. (2001). Development of a FLP/frt system for generating helper-dependent adenoviral vectors. *Mol. Ther.* **3,** 809–815.

37. Schiedner, G., Hertel, S. & Kochanek, S. (2000) Efficient transformation of primary human amniocytes by E1 functions of Ad5: generation of new cell lines for adenoviral vector production. *Hum. Gene Ther.* **11,** 2105–2116.

38. Palmer, D. and Ng, P. (2003) Improved system for production of helper-dependent adenoviral vector. *Mol. Ther.* **8,** 846–852.

39. Fallaux, F. J., Bout, A., van der Velde, I., et al. (1998) New helper cells and matched early region 1-deleted adenovirus vectors prevent generation of replication-competent adenoviruses. *Hum. Gene Ther.* **9,** 1909–1917.

40. Hartigan-O'Connor, D., Barjot, C., Crawford, R., and Chamberlain, J. S. (2002) Efficient rescue of gutted adenovirus genomes allows rapid production of concentrated stocks without negative selection. *Hum. Gene Ther.* **13,** 519–531.

41. Hitt, M., Bett, A. J., Addison, C. L., Prevec, L., and Graham, L. F. (1995) *Techniques for Human Adenovirus Vector Construction and Characterization. Methods in Molecular Genetics* (Adolph, K. W., ed.), Academic Press, San Diego, CA, vol. 7, pp. 13–30.

42. Ng, P., Parks, J. R., and Graham, L. F. (2002) *Preparation of Helper-Dependent Adenoviral Vectors,* 2nd ed. Methods in Molecular Medicine (Morgan, J. R., ed.), Humana Press, Totowa, NJ, vol. 69, pp. 371–388.

43. Huyghe, B. G., Liu, X., Sutjipto, S., et al. (1995) Purification of a type 5 recombinant adenovirus encoding human p53 by column chromatography. *Hum. Gene Ther.* **6,** 1403–1416.

44. Blanche, F., Cameron, B., Barbot, A., et al. (2000) An improved anion-exchange HPLC method for the detection and purification of adenoviral particles. *Gene Ther.* **7,** 1055–1062.

45. Vellekamp, G., Porter, F. W., Sutjipto, S., et al. (2001). Empty capsids in column-purified recombinant adenovirus preparations. *Hum. Gene Ther.* **12,** 1923–1936.

46. Maizel, J. V., Jr., White, D. O., and Scharff, M. D. (1968) The polypeptides of adenovirus. I. Evidence for multiple protein components in the virion and a comparison of types 2, 7A, and 12. *Virology* **36,** 115–25.

47. Mittereder, N., March, K. L., and Trapnell, B. C. (1996) Evaluation of the concentration and bioactivity of adenovirus vectors for gene therapy. *J. Virol.* **70,** 7498–7509.

48. Kreppel, F., Biermann, V., Kochanek, S., and Schiedner, G. (2002) A DNA-based method to assay total and infectious particle contents and helper virus contamination in high-capacity adenoviral vector preparations. *Hum. Gene Ther.* **13,** 1151–1156.

23

Adenovirus-Mediated Gene Transfer In Vivo

An Approach to Reduce Oxidative Stress

Yi Chu

Summary

Replication-deficient adenoviruses are used as vectors to study function of genes and to treat hypertension and cardiovascular diseases in preclinical studies. The purpose of this chapter is to provide an example of applications of the "first-generation," E1-deleted and partially E3-deleted, human adenovirus type 5 vector, to test the hypothesis that gene transfer of a primary antioxidant enzyme, human extracellular superoxide dismutase (ECSOD), reduces arterial pressure in a genetic animal model of hypertension.

Two concepts in application of gene transfer in vascular biology are illustrated. First, the liver, by iv injection of an adenoviral vector, can function as the source for abundant amounts of a transgene product, with profound vascular effects, when the transgene encodes a secreted protein. Second, the specific function of a domain of the transgene product can be studied by preparation and injection of isogenic vectors that express the identical product with or without a domain.

Key Words: Extracellular superoxide dismutase; heparin-binding domain; SHR; hypertension; adenoviral vector; intravenous gene transfer.

1. Introduction

Gene therapy is a much desired goal to treat hypertension and cardiovascular diseases, and replication-deficient adenoviruses have been used as vectors in preclinical studies *(1)*. Advantages of adenoviral vector are the ability to transduce nondividing as well as dividing cells with high efficiency, a relatively large cloning capacity to accommodate a variety of transgene inserts, and ease of production of high-concentration viral stocks. The major disadvantage is propensity of the virus to elicit a strong host immune response in adult animals, which leads to transient gene expression of the transgene. Immune responses to adenoviral vectors could be dramatically reduced by reduction of

From: *Methods in Molecular Medicine, Vol. 108: Hypertension: Methods and Protocols*
Edited by: J. P. Fennell and A. H. Baker © Humana Press Inc., Totowa, NJ

dose *(2)* and/or by the use of the helper-dependent or "gutted" vector *(3)*. The gutted vector eliminates all viral sequences except the inverted terminal repeats located on both ends of the viral genome and the packaging signal sequence located near the left inverted terminal repeat, which are required in *cis* for replication and packaging of the vector *(3)*.

The most frequently used adenoviral vectors are based on human adenoviruses type 2 and 5, with a linear double-stranded DNA genome of approximately 36 kb (assigned as a total of 100 map units). Several excellent protocols on adenoviral vector methodology have been published *(3–5)*. The purpose of this chapter is to provide an example of applications of the "first-generation" adenoviral vector (E1-deleted and partially E3-deleted) in a research setting. I will describe steps that were taken, using an adenoviral vector, to test the hypothesis that gene transfer of human extracellular superoxide dismutase (ECSOD) might reduce arterial pressure of spontaneously hypertensive rats (SHR) *(6)*. ECSOD is a secreted protein that binds plasma membrane or extracellular matrix through its positively charged heparin-binding domain.

I intend to illustrate two concepts in application of gene transfer in vascular biology. First, an adenoviral vector can be injected iv, cleared by the liver, and the liver then serves as the source for the protein of interest. This approach circumvents the problem that, when adenoviruses are injected iv, only a very small fraction of the virus transduces the vessel wall, and thus, it is difficult to alter vascular function by transduction of arteries directly. Second, this approach allows us to address an important question in vascular biology: what is the role of heparin-binding domain (HBD) in the function of ECSOD? By studying effects of a pair of adenoviral vectors, which are identical except for the HBD, we could study cardiovascular effects of ECSOD, with and without the HBD.

2. Materials

2.1. Reagents and Animals

1. Plasmid DNA containing human ECSOD cDNA (provided by Dr. James Crapo of the National Jewish Medical and Research Center at Denver, CO).
2. Shuttle plasmid pAdRSV4 DNA containing the left inverted terminal repeat (ITR) and viral packaging sequence (Ψ) of the human type 5 adenovirus followed in 5' to 3' order by RSV promoter, multiple cloning site (MCS), and SV40 polyadenylation sequence (polyA); Ad5 backbone DNA (based on Ad5 sub306, 9–100 map units, with deletion of E1 and partial E3 sequences (provided by University of Iowa Gene Transfer Vector Core, www.uiowa.edu/~gene).
3. Restriction enzymes, T4 DNA ligase, Taq DNA polymerase.
4. Oligodeoxynucleotide primers, deoxynucleotide triphosphates (dNTPs).
5. TA cloning vector, e.g., pCR3.1 (Invitrogen, Carlsbad, CA).

6. Cell culture medium: Dulbecco's modified Eagle's medium (DMEM)/high glucose containing 100 U/mL penicillin and 100 μg/mL streptomycin (pen/strep) with 10% or 2% fetal bovine serum (FBS).
7. HEK293, A549 cells (ATCC, Manassas, VA).
8. Male SHR and normotensive control WKY rats (20 wk of age, Harlan, Indianapolis, IN).
9. Anesthetics.

2.2. Equipment

1. Polymerase chain reaction (PCR) machine, e.g., GeneAmp System 2400 by ABI (Foster City, CA).
2. Horizontal agarose gel electrophoresis apparatus.
3. Vertical mini protein electrophoresis apparatus.
4. Water baths.
5. Microcentrifuge, e.g., Eppendorf 5415C (Brinkmann, Westbury, NY).
6. Ultracentrifuge, e.g., Optima LE-80K with SW28 and SW41Ti rotors by Beckman (Fullerton, CA).
7. Ultraviolet spectrophotometer, e.g., Beckmen DU640B.
8. Cell culture incubators and hood.
9. DNA sequencing equipment, e.g., ABI 3700 DNA analyzer with the use of Big Dye version 1 chemistry.
10. Animal surgical equipments.
11. Transducer and rodent ventilator.

3. Methods
3.1. Construction of Adenoviral Vectors

1. Plasmid pBlueScript (3.0 kb) with an insert of 1.4 kb human ECSOD cDNA was cleaved with Not I and Xho I. A 1.2-kb Not I-Xho I fragment containing ECSOD cDNA was purified using low-melting-point agarose gel electrophoresis, and ligated into pAdRSV4 vector that was cleaved with Not I and Xho I, flanked 5' by RSV promoter and 3' by a polyA sequence.
2. The RSV promoter sequence in the shuttle plasmid was then replaced by a CMV promoter/enhancer sequence (This additional step was required at the time; now a CMV promoter/enhancer-containing shuttle plasmid is available. *See* www. uiowa.edu/~gene). The CMVECSOD segment (Ad5/0-1 map unit-CMVpromoter/enhancer-ECSOD-polyA-Ad5/9-15 map units, in this 5'-3' order) was cotransfected with Ad5 backbone (9–100 map units, with deletion of E1 and partial E3 regions) DNA into HEK293 cells for homologous recombination.
3. Complementary DNA for human ECSOD with deletion of the heparin-binding domain (ECSODΔHBD) was amplified using the ECSOD plasmid as template, a sense primer that hybridizes the translation initiation signal/site with an upstream addition of a Not I site, and an antisense primer that hybridizes the cDNA sequence encoding the last amino acids prior to the RKKRRR basic amino acid

stretch that constitutes HBD, with a downstream addition of a translation stop codon (UGA) followed by an Xho I site. The sequences are 5'-ATAA GAATGCGGCCGCCTCCAGCCATGCTGGCGCTACTG-3' (sense primer) (see Note 1) and 5'-CTCGAGTCACTCTGAGTGCTCCCGCG-3' (antisense primer). The ECSODΔHBD PCR product (714 bp) was cloned into pCR3.1 and confirmed by sequencing (*see* **Note 2**). The ECSODΔHBD segment was then cleaved with Not I and Xho I, purified, and then ligated into the Ad5CMV shuttle vector that was created as described above. A general scheme from cloning of a transgene insert to homologous recombination is diagrammed in **Fig. 1**. All cloning recipes and reactions can be found in the classic **ref. 7** or its newer editions.

4. Materials for construction of a recombinant adenovirus as well as control adenoviral vectors such as AdCMVβgal can be obtained commercially (e.g., Clontech, Palo Alto, CA; PanVera, Madison, WI; and Stratagene, La Jolla, CA) or from vector cores/facilities (e.g., University of Iowa Gene Transfer Vector Core).

3.2. Identification, Propagation, Purification, and Titration of Adenoviral Vectors

1. Single plaques were picked from soft agarose-covered 293 cell lawn following homologous recombination, individually amplified on 293 cells, and the cell lysate was assayed for SOD enzymatic activity to identify AdCMVECSOD or AdECSODΔHBD.

2. Positive clones were propagated: 293 cells were seeded on 20 15-cm tissue culture plates, infected at a confluence of 80 to 90% with the vector at an estimated multiplicity of infection (MOI) of 5 plaque-forming units (PFU) per cell. Within a day, cytopathic effects were observed (i.e., cells becoming enlarged and about to round up). Cells were then harvested (around 30 h postinfection), and lysed by freezing on dry ice and thawing in 37°C waterbath. The cell lysate was loaded onto a cesium chloride (CsCl) cushion, centrifuged, and the virus band in the CsCl gradient was harvested. The virus was further purified with a second round of CsCl centrifugation. Purified virus was dialyzed against a buffer (e.g., 3% sucrose in phosphate-buffered saline, PBS) to remove CsCl. Physical titer of the virus was measured by optical density (1 $OD/_{260\,nm} = 1 \times 10^{12}$ particles/mL).

3. Biological titer (PFU/mL) of the purified virus was measured by plaque assay on 293 cells, as detailed below. (All steps are performed using sterile techniques in a culture hood.)
   a. Plate 293 cells, grown in DMEM containing 10% FBS and pen/strep, from two 10-cm plates with 100% confluency to ten 6-cm plates so that the 6-cm plates will be approx 80% confluent overnight.

Fig. 1. (*opposite page*) Construction of a recombinant adenovirus: from cloning gene of interest (in pTransgene) into a shuttle plasmid (pShuttle) to homologous recombination. X and Y are restriction enzymes (sites) that cleave to generate an intact DNA sequence for a transgene; A and B are restriction enzymes (sites) located in the multiple cloning site (MCS) that cleave pShuttle only once. X and A, and Y and B, are

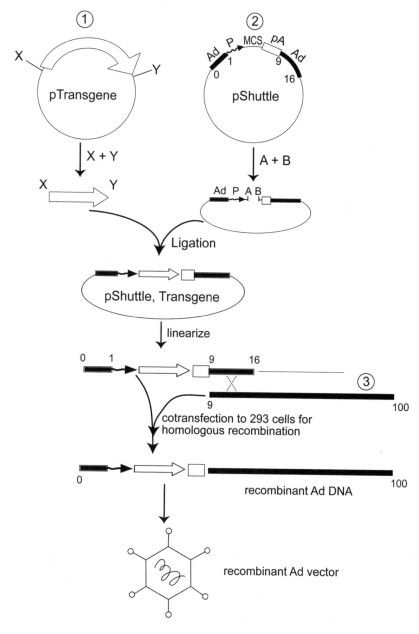

Fig. 1. (*continued*) compatible, respectively; if not present in either plasmid, a linker that contains the site needs to be put into place before digestions. Thick lines represent adenoviral sequences (Ad), with numbers indicating map unit; P represents promoter (most commonly from human CMV or RSV), MCS multiple cloning site, pA polyadenylation signal sequence.

b. Incubate the cells with the virus at three different dilutions in triplicate for overnight, in a volume of three mL of DMEM containing 2% FBS and pen/strep, among which 1 mL is the diluted virus (in the medium). The dilutions are $1/10^{11}$, $1/10^{10}$, and $1/10^{9}$, if the physical titer of the virus is in the range of 10^{12} particles/mL ($10^{-(n-1)}$ to $10^{-(n-3)}$ dilutions, with n being the exponential number of the physical titer). A remaining plate serves as uninfected cell control.

c. Prepare the overlay medium as follows. Sterilize 4% agarose in double-distilled H_2O (ddH_2O) (e.g., 40 mL in a 100-mL glass bottle) by autoclaving, and store it at 4°C. Liquidize the agarose by microwaving, and place the bottle in a 45°C water bath. Pipet 25 mL 2X DMEM, 1 mL FBS, 0.5 mL 100X pen/strep, and 13.5 mL ddH_2O into a sterile 50-mL tube and warm the tube in a 45°C water bath. When both the agarose and the medium reach 45°C equilibrium, pipet 10 mL of 4% agarose to the medium tube and mix by inverting the capped tube three times.

d. Aspirate the infectant from the plates, and overlay the overlay medium onto cells at 4 mL/plate. After solidification of the overlay medium in the culture hood, place the plates in a cell incubator.

e. Observe the plates briefly daily on an inverted-field microscope for cell morphology, and apply the overlay medium every 2–4 d at 1–2 mL/plate to keep cells healthy and viruses replicating in the cells. Plaques appear approx 6 d after the first application of overlay medium.

f. Count the number of plaques when they are sufficiently large (so that no false positives are counted), yet not overlapping (so that it is possible to obtain accurate numbers of plaques). Take the average of the most diluted triplicates (or the mid-diluted triplicates if the average is tighter, whereas no plaque has appeared in ≥ 1 plate of the most diluted triplicates) to calculate the titer: for example, if an average of 7 plaques is observed at the dilution of 10^{-11}, the biological titer of the virus is 7×10^{11} PFU/mL.

4. The ratio of particles to PFU generally ranges from 10 to 100:1. These assays are also described in detail elsewhere (*4,5*), and can be found from relevant websites (e.g., www.uiowa.edu/~gene).

3.3. Handling of Adenoviral Vector Stocks

1. Virus stocks should be aliquotted to avoid repeated thawing and freezing, and stored in a –80°C freezer, some of which should be saved for future comparisons, to examine reproducibility of effects.

2. After several rounds of propagation, or upon receipt of an adenoviral stock about which there is no information about wild-type adenovirus, the viral stock should be examined for wild-type adenovirus by performing plaque assay using A549 cells on which only wild-type virus can form plaques. Wild-type adenovirus may be generated during propagation by recombination between an adenoviral vector and the adenoviral sequence that is integrated in the genome of 293 cells, or by contamination, and has replication advantage over an adenoviral vector.

3. Wild-type adenovirus can also be detected using extracted DNA from a viral stock as template and primers for E1 genes in a regular PCR with a maximal sensitivity of 1 in a million viral genomes. A sensitive real-time PCR method is capable of detecting 1 wild-type adenovirus in a billion viral genomes *(8)*. If wild-type adenovirus is detected, plaque purification of the viral stock on 293 cells should be performed to isolate the adenoviral vector, and a new stock amplified.

3.4. In Vivo Gene Transfer to SHR and WKY Rats

1. Age-matched male SHR and WKY rats (around 20 wk old) were anesthetized with methohexital sodium intraperitoneally (50 mg/kg). Adenovirus (1×10^{12} particles/ml in 3% sucrose in PBS, vehicle) or vehicle was injected into the penile vein *(see* **Note 3**). The usual dose of adenovirus was 0.5 ml (5×10^{11} particles). Rats began to awaken within half an hour after injection.

2. The major target of systemic intravenous delivery of adenovirus is the liver in rats (which can be demonstrated easily by the use of an adenoviral vector that expresses β-galactosidase followed by X-gal histochemistry of different organs; for X-gal method, *see* **ref. 9**). Because the liver produces after respective transduction ECSOD and ECSODΔHBD, which are secreted proteins from the transduced cells, the transduction can be confirmed conveniently by assaying the enzymatic activity of the proteins in plasma with zymography *(10)*. Twenty microliters of plasma was loaded to a 10% native polyacrylamide gel (no SDS or reducing agents).

3. Electrophoresis was performed at a constant voltage of 100 V at 4°C for 4 h. The gels were then incubated in a solution containing 2.45 mmol/L nitroblue tetrazolium, 28 μmol/L riboflavin and 28 mmol/L TEMED, in the dark for 30 min. The gels were rinsed with tap water, and exposed to light for 10–20 min. Achromatic bands in the blue background developed, indicating the position of SOD activity. Plasma levels of human ECSOD or ECSODΔHBD peaked at 3 or 4 d after intravenous injection, and remained with gradual decrease up to approx 10 d after injection (**Fig. 2**).

3.5. Measurement of Mean Arterial Pressure in Anesthetized Rats

1. Rats were anesthetized with sodium pentobarbital (50 mg/kg ip) 3 d following intravenous injection of adenoviruses. A tracheostomy was performed, and the rats were ventilated.

2. The femoral artery was cannulated and arterial pressure was recorded directly. After 30–60 min of equilibration, MAP value was taken as an average of a 30–60-min recording. Body temperature and blood gases were monitored, and were normal in all groups. No heparin was used during the recording of arterial pressure. It was important to avoid heparin because heparin releases ECSOD from binding sites on cell surfaces. Gene transfer of ECSOD, but not ECSODΔHBD or control virus Adβgal, dramatically reduced arterial pressure of SHR, but not normotensive WKY rats (**Fig. 3A**).

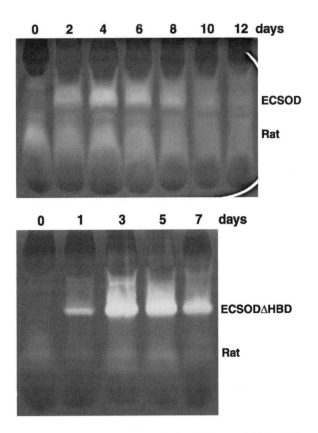

Fig. 2. Measurement of plasma SOD activity. Plasma SOD activity measured by in-gel zymography after native polyacrylamide gel electrophoresis in rats injected with AdECSOD (top panel) or AdECSODΔHBD (bottom panel). "Rat" indicates endogenous SOD activity in the plasma.

3.6. Measurement of Mean Arterial Pressure in Conscious Rats

1. To confirm the effect of ECSOD on arterial pressure in SHR, mean arterial pressure was also measured in conscious rats. A catheter (8 in of PE50 tubing with a 3.5-cm PE10 tip) was filled with heparinized saline (1000 U/mL) overnight.
2. Male SHR and WKY rats were anesthetized with sodium pentobarbital (50 mg/kg ip), and the tip of the catheter was inserted in a femoral artery and advanced into the abdominal aorta. The catheter was secured, tunneled, and exteriorized in the mid-scapular region. Patency of the catheter was maintained by filling with 0.1 mL of heparinized saline (1000 U/mL) daily after measurement of MAP.
3. Two days after instrumentation with the catheter, we injected either AdECSOD or Adβgal iv, and MAP was measured. Values are the average of the last 15 min from a 30–60-min recording obtained on the day of injection of the adenovirus

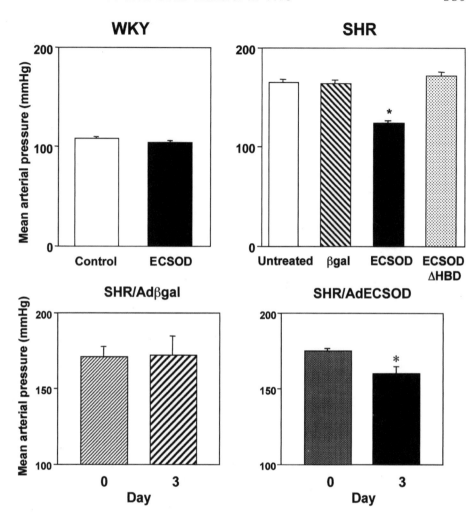

Fig. 3. Effects of adenovirus-mediated gene transfer on MAP. Effects of ECSOD and ECSODΔHBD overexpression on MAP of anesthetized SHR and WKY rats, 3 d after intravenous injection at 5×10^{11} particles/rat (top panel). Control WKY, $n = 6$; WKY after AdECSOD, $n = 5$. Untreated SHR, $n = 7$; SHR after Adβgal, $n = 8$; SHR after AdECSOD, $n = 7$; SHR after AdECSODΔHBD, $n = 5$. * = $p < 0.05$ vs SHR after Adβgal. Bottom panel: Effect of gene transfer of ECSOD on MAP of conscious SHR. Values are from SHR treated with Adβgal ($n = 5$) or AdECSOD ($n = 9$). * = $p < 0.05$ vs before injection of AdECSOD. (Reprinted with permission from **ref. 6**.)

and on the d 3 after injection of the virus. Gene transfer of ECSOD significantly reduced MAP in SHR, compared to the control virus (**Fig. 3B**). The effect on conscious SHR, however, is not as profound as in SHR under anesthesia.

3.7. Concluding Remarks

We have demonstrated an example in which first-generation adenoviral vectors were used to test the hypothesis that increased superoxide levels may contribute to hypertension in a genetic rat model, and gene transfer of human ECSOD reduces arterial pressure, with a strict requirement of the heparin-binding domain which mediates cellular binding. Methodology for such application of adenoviral vectors has been well established, and described in refs. *(4,5)*, and at websites of gene transfer vector cores.

Through the example, it is clear that the liver, by iv injection of the adenoviral vector, can function as the source for abundant amounts of a transgene product, with profound vascular effects, when the transgene encodes a secreted protein. The specific function of a domain of the transgene product can be studied by preparation and injection of isogenic vectors that express the identical product with or without a domain. New directions with adenovirus-mediated gene transfer include the use of the helper-dependent adenovirus *(3)*, creative ways to enhance transduction efficiency *(11)*, and design of the vector and the transgene to target and regulate expression *(12,13)*.

4. Notes

1. The 8-nucleotide sequence on the 5'-end is unnecessary for the sense primer, and is deleted from the ECSOD cDNA segment following *Not* I digestion. It was there for historical reasons. Because the template for the PCR is a single species DNA, design of the primers can be less stringent.
2. One may try to eliminate this step by cleaving the PCR product directly and then cloning it into the shuttle vector. We have found that the efficiency of accomplishing this procedure is poor, mainly because a restriction enzyme does not cleave well at the end of a DNA sequence. In contrast, restriction enzyme cleavage after cloning of the PCR product into a TA vector has 100% success rate.
3. A popular injection site for systemic intravenous delivery of viral vectors in rats is the tail vein. In our hands, it is much easier to inject adenoviral suspension into the penile vein than the tail vein in male rats.

Acknowledgments

Original studies, performed in the laboratory of Dr. Donald D. Heistad, were supported by National Institutes of Health (NIH) grants HL 16066, NS 24621, HL 62984, DK 54759, HL 14388, DK 15843, DK 52617, HL 55006, funds provided by the Veterans Affairs Medical Service, and a Carver Trust Research Program of Excellence. I would like to thank Dr. Heistad for guidance, encouragement and support, and critical reading of the manuscript. I would like to thank my colleagues, without whom the original work would have not been possible. We acknowledge the University of Iowa Gene Transfer Vector Core, supported in part by the NIH and the Roy J. Carver Foundation, for viral vector preparations.

References

1. Phillips, M. I. (2002) Gene therapy for hypertension: the preclinical data. *Meth. Enzymol.* 346, 3–13.
2. Gerdes, C. A., Castro, M. G., and Löwenstein P. R. (2000) Strong promoters are the key to highly efficient, noninflammatory and noncytotoxic adenoviral-mediated transgene delivery into the brain in vivo. *Mol. Ther.* **2,** 330–338.
3. Zhou, H., Pastore, L., and Beaudet, A. L. (2000) Helper-dependent adenoviral vectors. *Meth. Enzymol.* 346, 177–198.
4. Graham, F. L. and Prevec, L. (1991) Manipulation of adenoviral vectors. *Meth. Mol. Biol.* **7,** 109–128.
5. Gerard, R. D. and Meidell, R. S. (1995) Adenovirus vectors. In *DNA Cloning: A Practical Approach: Mammalian Systems*, (Hames, B. D. and Glover, D., eds.), Oxford University Press, Oxford, UK, pp. 285–307.
6. Chu, Y., Iida, S., Lund, D. D., et al. (2003) Gene transfer of extracellular superoxide dismutase reduces arterial pressure in spontaneously hypertensive rats: role of heparin-binding domain. *Circ. Res.* **92,** 461–468.
7. Maniatis, T., Fritsch, E. F., and Sambrook, J. (1982) *Molecular Cloning*. Cold Spring Harbor Laboratory Press, Cold Spring Harbor, NY.
8. Anderson, R. D., Haskell, R. E., Xia, H., and Davidson, B. L. (2000) A simple method for the rapid generation of recombinant adenovirus vectors. *Gene Ther.* **7,** 1034–1038.
9. Chu, Y. and Heistad, D. D. (2002) Gene transfer to blood vessels using adenovirus vectors. *Meth. Enzymol.* **346,** 263–276.
10. Beauchamp, C. and Fridovich, I. (1971) Superoxide dismutase: improved assays and an assay applicable to acrylamide gels. *Anal. Biochem.* **44,** 276–287.
11. Khurana, V.G., Weiler, D.A., Witt, T.A., et al. (2003) A direct mechanical method for accurate and efficient adenoviral vector delivery to tissues. *Gene Ther.* **10,** 443–452.
12. Work, L. M., Nicklin, S. A., White, S. J., and Baker, A. H. (2002) Use of phage display to identify novel peptides for targeted gene therapy. *Meth. Enzymol.* **346,** 157–176.
13. Thule, P. M. and Liu J. M. (2000) Regulated hepatic insulin gene therapy of STZ-diabetic rats. *Gene Ther.* **7,** 1744–1752.

24

Gene Therapy for Hypertension

Antisense Inhibition of the Renin–Angiotensin System

M. Ian Phillips and Birgitta Kimura

Summary

Despite excellent antihypertensive drugs on the market, about 70% of all hypertensive patients do not have their blood pressure under control. This is due to problems of compliance, largely because of having to take drugs daily and side effects. We propose an antisense therapy for hypertension because antisense treatment can provide long-lasting, highly specific control of blood pressure. Antisense to oligonucleotides can be designed to inhibit genes that produce proteins known to be overactive in hypertension and that are proven targets of current drug treatments. These include β1-receptors, angiotensin-converting enzyme (ACE), and angiotensin type 1 receptors (AT1R). Antisense oligonucleotides are short (12–20 bases), single strands of DNA. They are designed to hybridize to specific mRNA and prevent translation of the target protein. Antisense inhibition of ACE, angiotensinogen or AT1R genes components of the renin–angiotensin system effectively reduce high blood pressure in animal models of hypertension. These include a genetic model (SHR) a surgical model (2KIC), and an environmental model (cold-induced hypertension). In all models, a single systemic administration of antisense decreased blood pressure by about 25 mmHg, and the effect could last up to 1 mo. No toxic effects of repeated antisense treatment were found. The results indicate that antisense therapy could be used for human hypertension and provide long-term protection that would increase compliance of patients.

Key Words: Angiotensin; angiotensinogen; angiotensin-converting enzyme; antisense; hypertension; SHR; 2KIC.

1. Introduction

Antisense therapeutics can be applied to hypertension. Hypertension is a huge market, yet in spite of several excellent drugs being available for the treatment of hypertension, the number of patients with controlled hypertension is about 27% in the United States. In all other countries studied, even those like

From: *Methods in Molecular Medicine, Vol. 108: Hypertension: Methods and Protocols*
Edited by: J. P. Fennell and A. H. Baker © Humana Press Inc., Totowa, NJ

the United Kingdom and Canada where cost is not the major factor, patient compliance is even worse.

Part of the reason for these compliance problems is that current antihypertensive drugs must be taken daily. Some drugs, such as β-blockers, are selective but not highly specific, and side effects are a common reason for patients interrupting their treatment. Lack of control over 24 h exposes the patients to troughs and peaks of blood pressure. A common regimen of taking a pill in the morning increases the likelihood of stroke or heart attack at that time when control is at its weakest.

We have proposed an antisense therapy because antisense effects are long-lasting, highly specific, and therefore could provide prolonged control of blood pressure without peaks and troughs or side effects. Taking advantage of the targets that the pharmaceutical industry has long used, it is not necessary to analyze more candidate genes. We know that targeting β1-receptors, calcium receptors, and components of the renin–angiotensin system (RAS) can reduce blood pressure in hypertensive patients. We have developed antisense inhibition of these target genes for reducing high blood pressure. This chapter focuses on the proof-of-principle studies that have applied antisense inhibition to the RAS.

The RAS is important in blood pressure regulation, volume regulation, and vascular tissue growth. Angiotensin II (Ang II), an octapeptide, is the active peptide of the system. It is formed from angiotensin I (Ang I) by angiotensin-converting enzyme (ACE). Ang I is formed from angiotensinogen (AGT) by renin. Ang II is the ligand for angiotensin II type 1 receptors (AT1R) and angiotensin II type 2 receptors (AT2R). In addition, angiotensin II metabolites, Ang III, Ang IV, and Ang 1–7, are active and may have independent receptors. All the components of RAS are present in the brain as well as in the periphery, although renin levels in the brain are very low. Both the brain RAS and the blood-borne RAS are important for blood pressure regulation.

The brain RAS is also involved in drinking, salt intake, the baroreflex, and hormonal release from the paraventricular nucleus (PVN). The peripheral tissue RAS is involved in cardiac hypertrophy and hyperplasia. AT1 receptors have been shown to mediate the blood pressure and growth effects of Ang II *(1–4)*. The role of the AT2 receptor is still uncertain, although it has been implicated in apoptosis and has effects opposing those of the AT1 receptor *(4–7)*. However, mice with AT1 receptors but lacking AT2 receptors did not develop hypertrophy in response to Ang II infusion *(8)*, suggesting that the relationship between the two receptor types is more complex.

The rate-limiting step in the RAS cascade is the conversion to the decapeptide, Ang I. Increases in AGT production has been shown to have an effect on blood pressure both in humans and in experimental animals *(9–11)*. Transgenic mice that produce high levels of Ang II are hypertensive *(12–17)*, and hypertensive rat models have increased levels of Ang II *(18–22)*. The spontaneously hypertensive rat (SHR) also has increased density of Ang II receptors *(23,24)*.

Human genetic studies have shown that the AGT gene is linked to hypertension. In French and Utah (USA) populations, the AGT 235T variant is more frequent in hypertensives than in controls *(25–28)*. The ACE gene insertion/deletion variant has also been implicated, but the association of this gene with hypertension may depend both on the ethnic group and whether males or females are studied *(29,30)*. There is also some evidence for AT1 receptor gene polymorphism involvement in human hypertension and arterial stiffness *(1,3,31)*. The pressor effects of circulating Ang II have been known since the 1930s *(32)* and ACE inhibitors are one of the preferred classes of drugs used to treat high blood pressure. Both ACE inhibitors and the newer AT1 receptor antagonists decrease left ventricular hypertrophy (LVH) as well as hypertension *(2,4,33,34)*. However, these drugs have to be taken daily, and despite being effective in controlling hypertension, only 27% of patients with hypertension take the drugs consistently *(33–35)*. A shocking 73% of patient with hypertension do not comply with their drug treatment *(36)*. Cardiovascular disease is the leading cause of death in the United States and in Europe, and the World Health Organization (WHO) estimates that, worldwide, 17 million people die of cardiovascular disease every year (www.americanheart.org). Hodgson and Cai reported that the cost of hypertension in the United States in 1998 was $108.8 billion, and the American Heart Association estimated the direct and indirect costs of cardiovascular disease to be $329 billion in the United States in 2002 *(37)*. Clearly, new treatments for hypertension are needed. We propose that a gene therapy approach would offer several advantages that could increase compliance. One is that the treatment would be long-lasting (weekly, monthly or longer). Another is that because of the high specificity of gene targeting, there would be few side effects.

One approach is to target the mRNA of components involved in hypertension. Even though hypertension is a multifactorial disease, inhibition of the RAS is a promising strategy, as it is already known that pharmacological depression of the system decreases blood pressure. We propose antisense inhibition of well-documented drug targets such as ACE, AGT, and AT1R. Preclinically, we have tested antisense oligonucleotides (AS-ODN), plasmids, and viral vectors to decrease the levels of components of the RAS (**Tables 1** and **2**) *(33,34,38,39)*.

2. Antisense Oligonucleotides

Antisense oligonucleotides consist of short, 12–20 bases long, DNA sequences complementary to the mRNA producing the protein of interest. They bind to the mRNA and prevent translation of the specific protein encoded in

Table 1
Gene Therapy for Hypertension: AS Against Brain RAS Vasoconstrictor Genes

Target gene	Construct	Route of delivery	Animal model	Max Δ BP (mmHg)	Duration of effect	Reference
AT$_1$ receptor	AS-ODN	icv	SHR	-45	7 d	Gyurko et al., Gyurko et al., Piegari et al. (60,62,63)
AT$_1$ receptor	AS-ODN	icv	CIH	-35	4 d	Peng et al. (65)
AT$_1$ receptor (64)	AS-ODN	icv	2K1C chronic	-20	> 5 d	Kagiyama et al.
AT1 recepto	AAV	icv	SHR	-40	> 9 wk	Phillips et al. (54)
AGT	AS-ODN	icv	SHR	-35	n.d.	Gyurko et al., Wielbo et al., Kagiyama et al. (60,72,73)
AGT	AS-ODN	icv	CIH	-40	2 d	Peng et al. (65)
Renin	AS-ODN	icv	SHR	-20	3 d	Kubo et al. (84)
AGE 2	Decoy ODN	icv	SHR	-30	7 d	Nishii et al. (94)

Table 2
Gene Therapy for Hypertension: AS Against Peripheral RAS Vasoconstrictor Genes

Target gene	Construct	Route of delivery	Animal model	Max Δ BP (mmHg)	Duration of effect	Reference
AT$_1$ receptor	AS-ODN	ic	CIH	−35	n.d.	Peng et al. (*65*)
AT$_1$ receptor	AS-ODN	iv	2K1C acute	−30	> 7 d	Galli et al. (*68*)
AT$_1$ receptor	LNSV	ic in 5-d-old rats	SHR	−45	> 120 d	Iyer et al, Lu et al (*55,70*)
AT$_1$ receptor	LNSV	ic in 5-d-old rats	60% fructose	−20	> 2 wk	Katovich et al. (*95*)
AGT	AS-ODN	Portal vein	SHR	−20	4 d	Tomita et al. (*79*)
AGT	AS-ODN	iv	SHR	−30	7 d	Wielbo et al., Makino et al., Makino et al., Sugano et al. (*46,76–78*)
AGT	P AS-AGT	iv	SHR	−20	8 d	Tang et al. (*51*)
AGT	AAV	ic in 5-d-old rats	SHR	−25	6 mo	Kimura et al. (*53*)
AGE 2	Decoy ODN	Portal vein	SHR	−20	6 d	Morishita et al. (*96*)

the mRNA. To prevent breakdown in the circulation, the oligonucleotides are phosphorothioated, or otherwise modified, to increase stability. AS-ODNs can be administered by themselves, but delivery in liposomes, liposomes coupled to Sendai virus or to carrier molecules, increases uptake and prolongs the effect of AS-ODN *(40–47)*. In vitro experiments have shown that the AS-ODNs enter the cell and the nucleus *(48)*.

3. Plasmid Vectors

Full-length antisense mRNA can be manufactured in plasmid vectors under the control of a promotor *(49)*. Theoretically, plasmids should be effective longer than AS-ODNs; practically, however, the difference is negligible. There is also the problem of efficient uptake, but recent studies using liposomes and receptor-mediated uptake have shown adequate effects of antisense mRNA *(50,51)*. Plasmid vectors have the potential to express antisense mRNA in specific cell types if cell-specific promoters or cell-specific delivery systems are used *(52)*. Thus they would be advantageous when a transient expression is required.

4. Viral Vectors

Viral vectors containing cDNA in the antisense orientation can potentially integrate into the genome and express antisense mRNA for components of RAS. Our results show long-term attenuation of hypertension and cardiac hypertrophy (**Tables 1–3**) *(33,34,49,53,54)*. The adenoma-associated virus (AAV) was used because it is safe, stable, long-acting, and appropriate for gene therapy in adult models. Retroviruses preferentially infect dividing cells and integrate randomly into the genome *(33,34,49)*. They have been used in infant models in the study of the development of hypertension *(55–57)*. However, they are not suitable for adult gene therapy. Lentiviruses (based on HIV, SIV, or FIV) can infect nondividing cells and have a large carrying capacity. However, they integrate randomly, which may disrupt other genes and cause mutagenesis *(49,58,59)*. Adenoviruses have very good uptake and do not integrate into the host genome. They show high levels of short-term expression. Their major disadvantage for long-term therapy is the immune and inflammatory response they cause *(33,49,58,59)*.

Adeno-associated virus does not cause an immune response. It may integrate into the genome when it is modified and certainly has very long-lasting effects. The wild-type AAV does not cause any known diseases, and cannot proliferate without a helper virus. It is likely to be the safest of the viral vectors. The disadvantage of the AAV vector is its small carrying capacity for a vector delivering genes. AAV can only accommodate 4.4 kb, and thus the number of promoters, enhancers, and length of AS-mRNA is limited. In addi-

Table 3
AS to RAS: Effects on Growth

Target gene	Construct	Route of delivery	Animal model	Effect studied	Magnitude	Reference
AT_1	LNSV	ic in 5-d-old	TGR mRen2	Hypertrophy	90% decrease	Pachori et al. (*71*)
AGT	AS-ODN	iv	SHR	Hypertrophy	60% decrease	Makino et al. (*46*)
AGT	AS-ODN	iv	SHR	Media of aorta	32% decrease	Sugano et al. (*78*)
AGT	AAV	ic in 5-d-old	SHR	Hypertrophy	About 25% decrease	Kimura et al. (*53*)
ACE	AS-ODN	Into injured artery	SD balloon catheter injury	Neointima formation	Injured control: 0.24 mm² AS treated: 0.1 mm2	Morishita et al. (*18*)

369

tion, the deletion of the *rep* sequence removes the site-specific integration of the vector *(33,34,49,58)*. Nevertheless, one of the advantages of the antisense approach is that it is not necessary to have a full-length DNA and therefore shorter AS-DNA sequences can be used effectively in AAV.

4.1. RAS Gene Therapy

We began targeting AT1R and AGT for AS-ODNs in 1993 for hypertension gene therapy *(60)*. In the past 10 yr all of the components of the RAS have been targeted for gene therapy. Some studies have aimed at understanding the mechanisms of the actions of RAS, others to decrease hypertension, myocardial dysfunction, and growth effects of the RAS.

4.2. AT1 Receptors

Using antisense oligonucleotides in an intact animal showed that AT1 receptor antisense injected into the brain lateral ventricle of SHRs decreased blood pressure by about 25 mmHg within 24 h and caused a 16–40% decrease of AT1 receptors in the PVN and OVLT *(60)*. Subsequently these results have been corroborated by other studies from our laboratory as well as other researchers *(61–63)*. AT1 receptor AS-ODN applied to the central RAS can also attenuate blood pressure in non-genetic models of hypertension. These include the surgical model, two kidney one clip (2K1C) and the environmental model, cold-induced hypertension (CIH) *(64,65)*. The data are summarized in **Table 1**. In addition to the effect on blood pressure, spontaneous drinking and Ang II and isoproterenol-induced drinking is decreased by the AT1R antisense *(65–67)*. Saline (i.e., osmotic) induced drinking is not affected *(67)*. In early studies, AS-ODN applied to the peripheral circulation did not elicit a response. However, when they were mixed with liposomes, the uptake into peripheral organs increased and AT1ASODN were shown to decrease blood pressure by 25–35 mmHg and AT1 receptors in kidney and arteries in both CIH and 2K1C hypertensive rats *(65,68)*. The data are summarized in **Table 2**. AT1-AS-ODN administered before ischemia reperfusion in addition also protected against myocardial dysfunction *(69)*. The effects of AT1AS-ODN are transient, lasting for about 1 wk, with the maximum effect seen after 2–3 d.

Viral vectors, on the other hand, enabled very long-term expression of antisense. We have used AAV to deliver AT1AS mRNA both to the central and the peripheral system of SHRs and obtained attenuation of hypertension by approx 25 mmHg (*see* **Table 1**). The reduction in blood pressure lasts at least 9 wk *(54)*, and we have recorded normalization of blood pressure in double-transgenic mice for 6 mo. These mice have a gene for human rennin and a gene for human angiotensin. They therefore constantly overexpress Ang II and are hypertensive. AAV delivery of AS to AT1R dramatically reduces the blood pressure within a few days, and the effect persists for as long as the mice were tested. Our colleagues have used a lentiviral vector (LNSV) to deliver AT1AS mRNA to 5-d-old SHRs and obtained similar results (*see* **Table 2**) *(55,57,70)*. Indeed, the attenuation of hypertension as well as of hypertrophy could be shown to persist in offspring of the treated rats *(56,71)*.

4.3. Angiotensinogen

The earliest studies targeting AGT in the brain showed a substantial, up to 40 mmHg, blood pressure decrease in SHRs and a decrease of hypothalamic AGT *(60,72)*. Subsequent research has confirmed that intracerebroventricular (ICV) injections of AGT-AS-ODN decrease blood pressure in SHRs. Injections into the PVN did not affect blood pressure, although it did decrease vasopressin release *(73)*. The CIH and the 2K1C hypertensive models also respond to AGTAS-ODN CV treatment with a decrease in blood pressure *(64,65)*. The data are summarized in **Table 1**. The drinking response in CIH animals is also attenuated *(65)*. In a normotensive rat the drinking response to renin and isoproterenol is attenuated by ICV AGT-AS-ODN injection, while the drinking responses to carbachol, Ang II, and water depravation are unaffected *(74,75)*. Early studies reported no effect of AS-ODN injected into the peripheral circulation. This appears to have been due to failure to reach the target organs in sufficient numbers. We compared the effect of naked AS-ODN and liposome encapsulated AS-ODN directed against AGT on blood pressure, AGT and AngII concentration, and hepatic uptake. We found that naked AS-ODN was without effect, whereas with the liposome-encapsulated AS-ODN pressure was lowered in SHR. This was accompanied by lowered peripheral AGT, and Ang II in the liver after injection *(76)*. Similar results were obtained when AS-ODN was coupled to carrier molecules that targeted delivery to the liver (*see* **Table 2**) *(77–79)*. In addition to the effects on protein levels and blood pressure, AGT-AS-ODN also attenuated hypertrophy of the heart and the smooth muscle in the aorta (*see* **Table 3**) *(46,78)*. AGT-AS-ODNs attenuated hypertension for 4–5 d *(77,79)*. When a full-length AGT cDNA was inserted into a plasmid under the control of CMV promotor and injected with liposomes in SHRs, the blood pressure decrease lasted for 8 d *(51)*. The same construct delivered by AAV to 5-d-old SHRs caused a delay in the development of hypertension, attenuated hypertrophy, and reduced the degree of hypertension for at least 6 mo *(53)*.

4.4. Angiotensin-Converting Enzyme

AS-ODN directed against ACE mRNA has been used to lower the amount of vascular ACE and the formation of neointima after balloon catheter injury (**Table 3**) *(80)*. ACE-AS-ODN has also been shown to improve cardiac performance after ischemia-reperfusion injury *(81)*.

ACE is present at low to moderate levels in large areas of the brain and in high levels in the NTS and is likely to generate Ang II locally *(82)*. Increasing the levels of ACE in the brain by transfection with a plasmid containing the human ACE gene caused an increase in blood pressure, heart rate, Ang II, and ACE levels that lasted for 2 wk *(83)*. Unpublished results from our lab testing three different sequences of ACE-AS-ODN showed a decrease in blood pressure of hypertensive SHRs of 15–25 mmHg.

4.5. Renin

Renin-AS-ODN decreased blood pressure by about 20 mmHg for 2 d when injected into the lateral ventricle of SHRs. mRNA for renin was also suppressed by the treatment *(84)*. So far no studies have been done with renin-AS-ODN systemically. A complete study with β1-AS-ODN showed that renin release was inhibited and blood pressure decreased for up to 1 mo in SHRs *(43)*.

4.6. AT2

AT2-AS-ODN infused into the kidney of uninephrectomized normotensive rats increased blood pressure by about 20 mmHg throughout the infusion period *(85)*.

5. Discussion

The use of gene therapy to correct genetic abnormalities and to treat diseases is getting closer to being clinically relevant. At least one AS-ODN has been approved by the US Food and Drug Administration (FDA) to treat cytomegalovirus retinitis *(86,87)*, and AAVRPE65 has been used to restore sight in a canine model of blindness *(88)*. Adenovirus is being used in Phase I and Phase II clinical trials in cancer patients *(89–93)*. AS-ODNs and viral vectors have been introduced both into the periphery and the central system of the brain. For therapeutic uses, peripheral administration is more likely to be clinically acceptable. Preclinical studies described above have demonstrated that AS to AGT, AT1, and ACE can successfully lower blood pressure in hypertensive rats, and attenuate hypertrophy in adult animals when administered systemically. The decrease in blood pressure has been reported to vary between 15 and 40 mmHg *(46,51,53,65,76,79)*. While these effects would be highly advantageous clinically, it is probably not possible to achieve a "cure" for hypertension with AS-ODN, because the mechanism is a competition between copies of mRNA and the amount of ODN delivered to cells. Clearly, there is a dose-dependent effect. We found a correlation between dose of an AGT-AS producing plasmid and blood pressure, and there was also a large decrease in blood pressure found with AGT-AS-ODN using a carrier protein targeting the liver *(46,51)*. Another factor favoring the dose-dependant mechanism is that pharmacological drugs, both ACE inhibitors and AT1 receptor antagonists, are able to normalize blood pressure alone, although some new approaches have tried combinations.

The next step in research is to solve the problems to increase uptake of AS-ODNs and viral vectors, and, in the case of viral vectors, to ascertain that they do not cause adverse effects over a very long time, such as immune responses or tumor genesis. Nevertheless, AS gene therapy has the potential of providing extended protection against hypertension, cardiovascular disease, and a multitude of other diseases. Here we have reviewed its use on the RAS as a target system in hypertension and cardiovascular disease, but clearly any target with a known DNA sequence is a target for antisense inhibition.

References

1. Benetos, A., Gautier, S., Ricard, S., et al. (1996) Influence of angiotensin-converting enzyme and angiotensin II type 1 receptor gene polymorphisms on aortic stiffness in normotensive and hypertensive patients. *Circulation* **94,** 698–703.
2. Chung, O. and Unger, T. (1999) Angiotensin II receptor blockade and end-organ protection. *Am. J. Hypertens.* **12,** S150–S156.
3. Kurland, L., Melhus, H., Karlsson, J., et al. (2002) Polymorphisms in the angiotensinogen and angiotensin II type 1 receptor gene are related to change in left ventricular mass during antihypertensive treatment: results from the Swedish Irbesartan Left Ventricular Hypertrophy Investigation versus Atenolol (SILVHIA) trial. *J. Hypertens.* **20,** 657–663.
4. Unger, T. (2002) The role of the renin-angiotensin system in the development of cardiovascular disease. *Am. J. Cardiol.* **89,** 3A–9A.
5. De Paepe, B., Verstraeten, V. M., De Potter, C. R., et al. (2002) Increased angiotensin II type-2 receptor density in hyperplasia, DCIS and invasive carcinoma of the breast is paralleled with increased iNOS expression. *Histochem. Cell Biol.* **117,** 13–19.
6. De Paepe, B., Verstraeten, V. L., De Potter, C. R., et al. (2001) Growth stimulatory angiotensin II type-1 receptor is upregulated in breast hyperplasia and in situ carcinoma but not in invasive carcinoma. *Histochem. Cell Biol.* **116,** 247–254.
7. Schmieder, R. E., Erdmann, J., Delles, C., et al. (2001) Effect of the angiotensin II type 2-receptor gene (+1675 G/A) on left ventricular structure in humans. *J. Am. Coll. Cardiol.* **37,** 175–182.
8. Ichihara, S., Senbonmatsu, T., Price, E., Jr., et al. (2001) Angiotensin II type 2 receptor is essential for left ventricular hypertrophy and cardiac fibrosis in chronic angiotensin II-induced hypertension. *Circulation* **104,** 346–351.
9. Bloem, L. J., Foroud, T. M., Ambrosius, W. T., et al. (1997) Association of the Angiotensinogen Gene to Serum Angiotensinogen in Blacks and Whites. *Hypertension* **29,** 1078–1082.
10. Kim, H. S., Krege, J. H., Kluckman, K. D., et al. (1995) Genetic control of blood pressure and the angiotensinogen locus. *Proc. Natl. Acad. Sci. USA* **92,** 2735–2739.

11. Walker, W. G., Whelton, P. K., Saito, H., et al. (1979) Relation between blood pressure and renin, renin substrate, angiotensin II, aldosterone and urinary sodium and potassium in 574 ambulatory subjects. *Hypertension* **1**, 287–291.

12. Fukamizu, A., Sugimura, K., Takimoto, E., et al. (1993) Chimeric renin-angiotensin system demonstrates sustained increase in blood pressure of transgenic mice carrying both human renin and human angiotensinogen genes. *J. Biol. Chem.* **268**, 11617–11621.

13. Davisson, R. L., Ding, Y., Stec, D. E., et al. (1999) Novel mechanism of hypertension revealed by cell-specific targeting of human angiotensinogen in transgenic mice. *Physiol. Genom.* **1**, 3–9.

14. Merrill, D. C., Thompson, M. W., Carney, C. L., et al. (1996) Chronic hypertension and altered baroreflex responses in transgenic mice containing the human renin and human angiotensinogen genes. *J. Clin. Invest.* **97**, 1047–1055.

15. Morimoto, S., Cassell, M. D., Beltz, T. G., et al. (2001) Elevated blood pressure in transgenic mice with brain-specific expression of human angiotensinogen driven by the glial fibrillary acidic protein promoter. *Circ. Res.* **89**, 365–372.

16. Ohkubo, H., Kawakami, H., Kakehi, H., et al. (1990) Generation of transgenic mice with elevated blood pressure by introduction of the rat renin and angiotensinogen genes. *Proc. Natl. Acad. Sci. USA* **87**, 5153–5157.

17. Stec, D. E., Keen, H. L., and Sigmund, C. D. (2002) Lower blood pressure in floxed angiotensinogen mice after adenoviral delivery of cre-recombinase. *Hypertension* **39**, 629–633.

18. Morishita, R., Higaki, J., Miyazaki, M., et al. (1992) Possible role of the vascular reninangiotensin system in hypertension and vascular hypertrophy. *Hypertension* **19**, II62–II67.

19. Morton, J. J. and Wallace, E. C. (1983) The importance of the renin-angiotensin system in the development and maintenance of hypertension in the two-kidney oneclip hypertensive rat. *Clin. Sci. (Lond.)* **64**, 359–370.

20. Phillips, M. I. and Kimura, B. K. (1986) Levels of brain angiotensin in the spontaneously hypertensive rat and treatment with ramiprilat. *J. Hypertens. Suppl.* **4**, S391–S394.

21. Phillips, M. I. and Kimura, B. (1988) Brain angiotensin in the developing spontaneously hypertensive rat. *J. Hypertens.* **6**, 607–612.

22. Navar, L. G., Von Thun, A. M., Zou, L., et al. (1995) Enhancement of intrarenal angiotensin II levels in 2 kidney 1 clip and angiotensin II induced hypertension. *Blood Press. Suppl.* **2**, 88–92.

23. Brown, L., Passmore, M., Duce, B., et al. (1997) Angiotensin receptors in cardiac and renal hypertrophy in rats. *J. Mol. Cell Cardiol.* **29**, 2925–2929.

24. Gutkind, J. S., Kurihara, M., and Saavedra, J. M. (1988) Increased angiotensin II receptors in brain nuclei of DOCA-salt hypertensive rats. *Am. J. Physiol.* **255**, H646–H650.

25. Atwood, L. D., Kammerer, C. M., Samollow, P. B., et al. (1997) Linkage of Essential hypertension to the angiotensinogen locus in mexican americans. *Hypertension* **30**, 326–330.

26. Corvol, P. and Jeunemaitre, X. (1997) Molecular Genetics of human hypertension: role of angiotensinogen. *Endocr. Rev.* **18**, 662–677.

27. Jain, S., Tang, X., Narayanan, C. S., et al. (2002) Angiotensinogen gene polymorphism at –217 affects basal promoter activity and is associated with hypertension in African-Americans. *J. Biol. Chem.* **277**, 36,889–36,896.

28. Niu, T., Xu, X., Rogus, J., et al. (1998) Angiotensinogen gene and hypertension in Chinese. *J. Clin. Invest.* **101**, 188–194.

29. Agerholm-Larsen, B., Nordestgaard, B. G., and Tybjarg-Hansen, A. (2000) ACE gene polymorphism in cardiovascular disease: meta-analyses of small and large studies in whites. *Arterioscler. Thromb. Vasc. Biol.* **20**, 484–492.

30. O'Donnell, C. J., Lindpaintner, K., Larson, M. G., et al. (1998) Evidence for association and genetic linkage of the angiotensin-converting enzyme locus with hypertension and blood pressure in men but not women in the framingham heart study. *Circulation* **97**, 1766–1772.

31. Bonnardeaux, A., Davies, E., Jeunemaitre, X., et al. (1994) Angiotensin II type 1 receptor gene polymorphisms in human essential hypertension. *Hypertension* **24**, 63–69.

32. Phillips, M. I. and Schmidt-Ott, K. M. (1999) The discovery of renin 100 years ago. *News Physiol. Sci.* **14**, 271–274.

33. Phillips, M. I. (2001) Gene therapy for hypertension: sense and antisense strategies. *Expert. Opin. Biol. Ther.* **1**, 655–662.

34. Phillips, M. I. (2001) Gene therapy for hypertension: the preclinical data. *Hypertension* **38**, 543–548.

35. Phillips, M. I. (2000) Somatic gene therapy for hypertension. *Braz. J. Med. Biol. Res.* **33**, 715–721.

36. Kaplan, N. M. (1998) *Clinical Hypertension*. Williams & Williams, Baltimore.

37. Hodgson, T. A. and Cai, L. (2001) Medical care expenditures for hypertension, its complications, and its comorbidities.*Med. Care* **39**, 599–615.

38. Kagiyama S, Kagiyama T, Phillips MI. (2001) Antisense oligonucleotides strategy in the treatment of hypertension. Curr Opin Mol Ther. 3, 258-264.

39. Phillips, M. I., Wielbo, D., and Gyurko, R. (1994) Antisense inhibition of hypertension: a new strategy for renin-angiotensin candidate genes. *Kidney Int.* **46**, 1554–1556.

40. Dzau, V. J., Mann, M. J., Morishita, R., et al. (1996) Fusigenic viral liposome for gene therapy in cardiovascular diseases. *Proc. Natl. Acad. Sci. USA* **93**, 11421–11425.

41. Fillion, P., Desjardins, A., Sayasith, K., et al. (2001) Encapsulation of DNA in negatively charged liposomes and inhibition of bacterial gene expression with fluid liposome-encapsulated antisense oligonucleotides. *Biochim. Biophys. Acta* **1515**, 44–54.

42. Hughes, J. A., Bennett, C. F., Cook, P. D., et al. (1994) Lipid membrane permeability of 2'-modified derivatives of phosphorothioate oligonucleotides. *J. Pharm. Sci.* **83**, 597–600.

43. Zhang, Y. C., Bui, J. D., Shen, L., et al. (2000) Antisense inhibition of beta(1)-adrenergic receptor mRNA in a single dose produces a profound and prolonged reduction in high blood pressure in spontaneously hypertensive rats. *Circulation* **101,** 682–688.

44. Zhang, Y. M., Rusckowski, M., Liu, N., et al. (2001) Cationic liposomes enhance cellular/nuclear localization of 99mTc-antisense oligonucleotides in target tumor cells. *Cancer Biother. Radiopharm.* **16,** 411–419.

45. Morishita, R., Gibbons, G. H., Ellison, K. E., et al. (1993) Single intraluminal delivery of antisense cdc2 kinase and proliferating-cell nuclear antigen oligonucleotides results in chronic inhibition of neointimal hyperplasia. *Proc. Natl. Acad. Sci. USA* **90,** 8474–8478.

46. Makino, N., Sugano, M., Ohtsuka, S., et al. (1999) Chronic antisense therapy for angiotensinogen on cardiac hypertrophy in spontaneously hypertensive rats. *Cardiovasc. Res.* **44,** 543–548.

47. Clare, Z. Y., Kimura, B., Shen, L., et al. (2000) New beta-blocker: prolonged reduction in high blood pressure with beta(1) antisense oligodeoxynucleotides. *Hypertension* **35,** 219–224.

48. Li, B., Hughes, J. A., and Phillips, M. I. (1997) Uptake and efflux of intact antisense phosphorothioate deoxyoligonucleotide directed against angiotensin receptors in bovine adrenal cells. *Neurochem. Int.* **31,** 393–403.

49. Mohuczy, D. and Phillips, M. I. (2000) Designing antisense to inhibit the renin-angiotensin system. *Mol. Cell Biochem.* **212,** 145–153.

50. Merdan, T., Kopecek, J., and Kissel, T. (2002) Prospects for cationic polymers in gene and oligonucleotide therapy against cancer. *Advanced Drug Delivery Rev.* **54,** 715–758.

51. Tang, X., Mohuczy, D., Zhang, Y. C., et al. (1999) Intravenous angiotensinogen antisense in AAV-based vector decreases hypertension. *Am. J. Physiol.* **277,** H2392–H2399.

52. Zhang, Y., Jeong, L. H., Boado, R. J., et al. (2002) Receptor-mediated delivery of an antisense gene to human brain cancer cells. *J. Gene Med.* **4,** 183–194.

53. Kimura, B., Mohuczy, D., Tang, X., et al. (2001) Attenuation of hypertension and heart hypertrophy by adeno-associated virus delivering angiotensinogen antisense. *Hypertension* **37,** 376–380.

54. Phillips, M. I., Mohuczy-Dominiak, D., Coffey, M., et al. (1997) Prolonged reduction of high blood pressure with an in vivo, nonpathogenic, adeno-associated viral vector delivery of AT1-R mRNA antisense.PG -. *Hypertension* **29,** 374–380.

55. Lu, D., Raizada, M. K., Iyer, S., et al. (1997) Losartan versus gene therapy: chronic control of high blood pressure in spontaneously hypertensive rats. *Hypertension* **30,** 363–370.

56. Metcalfe, B. L., Raizada, M., and Katovich, M. J. (2002) Genetic targeting of the renin angiotensin system for long-term control of hypertension. *Curr. Hypertens. Rep.* **4,** 25–31.

57. Wang, H., Lu, D., Reaves, P. Y., et al. (2000) Retrovirally mediated delivery of angiotensin II type 1 receptor antisense in vitro and in vivo. *Meth. Enzymol.* **314,** 581–590.

58. Hauswirth, W. W. and McInnes, R. R. (1998) Retinal gene therapy 1998: summary of a workshop. *Mol. Vis. 4,* 11.
59. Sinnayah, P., Lindley, T. E., Staber, P. D., et al. (2002) Selective gene transfer to key cardiovascular regions of the brain: comparison of two viral vector systems. *Hypertension* **39,** 603–608.
60. Gyurko, R., Wielbo, D., and Phillips, M. I. (1993) Antisense inhibition of AT1 receptor mRNA and angiotensinogen mRNA in the brain of spontaneously hypertensive rats reduces hypertension of neurogenic origin. *Regul. Pept.* **49,** 167–174.
61. Ambuhl, P., Gyurko, R., and Phillips, M. I. (1995) A decrease in angiotensin receptor binding in rat brain nuclei by antisense oligonucleotides to the angiotensin AT1 receptor. *Regul. Pept.* **59,** 171–182.
62. Gyurko, R., Tran, D., and Phillips, M. I. (1997) Time course of inhibition of hypertension by antisense oligonucleotides targeted to AT1 angiotensin receptor mRNA in spontaneously hypertensive rats. *Am. J. Hypertens.* **10,**56S–62S.
63. Piegari, E., Galderisi, U., Berrino, L., et al. (2000) In vivo effects of partial phosphorothioated AT1 receptor antisense oligonucleotides in spontaneously hypertensive and normotensive rats. *Life Sci.* **66,** 2091–2099.
64. Kagiyama, S., Varela, A., Phillips, M. I., et al. (2001) Antisense inhibition of brain reninangiotensin system decreased blood pressure in chronic 2-kidney, 1 clip hypertensive rats. *Hypertension* **37,** 371–375.
65. Peng, J. F., Kimura, B., Fregly, M. J., et al. (1998) Reduction of cold-induced hypertension by antisense oligodeoxynucleotides to angiotensinogen mRNA and AT1-receptor mRNA in brain and blood.PG -. *Hypertension* **31,** 1317–1323.
66. Meng, H., Wielbo, D., Gyurko, R., et al. (1994) Antisense oligonucleotide to AT1 receptor mRNA inhibits central angiotensin induced thirst and vasopressin. *Regul. Pept.* **54,** 543–551.
67. Sakai, R. R., Ma, L. Y., He, P. F., et al. (1995) Intracerebroventricular administration of angiotensin type 1 (AT1) receptor antisense oligonucleotides attenuate thirst in the rat. *Regul. Pept.* **59,** 183–192.
68. Galli, S. M. and Phillips, M. I. (2001) Angiotensin II AT(1A) receptor antisense lowers blood pressure in acute 2-kidney, 1-clip hypertension. *Hypertension* **38,** 674–678.
69. Yang, B., Li, D., Phillips, M. I., et al. (1998) Myocardial angiotensin II receptor expression and ischemia-reperfusion injury. *Vasc. Med.***3,** 121–130.
70. Iyer, S. N., Lu, D., Katovich, M. J., et al. (1996) Chronic control of high blood pressure in the spontaneously hypertensive rat by delivery of angiotensin type 1 receptor antisense. *Proc. Natl. Acad. Sci. USA* **93,** 9960–9965.
71. Pachori, A. S., Numan, M. T., Ferrario, C. M., et al. (2002) Blood pressure-independent attenuation of cardiac hypertrophy by AT(1)R-AS gene therapy. *Hypertension* **39,** 969–975.
72. Wielbo, D., Sernia, C., Gyurko, R., et al. (1995) Antisense inhibition of hypertension in the spontaneously hypertensive rat. *Hypertension***25,** 314–319.
73. Kagiyama, S., Tsuchihashi, T., Abe, I., et al. (1999) Antisense inhibition of angiotensinogen attenuates vasopressin release in the paraventricular hypothalamic nucleus of spontaneously hypertensive rats. *Brain Res.* **829,** 120–124.

74. Sinnayah, P., Kachab, E., Haralambidis, J., et al. (1997) Effects of angiotensinogen antisense oligonucleotides on fluid intake in response to different dipsogenic stimuli in the rat. *Brain Res. Mol. Brain Res.* **50,**43–50.

75. Sinnayah, P., McKinley, M. J., and Coghlan, J. P. (1997) Angiotensinogen antisense oligonucleotides and fluid intake. *Clin. Exp. Hypertens.* **19,** 993–1007.

76. Wielbo, D., Simon, A., Phillips, M. I., et al. (1996) Inhibition of hypertension by peripheral administration of antisense oligodeoxynucleotides. *Hypertension* **28,** 147–151.

77. Makino, N., Sugano, M., Ohtsuka, S., et al. (1998) Intravenous injection with antisense oligodeoxynucleotides against angiotensinogen decreases blood pressure in spontaneously hypertensive rats. *Hypertension* **31,** 1166–1170.

78. Sugano, M., Tsuchida, K., Sawada, S., et al. (2000) Reduction of plasma angiotensin II to normal levels by antisense oligodeoxynucleotides against liver angiotensinogen cannot completely attenuate vascular remodeling in spontaneously hypertensive rats.PG -. *J. Hypertens.* **18,** 725–731.

79. Tomita, N., Morishita, R., Higaki, J., et al. (1995) Transient decrease in high blood pressure by in vivo transfer of antisense oligodeoxynucleotides against rat angiotensinogen. *Hypertension* **26,** 131–136.

80. Morishita, R., Gibbons, G. H., Tomita, N., et al. (2000) Antisense oligodeoxynucleotide inhibition of vascular angiotensin-converting enzyme expression attenuates neointimal formation: evidence for tissue angiotensin-converting enzyme function. *Arterioscler. Thromb. Vasc. Biol.* **20,** 915–922.

81. Chen, H., Mohuczy, D., Li, D., et al. (2001) Protection against ischemia/reperfusion injury and myocardial dysfunction by antisense-oligodeoxynucleotide directed at angiotensin-converting enzyme mRNA. *Gene Ther.* **8,** 804–810.

82. Phillips, M. I. and Kimura, B. (1999) Central nervous system and angiotensin in the development of hypertension. In *Development of the Hypertensive Phenotype: Basic and Clinical Studies*, (McCarty, R., Blizard, D. A., Chevalier, R. L., eds.), Elsevier, pp. 383–411.

83. Nakamura, S., Moriguchi, A., Morishita, R., et al. (1999) Activation of the brain angiotensin system by in vivo human angiotensin-converting enzyme gene transfer in rats. *Hypertension* **34,** 302–308.

84. Kubo, T., Ikezawa, A., Kambe, T., et al. (2001) Renin antisense injected intraventricularly decreases blood pressure in spontaneously hypertensive rats. *Brain Res. Bull.* **56,** 23–28.

85. Moore, A. F., Heiderstadt, N. T., Huang, E., et al. (2001) Selective inhibition of the renal angiotensin type 2 receptor increases blood pressure in conscious rats. *Hypertension* **37,** 1285–1291.

86. Orr, R. M. (2001) Technology evaluation: fomivirsen, Isis Pharmaceuticals Inc/ CIBA vision. *Curr. Opin. Mol. Ther.* **3,** 288–294.

87. de Smet MD, Meenken CJ, van den Horn GJ. (1999) Fomivirsen—a phosphorothioate oligonucleotide for the treatment of CMV retinitis. *Ocul. Immunol. Inflamm.* **7,** 189–198.

88. Acland, G. M., Aguirre, G. D., Ray, J., et al. (2001) Gene therapy restores vision in a canine model of childhood blindness. *Nat. Genet.* **28,** 92–95.

89. Freytag, S. O., Khil, M., Stricker, H., et al. (2002) Phase I study of replication-competent adenovirus-mediated double suicide gene therapy for the treatment of locally recurrent prostate cancer. *Cancer Res.* **62,** 4968–4976.

90. Reid, T., Galanis, E., Abbruzzese, J., et al. (2001) Intra-arterial administration of a replication-selective adenovirus (dl1520) in patients with colorectal carcinoma metastatic to the liver: a Phase I trial. *Gene Ther.* **8,** 1618–1626.

91. Harvey, B. G., Maroni, J., O'Donoghue, K. A., et al. (2002) Safety of local delivery of low-and intermediate-dose adenovirus gene transfer vectors to individuals with a spectrum of morbid conditions. *Hum. Gene Ther.* **13,** 15–63.

92. The, B. S., Aguilar-Cordova, E., Kernen, K., et al. (2001) Phase I/II trial evaluating combined radiotherapy and in situ gene therapy with or without hormonal therapy in the treatment of prostate cancer,Äîa preliminary report. *Int. J. Radiat. Oncol. Biol. Phys.* **51,** 605–613.

93. Lamont, J. P., Nemunaitis, J., Kuhn, J. A., et al. (2000) A prospective phase II trial of ONYX-015 adenovirus and chemotherapy in recurrent squamous cell carcinoma of the head and neck (the Baylor experience). *Ann. Surg. Oncol.* **7,** 588–592.

94. Nishii, T., Moriguchi, A., Morishita, R., et al. (1999) Angiotensinogen gene-activating elements regulate blood pressure in the brain. *Circ. Res.* **85,** 257–263.

95. Katovich, M. J., Reaves, P. Y., Francis, S. C., et al. (2001) Gene therapy attenuates the elevated blood pressure and glucose intolerance in an insulin-resistant model of hypertension. *J. Hypertens.* **19,** 1553–1558.

96. Morishita, R., Higaki, J., Tomita, N., et al. (1996) Role of transcriptional *cis*-elements, angiotensinogen gene-activating elements, of angiotensinogen gene in blood pressure regulation. *Hypertension* **27,** 502–507.

25

Modulation of Gene Expression by RNAi

Cezary Wójcik, Rosalind Fabunmi, and George N. DeMartino

Summary

RNA interference (RNAi) is a form of posttranscriptional gene silencing in which the presence within the cell of double-stranded RNA (dsRNA) leads to the specific degradation of mRNA with a complimentary sequence. RNAi is a natural phenomenon that can be exploited as a powerful tool to study gene function by generating gene "knockdowns" in various cell types. RNAi is mediated by short interfering RNAs (siRNAs), which are generated within cells from long dsRNAs. To avoid generalized toxic effects, mammalian cells are transfected directly with 21–23-bp-long siRNAs generated either by chemical synthesis or obtained by a series of enzymatic reactions. The present chapter deals with siRNA design, synthesis, transfection, and readout of efficiency in a mammalian cell culture system. The general principle is illustrated by the functional knockdown of p97/VCP (valosin-containing protein) in HeLa cells using five different siRNA sequences.

Key Words: RNA interference; siRNA synthesis; HeLa cells; Cell culture; cell transfection; gene knockdown; p97; VCP.

1. Introduction

1.1. Overview

RNAi interference (RNAi) is a form of posttranscriptional gene silencing in which the presence within the cell of double-stranded RNA (dsRNA) leads to the specific degradation of mRNA with a complimentary sequence (*1*). RNAi is a normal mechanism, which can be exploited as a powerful tool to study gene function. RNAi is faster to perform and much cheaper than traditional knockout approaches. It can be used to reduce the expression of essential genes in preexisting populations of cells (*2*). Gene expression is seldom knocked out completely by RNAi, however, and hence the response has been termed *knockdown*. The degree of knockdown can be sufficient to provide important insights into a gene's function, but caution must be advised about drawing

From: *Methods in Molecular Medicine, Vol. 108: Hypertension: Methods and Protocols*
Edited by: J. P. Fennell and A. H. Baker © Humana Press Inc., Totowa, NJ

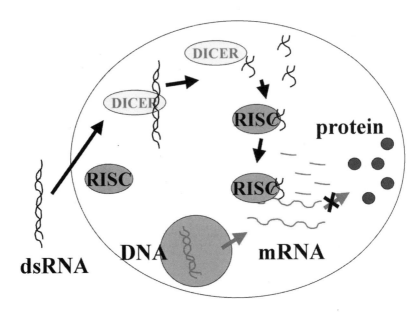

Fig. 1. Simplified schematic representation of the RNA interference (RNAi) pathway. Long stretches of double-stranded RNA are delivered to the cell or synthesized within it. They are recognized by a complex RNAse type III enzyme called Dicer, which cleaves the dsRNA into short 19–21-bp-long stretches called small interfering RNAs. siRNAs bind several proteins, forming the active RISC complex, which specifically recognizes mRNAs complementary to either of the siRNA strands. Once recognized, the mRNA is cleaved into small fragments and therefore the synthesis of its given protein is prevented.

negative conclusions, since the protein remaining after RNAi may still be sufficient to perform its function(s).

RNAi is an ancient mechanism, which probably evolved as a defense against certain viruses and retrotransposons. It was first described in *Caenorhabditis elegans*, where introduction of long dsRNAs (300–1000 bp) induces specific RNAi *(3)*. In contrast, introduction of long dsRNAs into mammalian cells (with the notable exception of oocytes and early embryos *[4]*) triggers a cascade of sequence-independent events resulting in a generalized cytotoxic response *(5,6)*. However, the molecular dissection of RNAi mechanism (**Fig. 1**) allowed the development of RNAi in mammalian cells as well. "Science" designated this achievement "the breakthrough of the year for 2002" *(7)*. Long dsRNAs are converted within cells into 21–23-bp-long dsRNA fragments called siRNAs (small interfering RNAs) by the RNAse III enzyme Dicer *(8)*. siRNAs mediate the specific cleavage of targeted mRNAs in both invertebrate and mammalian cells *(9)*, but unlike long dsRNAs, they do not elicit a cytotoxic response in mammalian cells. Therefore, the direct use of short siRNAs in mammalian cells bypasses the initial step of the RNAi pathway, circumventing the nonspecific effects of long dsRNAs *(10)*.

siRNAs for experimental use can be generated either by a series of enzymatic reactions such as the one performed with the use of the Silencer™ (Ambion, Austin, TX) kit or by direct chemical synthesis (by in-house facility or from a commercial provider). For alternative approaches, *see* **Notes 1** and **2**. Because siRNAs must be transfected into mammalian cells with the aid of a specific transfection reagent, the success of the technique is largely dependent on the transfection efficiency. We do not endorse products from any particular company, but the methods outlined below have worked well in our laboratory with the use of the indicated suppliers.

2. Materials

1. Chemically synthesized siRNAs (Dharmacon, Lafayette, CO; Qiagen, Hilden, Germany; Ambion, Austin, TX, etc.).
2. Silencer kit (Ambion, Austin, TX).
3. Oligofectamine™ (Invitrogen, Carlsbad, CA).
4. OptiMEMÔ™ medium, high-glucose Dulbecco's modified Eagle's medium (DMEM), antibiotic/antimycotic 100X solution, phosphate-buffered saline (PBS), trypsin-EDTA (Invitrogen, Carlsbad, CA).
5. Cell culture flasks and dishes (Nalgene Nunc, Rochester, NY).
6. Eppendorf centrifuge tubes (Hamburg, Germany).
7. Gilson pipetters (Villiers Le Bel, France).
8. Temperature-controlled water bath.
9. Cell-culture incubator and hood.
10. Inverted microscope.
11. Temperature-controlled incubator.
12. PC or Mac computer with fast Internet access.
13. UV-transparent cuvets and spectrophotometer.

All solutions should be made to the standard required for molecular biology grade and should be RNAse-free, where required.

3. Methods

We have found that the Silencer kit is a useful and cost-effective means for initial screening for RNAi efficiency or whenever siRNA is needed for only a few experiments, whereas chemical synthesis is desirable for siRNAs of known efficiency and whenever multiple experiments are expected. The methods described below include (1) the design of siRNAs, (2) synthesis of siRNAs with the use of Silencer kit, (3) transfection of mammalian cells with RNAi prepared by either the Silencer kit or chemical synthesis methods, and (4) analysis of the results.

3.1. Design of the siRNAs

Design of the siRNAs is probably the most important step for this methodology and is critical to the success of the experiment.

1. Identify the mRNA sequence of interest. Keep in mind that mammalian cells contain multiple mRNAs coding for the same or similar products that have been reported in databanks such as Genbank (*see* **Notes 3** and **4**). Some of these may represent real differences, but many are artifacts and represent multiple reporting of the same gene.
2. In principle, any 21-bp-long stretch of mRNA will mediate RNAi; nevertheless, it is wise to avoid sequences of potential higher complexity or regions that may bind transcription factors, because complex tertiary structures of the mRNA may prevent binding of RNAi machinery.
3. Albeit not an absolute requirement, it is advisable to select sequences with approximately equal content of purines and pyrimidines.
4. Avoid stretches of more than four or five identical nucleotides.
5. Following the algorithm proposed originally by Elbashir et al. *(10)*, identify the cDNA or mRNA sequence for target, move 70 bp downstream from the ATG start-codon, then find the first AA doublet. Record 19 bp after the AA doublet and perform BLAST on the whole 21-bp sequence
6. A BLAST search should identify the specific target gene, which may appear under several different names either as a whole sequence or as a piece of a sequence. If a different gene is specifically identified by the BLAST search or if there are doubts regarding a sequence, then it is better to abandon this sequence and repeat the procedure from **step 3**, searching for another AA downstream. Sometimes it is necessary to repeat the search several times.
7. As a practical rule, consider an siRNA to be specific when it identifies the gene of interest by BLAST search with a specificity of 100%, and any other gene with a specificity less than or equal to 17 of 21 bp. Whenever the BLAST search identifies another gene with a specificity higher than 17 of 21 bp, there is a chance that this gene will be silenced in addition to the targeted gene, therefore such sequence should not be used for siRNA design.
8. Even if all design rules are strictly followed, there is no guarantee that a given sequence will be effective for siRNA. Therefore we recommend the design and synthesis of at least two different siRNAs.

3.2. Synthesis of siRNAs Using the Silencer Kit

All siRNA synthesis was carried out according to the manufacturer's protocol, with minor modifications.

1. When ordering the oligonucleotides for this method of siRNA synthesis, the total oligonucleotide length must be 29 nucleotides, i.e., the 21 nucleotides designed as above (*see* **Subheading 3.1.**) plus an additional stretch of 8 nucleotides at the

3'-end (5'-CCT GTC TC-3'). This additional sequence is complementary to the T7 promoter primer provided with the kit. 50-nmol synthesis scale provides sufficient template for siRNA synthesis. There is no need for further purification of oligonuclotides after desalting.

2. Dissolve both sense and antisense oligonucleotides into an appropriate volume of RNAse free water to generate a 1 mM stock solution. Keep in mind that the scale of synthesis does not reflect the amount of oligonucleotides present in the vial. This is usually indicated on the data sheet provided by the oligonucleotide manufacturer.

3. Measure the OD_{260} of the 1 mM oligonucleotide solution diluted 1:200 in ultrapure water. Obtain the oligonucleotide concentration in the original stock by the following calculation: [oligonucleotide] = OD_{260} × 200 (dilution factor) × 20 (OD_{260} of 1 indicates 20-μg/mL concentration of oligonucleotides).
Convert the concentration from μg/mL into molarity. The molecular weight of a 29-mer oligonucleotide is approx 8750 daltons. The actual micromolar oligonucleotide concentration calculated by this method will vary from the expected 1000 μM value.

4. Prepare 100 μL of a 100 μM oligonucleotide stock by diluting the "1000 μM" stock with RNAse-free water provided with the kit. Keep in mind that this is not a simple 1:10 dilution because for all calculations, the actual micromolar concentration calculated from OD260 measurement should be used.

5. Thaw the DNA hybridization buffer, T7 reaction buffer, T7 promoter primer solution, 10X Klenow reaction buffer, 10X dNTP mix, 2X dNTP mix provided in the kit at room temperature (RT). Briefly vortex and tap-spin before use.

6. For both sense and antisense oligonucleotide forming a pair that will be used to make a single siRNA, mix in an PCR tube 1 μL of the T7 promoter primer, 3 μL of the DNA hybridization buffer, and 1 μL of a given oligonucleotide (out of the 100 μM stock). Keep the 100 μM stock frozen at –20°C for future use.

7. Heat the mix for 5 min at 70°C in a thermocycler and then leave at RT for 5 min.

8. Immediately add to each tube the following reagents provided in the kit: 1 μL of the 10X Klenow buffer, 1 μL of 10X dNTP mix, 2 μL of RNAse-free water, and 1 μL of the Exo-Klenow enzyme.

9. Mix gently by pipetting and incubate in the thermocycler at 37°C for 30 min.

10. Use an RNAse-free Eppendorf tube for each of the oligonucleotides. To each tube add 2 μL of the product obtained in the previous reaction (the rest can be stored at –20°C for future use), 4 μL of RNAse-free water, 10 μL of 2X dNTP mix (take caution not to confuse with the 10X dNTP mix), 2 μL of 10X T7 reaction buffer, and 2 μL enzyme mix.

11. Incubate for 2 h at 37°C in a cabinet incubator.

12. Mix sense and antisense reaction into one tube and continue incubation at 37°C overnight.

13. The following day, thaw the digestion buffer at RT and mix the contents of the vial thoroughly by vortexing.

14. To the overnight reaction, add the following components provided with the kit in the following order: 6 μL digestion buffer, 48.5 μL nuclease-free water, 3 μL RNAse, and 2.5 μL DNAse.

15. Mix gently by pipetting and incubate at 37°C for 1 h in the cabinet incubator.

16. Preheat RNAse-free water to 75°C in a water bath.

17. For each siRNA synthesized, place the minicolumn provided in the kit into a collection Eppendorf tube and prewet the column with 100 μL of the siRNA wash buffer (provided with the kit).

18. Add the product of **step 15** to the tube and centrifuge it at maximum speed for 1 min in a benchtop microcentrifuge.

19. Lift the column, discard the flow through and place it back into the collection tube.

20. Apply 500 μL of the siRNA wash buffer to the column and centrifuge at maximum speed for 1 min.

21. Discard the flow through and repeat the wash from the previous step.

22. Transfer the minicolumn to a new tube and add 100 μL of the RNAse-free water preheated to 75°C.

23. After 2 min, spin the tube with the minicolumn at maximum speed for 1 min.

24. Your synthesized siRNA will be in the flowthrough; this time, discard the minicolumn.

25. Dilute the siRNA 1:200 in ultrapure water in a cuvet and measure OD_{260} using the same water as a blank.

26. Calculate the concentration of siRNA using the following formula: [siRNA] = OD_{260} × 200 (dilution) × 40 (OD_{260} of 1 is equivalent to 40 μg/mL concentration of siRNA).

27. Convert the concentration of siRNA from μg/mL to μM by dividing it by 14 (Note: there are 14 μg of RNA in 1 nmol of an average 21-mer of double-stranded RNA).

28. Dilute the siRNA stock with RNAse-free water to obtain a final concentration of 2 μM. Store in 50–100-μL aliquots in PCR tubes at –20°C. siRNAs remain stable for over 1 yr under those conditions.

3.3. Transfection of Mammalian Cells

3.3.1. Experimental Setup

After siRNA administration, the cellular levels of the targeted mRNA decline rapidly (1); however, a change in phenotype depends on the downregulation of the targeted protein, which, in turn, depends on the proteins' half-life. For short-lived proteins, efficient knockdown is observed in as little as 24 h following the initial transfection with siRNA. Downregulation of long-lived proteins requires a slightly different approach, because the protein levels will often not decrease significantly until 72 h posttransfection or longer. **Figure 2** gives an example of how slow the downregulation of a long-lived protein might be, in that case showing the RNAi of a ubiquitous cellular

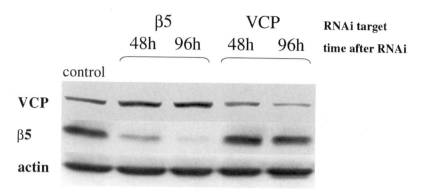

Fig. 2. Time dependence of RNAi-mediated knockdown of long-lived proteins. HeLa cells were treated with siRNA, targeting either the β5 subunit of the proteasome or the VCP/p97 protein. Cells were collected after 48 h or subjected to a second round of RNAi and collected 96 h after the first RNAi treatment. Whole cell lysates were run on SDS-PAGE and Western blotted with the indicated antibodies. RNAi induced a specific decrease of the levels of each protein, which was more pronounced after 96 h. Note that the levels of the untargeted protein and actin remain unchanged, demonstrating the specificity of the response.

ATPase of the AAA family called p97/VCP (valosin-containing protein). In the case of targets essential for growth, such as proteasome subunits, the long half-life poses a real problem, because the transfection efficiency never reaches 100% with the methods used. The remaining subpopulation of untransfected "wild-type" cells may take over the subpopulation of growth-impaired transfected cells, constituting the majority of cells after 72 h or longer incubation times. To circumvent these negative effects, we recommend the use of a second transfection 48 h after the initial transfection, in order to improve RNAi efficiency and reduce the number of wild type cells. We have used this protocol successfully to downregulate the expression of several long-lived proteins in mammalian cells *(11)*.

The following protocol has been designed for 1 well on a standard 6-well plate (32 mm in diameter). The amount of reagents for use can be adapted to the surface area of the tissue culture vessel. We have typically used HeLa cells for our RNAi experiments, but the method can be adapted to most mammalian cell types (e.g., CHO, HEK-293 *[12]*, COS7m NIH/3T3, A549, HT-29, MCF-7 *[13]*, JURKAT, and primary T human cells *[14]*, *see* **Note 3**), and it has even been used in whole animals in vivo *(15)* (*see* **Note 2**).

Whereas the siRNA obtained by enzymatic synthesis should be kept as 2 μ*M* stock at –20°C (*see* **Subheading 3.3.1.**, **step 28**), chemically synthesized siRNA should be dissolved in RNAse-free water to a stock concentration of

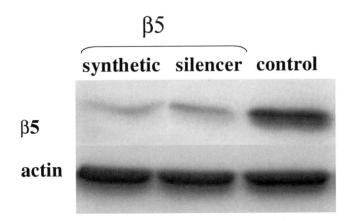

Fig. 3. RNAi of the same target with siRNAs of the same sequence, which have been synthesized either by chemical synthesis or with the use of Ambion's Silencer kit. HeLa cells have been treated with siRNA targeting β5 subunit of the proteasome obtained either by chemical synthesis (synthetic) or with the use of Ambion's Silencer kit. The concentration of the siRNA obtained with the Silencer kit was one-tenth of the concentration of the siRNA obtained by chemical synthesis, but the efficiency of protein knockdown is comparable. Whole-cell lysates obtained 96 h from the initial treatment were run on SDS-PAGE and Western blotted with the indicated antibodies.

20 μ*M*. We recommend the 10X higher concentration, because chemically synthesized siRNA is less potent than the siRNA of the same sequence synthesized by the Silencer kit *(13)*. **Figure 3** shows the almost identical effectiveness of a 10X lower concentration of an siRNA targeting the β5-subunit of the proteasome compared with the siRNA of the same sequence obtained by means of chemical synthesis.

3.3.2. Protocol for Transfection

1. Plate cells 1 d in advance at a density dependent on whether you are studying long-lived or short-lived proteins, i.e., whether you wish to harvest the cells after 24–48 h for short-lived proteins or whether you want to perform a second RNAi and harvest the cells 4 d after the initial RNAi for long-lived proteins. We have observed efficient RNAi when the cells have been plated the same day the experiment is performed, at least 3 h in advance. If it is expected that the knockdown of the target protein will impair cell growth and/or induce apoptosis a higher plating density is preferred. For short experiments, 40% cell density is good; whereas for longer experiments it should be less than 40%. HeLa cells can be plated as low as 10% confluency.
2. Thaw the siRNA stock aliquot on ice.

3. Working under the cell culture hood, mix in a sterile Eppendorf tube 5 μL of the siRNA stock and 87.5 μL of OptiMEM. It is recommended that you do not add antibiotics to the OptiMEM, as it may interfere with transfection efficiency. Other serum-free media can also be used instead.

4. In another Eppendorf tube, mix 1.5 μL oligofectamine (*see* **Note 5**) and 6 μL OptiMEM, wait 5 min (if you have various siRNAs to transfect, you can mix oligofectamine in a single tube).

5. Add 7.5 μL of the oligofectamine/OptiMEM mix to the 92.5 μL siRNA/ OptiMEM mix.

6. Wait at least 20 min (you can leave this mix for maximum of 2 h).

7. Aspirate old media from the cells, wash the cells with OptiMEM once, aspirate media again, and add 500 μL OptiMEM per well.

8. Add 95 μL of the siRNA mix to the well.

9. Swirl gently, place in incubator.

10. After 3–6 h, add 1.5 mL of normal growth medium with antibiotics per well (we use DMEM high glucose).

11. Harvest the cells after 24–48 h if you are targeting a short-lived protein; otherwise repeat the transfection after 2 d and harvest the cells 4 d after the initial transfection.

3.4. Analysis of the RNAi Experiments

Efficient RNAi implies almost complete degradation of mRNA complementary to the siRNAs used in the experiment, therefore its efficiency can be monitored directly by the measurement of mRNA levels by Northern blotting, semiquantitative reverse-transcription PCR (RT-PCR) or real-time RT-PCR (*see* **Note 6**). As a consequence of the degradation of target mRNA, the levels of target protein also decrease and can be documented by Western blotting with a specific antibody. Depending on the function of the targeted protein, the efficiency of RNAi may also be measured indirectly by the quantification of the induced phenotype. For example, if you are targeting the proteasome ubiquitin system, analysis would include the accumulation of ubiquitinated protein, induction of apoptosis, block in the cell cycle, and change in enzymatic activity. The method of choice should be adapted for each particular case. It is important to distinguish methods that deal with the whole population of cells from those that deal with individual cells. Methods that measure physiological effects in a population of cells (e.g., Western blotting) will be biased by the amount of nontransfected cells, which may contribute a significant signal and obscure the outcome of the experiment. In contrast, methods that deal with individual cells (e.g., immunocytochemistry) will allow you to distinguish cells that have been transfected from those that have not, if there is a clearly visible feature such as immunolabeling with an antibody detecting the targeted protein.

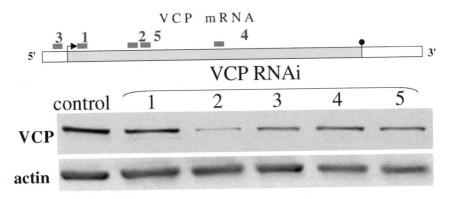

Fig. 4. Effect of five different siRNAs targeting different regions of the mRNA. The targeted regions are highlighted below in a diagramatic representation of VCP/ p97 mRNA. The different siRNAs have been arbitrarily numbered from 1 to 5. siRNA 1 was obtained by chemical synthesis, while siRNAs 2–5 were obtained with the use of the Ambion's SILENCER kit. Whole cell lysates obtained 96 h after the initial treatment were run on SDS-PAGE and Western blotted with the indicated antibodies. Note the different degree of knockdown for the five different siRNAs.

In every experiment it is very important to have appropriate controls. A positive control in RNAi experiments should consist of the use of an siRNA of known efficiency targeting the same gene as the siRNA under study. In many instances, a positive control is not available, so at least two or more different siRNAs targeting the same gene should be compared: the more comparisons, the better. **Figure 4** shows an example of differential effects of five different siRNAs targeting the same gene (human VCP/p97). Other examples can be found in **refs.** *12* and *13*. The negative control consists of a scrambled sequence siRNA with the same nucleotide content as the experimental siRNA. It is important to verify that scrambled siRNA does not affect any other gene. It can be expensive to generate scrambled counterparts for each siRNA tested, so an acceptable control is an siRNA that knocks down a different gene product, ideally one that does not affect cellular phenotype and does not interfere with the same pathway as the gene of interest. Such siRNA may serve as a negative control of any nonspecific RNAi effects on one hand, while on the other it will serve to assess the efficiency of the whole RNAi procedure. Another negative control is an inefficient siRNA targeting another gene. Finally, it is also important to include a control consisting of the transfection reagent alone.

4. Notes

1. In addition to the methods described in this chapter, there are also at least two other methods used to induce RNAi in mammalian cells. One consists of trans-

fection with a mix of multiple siRNAs rather than a single siRNA. Such a mix is obtained in vitro from long dsRNAs with the use of recombinant Dicer *(16)*. A second method consists of the construction of specific vectors such as the pSUPER series, which are engineered in such a way that they express hairpin siRNAs under the control of the RNA polymerase III promoter *(17)*. These methods will not be discussed in detail here.

2. RNAi has been perfomed successfully in vivo with the use of both siRNAs *(15)* and pSUPER-type vectors *(18)*.

3. When working with multiple cell lines, keep in mind that RNAi is species-specific, because the mRNA sequences differ even in closely related species that have the same amino acid sequence of target protein. Each species requires the design of its own siRNAs.

4. When studying a new protein of uncertain function, we have found it very informative to perform the RNAi of its *Drosophila* homolog in the Schneider-2 cell culture system using the methodology originally developed by the Dixon laboratory *(2)*. Schneider-2 (S-2) cells are easy to grow and RNAi can be performed using long dsRNAs, which are much cheaper to synthesize than short siRNAs. Moreover, S-2 cells do not require the use of transfection reagents because they readily take up dsRNA from media. Detailed description of these experiments can be find in our published papers *(11,18)*.

5. We have obtained good results with the use of oligofectamine as the transfection reagent for HeLa cells, but several companies now offer transfection reagents designed specifically for transfection with siRNAs (such as Ribojuice from Novagen, Madison, WI; Nucleofector from Amaxa, Cologne, Germany; GeneSilencer from Gene Therapy Systems, San Diego, CA; sPORT reagents from Ambion, Austin, TX), which may be useful especially for work with cell lines that are difficult to transfect.

6. The transfection efficiency with siRNAs can be monitored by two different methods. The indirect method relies on contransfection of a plasmid carrying a marker such as GFP or β-galactosidase and requires the use of a transfection reagent other than oligofectamine that is suitable for both oligonucleotides and vectors, such as lipofectamine 2000 (Invitrogen, Carlsbad, CA). The direct method consists of the use of siRNAs that have been labeled with a fluorescent marker such as, e.g., Cy3. Ambion (Austin, TX) offers labeling of siRNAs they synthesize and sells a Silencer siRNA labeling kit that may be used to label siRNAs from other source *(20)*.

Acknowledgments

Research with the use of RNAi in GDM laboratory is supported by the Welch Foundation and National Institutes of Health. We acknowledge the helpful comments of other members of the DeMartino lab.

References

1. Hannon, G. J. (2002) RNA interference. *Nature* **418**, 244–251.

2. Clemens, J. C., Worby, C. A., Simonson-Leff, et al. (2000) Use of double-stranded RNA interference in Drosophila cell lines to dissect signal transduction pathways. *Proc. Natl. Acad. Sci. USA* **97,** 6499–6503.

3. Fire, A., Xu, S., Montgomery, M. K., Kostas, S. A., Driver, S. E., and Mello, C. C. (1998) Potent and specific genetic interference by double-stranded RNA in *Caenorhabditis elegans. Nature* **391,** 806–811.

4. Wianny, F. and Zernicka-Goetz, M. (2000) Specific interference with gene function by double-stranded RNA in early mouse development. *Nat. Cell Biol.* **2,** 70–75.

5. Manche, L., Green, S. R., Schmedt, C., and Mathews, M. B. (1992) Interactions between double-stranded RNA regulators and the protein kinase DAI. *Mol. Cell Biol.* **12,** 5238–5248.

6. Minks, M. A., West, D. K., Benvin, S., and Baglioni, C. (1979) Structural requirements of double-stranded RNA for the activation of 2',5'-oligo(A) polymerase and protein kinase of interferon-treated HeLa cells *J. Biol. Chem.* **254,** 10, 180–10,183.

7. Couzin, J. (2002) Breakthrough of the year. Small RNAs make big splash. *Science* **298,** 2296–2297.

8. Bernstein, E., Caudy, A. A., Hammond, S. M., and Hannon, G. J. (2001) Role for a bidentate ribonuclease in the initiation step of RNA interference. *Nature* **409,** 363–366.

9. Elbashir, S. M., Lendeckel, W., and Tuschl, T. (2001) RNA interference is mediated by 21- and 22-nucleotide RNAs. *Genes Dev.* **15,** 188–200.

10. Elbashir, S. M., Harborth, J., Lendeckel, W., Yalcin, A., Weber, K., and Tuschl, T. (2001) Duplexes of 21-nucleotide RNAs mediate RNA interference in cultured mammalian cells. *Nature* **411,** 494–498.

11. Wojcik, C., Yano, M., and DeMartino, G. N. (2004) RNA interference of Valosin-Containing protein (VCP/p97) reveals multiple cellular roles linked to ubiquitin-proteasome dependent proteolysis. *J. Cell Sci.* **117,** 281–292.

12. Hayes, S. and Bruggink, F. (2002) Targeted suppression of gene expression using siRNA and Ribojuice siRNA transfection reagent. *inNovations* **14,** 9–11.

13. Brown, D., Jarvis, R., Pallotta, V., Byrom, M., and Ford, L. (2002) RNA Interference in mammalian cell culture: design, execution and analysis of the siRNA effect. *Ambion Technotes Newslett.* **9,** 3–6.

14. Lun, K. (2002) Delivery of siRNA and DNA oligonucleotides into primary cells and hard-to-transfect cell lines with the Nucleofector technology. *Amaxa Technotes* 1–5.

15. McCaffrey, A. P., Meuse, L., Pham, T. T., Conklin, D. S., Hannon, G. J., and Kay, M. A. (2002) RNA interference in adult mice. *Nature* **418,** 38–39.

16. Myers, J. W., Jones, J. T., Meyer, T., and Ferrell, J. E. (2003) Recombinant Dicer efficiently converts large dsRNAs into siRNAs suitable for gene silencing. *Nat. Biotechnol.* **21,** 324–328.

17. Brummelkamp, T. R., Bernards, R., and Agami, R. (2002) A system for stable expression of short interfering RNAs in mammalian cells. *Science* **296,** 550–553.

18. Brummelkamp, T. R., Bernards, R., and Agami, R. (2002) Stable suppression of tumorigenicity by virus-mediated RNA interference. *Cancer Cell* **2,** 243–247.
19. Wojcik, C. and DeMartino, G. N. (2002) Analysis of *Drosophila* 26 S proteasome using RNA interference. *J. Biol. Chem.* **277,** 6188–6197.
20. Byrom, M., Palotta, V., Brown, D., and Ford, L. (2002) Visualizing siRNA in mammalian cells. *Ambion Technotes Newsletter* **9,** 6–8.

26

In Vivo Biopanning

A Methodological Approach to Identifying Novel Targeting Ligands for Delivery of Biological Agents to the Vasculature

Lorraine M. Work, Campbell G. Nicol, Laura Denby, and Andrew H. Baker

Summary

In order for gene delivery to be clinically acceptable, a number of crucial developments need to be made to existing vectors. Significant advances have been made in the identification of novel platform vectors that possess modified tropism to the native vector, directing infectivity away from nontarget tissues such as the liver. In order to fully optimize these detargeted platform vectors, they need to be retargeted toward a chosen, defined site, which will be defined according to the disease studied. The successful transition of targeting peptides identified using in vitro screening protocols to an in vivo disease model may be compromized by the complexity of delivery into an intact biological system. To this end, peptides identified using in vivo biopanning may prove to be of greater clinical significance given that they were identified in the disease model of choice and so should translate more successfully to the intact preclinical model. Exploitation of the heterogeneity of the vascular endothelium using such an approach will go a long way toward improving the efficiency and achieving site-specific gene expression, with important clinical implications for the systemic application of gene delivery.

Key Words: gene therapy; phage display; adenoviruses; peptides; targeting; endothelium; in vivo models of disease.

1. Introduction

There are a number of diseases and disorders that are currently refractory to standard pharmacological intervention; for these, and many others, gene therapy represents an attractive intervention strategy. Transient or sustained gene delivery and expression at target sites following systemic administration of the chosen gene delivery vector remains the "holy grail" of gene therapy. To date, progress in this area has been hampered by the native tropism of existing

From: *Methods in Molecular Medicine, Vol. 108: Hypertension: Methods and Protocols*
Edited by: J. P. Fennell and A. H. Baker © Humana Press Inc., Totowa, NJ

vector systems toward, in particular, the liver. In recent years a great deal of research attention has focused on the identification of native receptors and co-receptors for the most commonly applied viral vector systems, and progress has been made in understanding basic vector biology. The major limiting factor for the targeted delivery of gene therapy vectors presently, therefore, remains the identification of novel targeting ligands for specific target sites. Pioneering studies performed in the late 1990s by Rajotte et al. *(1)* described the existence of a so-called address system in the mouse, whereby the endothelium resident within different organs expressed a number of unique receptors that could be identified by small peptides displayed on the coat protein of bacteriophage. These peptides could then be used to specifically target phage populations to chosen target sites following systemic administration. Since then, a number of organs and tumor models have been targeted successfully using ligands identified by in vivo biopanning, and recently the approach was described in a human subject with a similar "address system" evident *(2)*. In this chapter we will summarise the successful applications of in vivo biopanning and its identified ligands to date and describe the methods required to perform in vivo biopanning using our experience with a rat. However, the method can be applied to any preclinical model.

In vivo biopanning applies the theory proven on many occasions to be successful in vitro (reviewed in **ref. 3**), to in vivo models of disease. A bacteriophage or phage is a virus whose host is a bacterium. Phage display of peptide libraries is based on the concept that insertion of a random oligonucleotide encoding a peptide within a structural gene of the phage will lead to the display of the peptide on the surface of the phage *(4–8)*. Derivatives of Ff (F-pilus-dependent) filamentous *Escherichia coli* bacteriophages, such as M13 or fd, are most commonly used as vectors for phage display. Using filamentous bacteriophage, Smith first demonstrated that exogenous peptides could be displayed on the phage surface as fusions with the coat proteins pIII or pVIII *(8)*. Briefly, phage display libraries are infused systemically (usually intravenously) and allowed to circulate for a predetermined time prior to phage recovery from the target organ, amplification, and reinfusion over a further two or three rounds (**Fig. 1**). The encoded peptide insert of a number of phage clones homing to the target (and nontarget) organ are then sequenced and consensus motifs or sequences identified. Early studies by Pasqualini and Ruoslahti *(9)* were the first to describe the use of phage display technology to differentiate between the endothelial layer in the brain and kidney of Balb/c mice. Peptides containing consensus motifs displayed as homogenous populations of phages were infused and shown to be selective for the organ from which they were isolated, demonstrating proof of principle and opening the door to a number of subsequent studies utilizing in vivo biopanning.

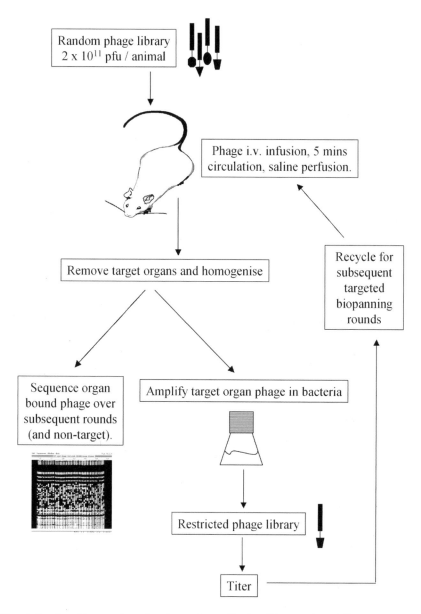

Fig. 1. In vivo biopanning. Random phage display library (2×10^{11} PFU/animal) is infused via the femoral vein and allowed to circulate for 5 min before saline perfusion through the heart under physiological pressure. This removes unbound phage which may be present in the target organ at the time of harvest. Phage are recovered and amplified back to the original titer before restricted populations are reinfused over subsequent rounds. Phage clones are selected after each round for sequencing of the encoded peptide insert.

In vitro biopanning has also been used to identify peptides subsequently shown to be capable of directing organ- and tissue-specific binding in vivo, many of these studies have used cancer models as a platform for intervention. Of the first peptides identified and shown to be successful in retargeting to a number of cell types and cancer models were peptides containing the Arg-Gly-Asp (RGD) motif, known to target many integrins *(10)*. Initial studies found that GACRGDCLGA, which contained one disulfide bond and so displayed the peptide in a constrained conformation, was 10 times more efficient than linear RGD-containing peptides in binding assays *(11)*. Later studies by the same group found RGD-4C (CGCRGDCFC), which contained two disulfide bonds, to be further efficient and selective for the α_v integrins *(12)*. In vivo experiments whereby the RGD-4C peptide was administered intravenously in tumor-bearing mice demonstrated selective phage binding to tumor vasculature compared to nontarget organs (brain and kidney) *(13)*. Furthermore, this peptide was used to enhance the efficacy and reduce the toxicity associated with a chemotherapeutic agent, given systemically, to target drug delivery to the tumor vasculature in a mouse model with human breast cancer xenografts *(14)*. Subsequently, many groups have used the RGD-4C peptide in conjunction with gene delivery vectors to target cancer cells, improve transduction into cells refractory to viral infection but known to express the α_v integrins, and attempt to alter systemic distribution of viruses (reviewed by **refs. 15** and **16**). While RGD-4C has been shown to be efficient at retargeting, it lacks selectivity, as many cells express the α_v integrins; further in vivo biopanning studies have identified potentially selective peptides for a number of targets.

Parallel studies by Arap et al. *(14)* demonstrated that phage displaying peptides containing the Asn-Gly-Arg (NGR) motif were further able to direct drug delivery to tumor vasculature *(14)*. The tumor-targeting effect was found to be dependent on the presence of a disulfide bridge constraint within the NGR-containing peptide sequence *(17)*. Subsequently, aminopeptidase N (CD13) was identified as the receptor for this tumor-homing peptide *(18)* and an isoform of CD13 shown to be present on tumor vasculature *(19)*. Given the role of aminopeptidase N in angiogenesis, this highlights a potential new target for both inhibiting angiogenesis and tumor-targeting.

Using the rat homolog of human melanoma proteoglycan, NG2, random phage libraries were screened in vitro and two specific NG2-binding peptides were identified. Intravenous injection of homogenous phages containing each peptide resulted in selective homing to tumor vasculature *(20)*. A peptide mimetic of E-selectin isolated by in vitro biopanning bound to the selectins reduced cell adhesion and inhibited lung colonization by sialyl-lewis X-expressing tumor cells in vivo *(21)*. Koivunen et al. *(22)* isolated peptides targeted to matrix metalloproteinase-2 and -9, proteolytic enzymes associated with cancer cell invasion and metastasis. These peptides were able to inhibit endothelial and tumor cell migration in vitro and, more important, prevent tumor growth and invasion in vivo in mouse models of human carcinoma *(22)*. This study therefore demonstrated isolation of phage that encode peptides with distinct and selective biological activity. A combined ex vivo and in vivo biopanning approach was described by Porkka et al. *(23)* using a cDNA phage display library. Phage libraries were incubated for two rounds ex vivo with progenitor cell-enriched bone marrow cells before two in vivo rounds in mice bearing a HL-60 xenograft tumor. This gave a cDNA fragment encoding an N-terminal fragment of human high-mobility group protein 2 (HMGN2), which homed to tumors when administered intravenously *(23)*.

Targeting vascular endothelial growth factor (VEGF)-induced angiogenesis peptides that blocked the VEGF-kinase domain receptor (KDR) interaction were identified in vitro and found to inhibit VEGF-induced endothelial cell proliferation in vitro. When administered in vivo, in a rabbit corneal angiogenesis model, VEGF-mediated angiogenesis was selectively blocked *(24)*. Similarly, Hetian et al. *(25)* identified a novel peptide which interfered with the VEGF-KDR interaction in vitro. The peptide both inhibited endothelial cell proliferation in vitro and was antiangiogenic as determined using the chick embryo chorioallantoic membrane in vivo angiogenesis model. Importantly, the peptide also inhibited solid tumor growth and metastases in vivo *(25)*.

Many reports have also identified targeting ligands by using in vivo biopanning for the treatment of cancers. Using an angiogenic mouse model whereby angiogenesis was induced using the dorsal air sac method, phage were administered intravenously and those phage displaying peptides that homed to the angiogenic vessels isolated *(26,27)*. A number of 15-mer targeting peptides were identified and found to inhibit VEGF-induced migration of endothelial cells in vitro and angiogenesis in vivo. Using exogenous fragment peptides, the essential epitope driving tumor homing in vivo was determined to be a pentapeptide HWRPW motif *(26)*. In a similar study from the same group *(27)*, an alternative identified pentapeptide was synthesised and used to target liposomes in vivo, resulting in a marked accumulation of peptide-modified liposomes in implanted tumors. Conjugation of a chemotherapeutic agent to the peptide–liposome complex resulted in marked tumor growth suppression and angiogenesis in vivo *(27)*. Cancer of the prostate has also been successfully targeted for destruction using ligands identified by in vivo biopanning. Phage localizing to the vasculature of the prostate in mice were recovered and one of the peptide sequences displayed was shown to home to the prostate 10–15-fold above other organs. Systemic administration of the synthetic peptide linked to a pro-apoptotic peptide resulted in tissue disruption in the prostate alone and delayed the development of prostate cancers in transgenic adenocarcinoma of the mouse prostate (TRAMP) mice *(28)*. For a breast cancer model, in vivo biopanning was performed in mice and phage homing to mammary tissue isolated with a nonapeptide enriched over the four rounds of biopanning were identified. Homogenous phage populations displaying the peptide localized to the vasculature of normal breast and mammary carcinoma and was not detected in nontarget organs (brain and pancreas). Competition studies and results of homology searches identified the receptor for the breast-homing phage as aminopeptidase P *(29)*.

Moving from the field of cancer therapy, there is only one example of successful in vivo biopanning with targeting ligand identification being then demonstrated in vivo *(30)*. Human synovium and skin were transplanted into severe combined immunodeficient (SCID) mice before a constrained 7-mer library was administered intravenously. Phage homing to the synovium were recovered and three further rounds of biopanning performed. One peptide isolated maintained homing specificity to the synovium when displayed on the phage or as a free peptide in vivo *(30)*. There are, however, reports of ligands identified ex vivo and in vivo that have been successful when applied in an in vitro setting.

Biopanning ex vivo on microdissected intact proximal convoluted tubule (PCT) segments from rats identified two PCT-specific ligands that resulted in a 13- to 17-fold increase in phage homing to PCT compared to other parts of the kidney or control, unselected phage *(31)*. A combined in vitro and in vivo approach was used by Michon et al. *(32)* to identify peptides targeting restenotic smooth muscle cells (SMC). Following three rounds of in vitro biopanning on rat aortic SMC, selected phage were administered intravenously to animals subjected to denudation of the carotid artery 7 d previously. Phage were then recovered from the injured carotid artery and put through three further rounds of in vivo biopanning. Analysis of peptide sequences identified two sequences that bound selectively to SMC in vitro and, in particular, proliferating SMC compared to those which had been growth-arrested, which led the authors to propose a use for targeting restenotic lesions where the SMC are actively proliferating *(32)*.

The lack of reports of in vivo biopanning from application to therapeutic outcome or indeed demonstration of targeting fidelity in vivo out with the field of tumor biology demonstrates the technical difficulties and complexity of the approach relative to the disease or disorder studied. Clearly, the identification of novel, specific targeting ligands is one step in the search for a systemically injectable gene delivery vector or, indeed, drug delivery system. Improvement in vector biodistribution profiles detargeting from nontarget tissue coupled with the introduction of a novel targeting ligand could direct gene transfer to desired sites, which is essential before gene therapy can be considered clinically for systemic administration.

2. Materials

All the microbiological reagent compositions were obtained from *Molecular Cloning: A Laboratory Manual (33)*.

1. PhD Phage Display Peptide Library Kit (New England Biolabs, Beverley, MA).
2. Luria-Bertani (LB) medium. Per liter: 10 g bacto-tryptone, 5 g yeast extract, 5 g NaCl, pH 7.5. Autoclave and store at room temperature.
3. LB agar. As for LB medium, + 15 g bacto-agar. Autoclave, cool to <70°C. Store plates at 4°C.
4. Agarose top, (per liter): 10 g bactro-tryptone, 5 g yeast extract, 5 g NaCl, 1 g MgCl·6H$_2$O, 7 g agarose. Autoclave, dispense into 25–50-mL aliquots. Store solid at room temperature and melt in microwave as required.
5. Dulbecco's Modified Eagle's Medium (1000 mg/L glucose) (DMEM)/1% bovine serum albumin (BSA). Filter sterilize and store 4°C.
6. DMEM-PI. DMEM/1% BSA, 1-µg/mL leupeptin hemisulfate , 2-µg/mL aproprotin, 1 mM phenylmethylsulfonylfluride (PMSF). Make up fresh each time. Store on ice before use.
7. Tetracycline: 10 mg/mL in deionized H$_2$O. Filter-sterilize. Store at –20°C. Protect from light.
8. Polyethylene glycol/NaCl: 20% (w/v) polyethylene glycol-8000 (PEG), 2.5 M NaCl. Autoclave and store at room temperature.
9. Isopropyl thiogalactoside (IPTG)/5-Bromo, 4-chloro-3-indoly-β-D-galacto-pyranoside (X-gal): 50-mg/mL IPTG, 40-mg/mL X-gal diluted in dimethyl formamide (DMF). Toxic, must be made up in fume hood. Protect from light. Store at –20°C.
10. Tris-buffered saline (TBS): 150 mM NaCl, 50 mM Tris-HCl, pH 7.6. Autoclave and store at room temperature.
11. TBS/Na$_2$N$_3$: As for TBS, + 0.02% Na$_2$N$_3$. Sterile filter and store at room temperature.

3. Methods

At present, there are several phage display libraries available from commercial sources utilizing different types of bacteriophage (e.g., M13, fd, f1, T7, T4). The most common phage used is the non-lytic filamentous M13 strain. Libraries constructed using this can contain peptides (usually between 7-mer and 20-mer amino acids in length) displayed in a linear or constrained manner (*see* **Note 1**).

The methods discussed apply to the commercially available linear and constrained 7-mer libraries (New England Biolabs). These consist of randomized

7-mer peptides, fused to the coat protein pIII of M13 via a flexible linker (*see* **Note 2**). The constrained library contains two additional cysteine residues, which flank the 7-mer and consequently form a disulfide bond, resulting in the peptide being constrained in a loop (*see* **Note 3**). The same in vivo biopanning strategy is followed for both phage display libraries used and is modified from that described by Pasqualini et al. *(34)*. The main difference occurs at the amplification step between rounds of panning which will be discussed later. It is recommended that linearly presented libraries be used initially, as these are easier and less time-consuming for any preliminary explorations.

3.1. Titering the Phage Library

Initially, the titer of the phage library (stored at –20°C) obtained from its commercial source is checked to ensure that it has not been lowered during delivery. The bacteriophage host strain *Escherichia coli* ER2738 is supplied with the New England Biolab's PhD Phage Display Library Peptide Kit (www.neb.com). ER2738 maintains the F' pilus, which is essential to allow M13 phage infection into the bacterium. Phage in this library carry the lacZα gene and when they infect an α-complementing bacterial strain (e.g., ER2738), the resulting phage plaques appear blue on plates containing X-gal/IPTG (*see* **Note 4**). Due to the importance of the infection step, the bacteria must be grown on selective media containing tetracycline to ensure the F' episome is retained in all progeny (*see* **Note 5**). To maintain optimal infectivity, it is recommended that a fresh plate be streaked every 2 wk from glycerol stocks of ER2738.

1. Streak an LB-tetracycline plate (12.5 μg tetracycline/mL LB agar) with *E. coli* ER2738. Invert the plate and place in a dark incubator (tetracycline is inactivated by light) at 37°C overnight until single colonies appear (*see* **Note 6**).
2. Transfer a single colony of ER2738 into a sterile UC containing 10 mL aliquots of LB broth (without tetracycline—*see* **Note 7**).
3. Grow with agitation (180 rpm) at 37°C for 4–4.5 h (not overnight—*see* **Note 8**) until the culture is in the mid-log phase (OD_{600} = 0.5–1.0). This will be used to titer the phage. Place enough LB plates (containing X-gal/IPTG) in an incubator (37°C) 2 h before to titering the phage. Heat a water bath to 45°C (*see* **Note 9**).
4. Melt agarose tops and quickly aliquot out 3 mL into 5-mL polystyrene tubes so that there is one per plate (*see* **Note 10**).
5. Place these tubes in the water bath and allow them sufficient time to equilibrate to 45°C (prolonged incubation at this temperature is not recommended, as the agar may begin to set).
6. Aliquot 200 μL of bacterial culture into sterile Eppendorfs, allowing one per phage dilution to be plated. At least three dilutions should be plated out for each sample (*see* **Note 11**). Set up one bacterial aliquot as an uninfected control (*see* **Note 12**).

7. Prepare serial dilutions of the library in sterile Eppendorfs –2 μL of library added to 18 μL of PBS to make 10^{-1} dilution (vortex well to mix), followed by 100-fold serial dilutions in LB broth until a dilution corresponding to what the titer is supposed to be is obtained.
8. Add 10 μL of the serial dilution to 200 μL of bacterial culture and vortex briefly. Allow the tube to sit for 5 min at room temperature (*see* Note **13**). Starting with the control, remove the entire bacteria/phage mixture and immediately add to an aliquot of top agar (*see* Note **14**). Quickly pour this onto a warmed agar plate and, by tilting and turning the plate, spread the agar evenly over the plate surface.
9. Allow to set (10–15 min), invert the plates, and incubate at 37°C overnight to allow the lawn of bacteria to grow.
10. Remove the plates from the incubator and check that the control plate is free from phage plaques. If the control plate contains any clear/blue plaques, then all plates should be discarded (the plating out should be repeated with fresh culture from a freshly streaked plate). If it is contains no clear/blue plaques, count the serial dilution plates that contain around 100 blue plaques and calculate the titers (*see* Note **15**).

The method for titering the phage library is also used to establish the number of phage recovered after a round of biopanning, before and after the amplification step.

3.2. First-Round Biopanning on Target Tissue In Vivo

In vivo biopanning precludes the use of a preclearing step such as that applied in vitro (*3*). The nontarget tissues in the animal model used reduces the number of phage-displayed peptides from the primary library that bind to all tissues (e.g., to ubiquitous cell receptors) or that bind to nontarget tissues with a greater prevalence.

An initial input titer of phage library of 2×10^{11} plaque-forming units (PFU) phage per animal is used in the in vivo experiments (*see* Note **16**). The method described here refers to in vivo biopanning in the rat and may need to be modified or optimized for use in other animal models.

1. On the day of the procedure, aliquot DMEM/PI (*see* Note **17**) into labeled tubes—one for each organ or tissue being removed (a volume sufficient to completely immerse the tissue). Place these on ice to keep the solution chilled.
2. Remove the library aliquot from the freezer and vortex briefly to mix. Remove 2×10^{11} phage and dilute in PBS to a volume of no more than 250 μL. This ensures that as much of the phage will get into the animal as possible.
3. Maintain rats (10–12 wk of age) under terminal anesthesia with a halothane/O_2 mixture throughout the procedure.
4. Expose the femoral vein and inject phage using a gauge needle (we recommend using insulin needles to minimize the amount of dead space in the needle). Begin timing.

5. After 3.5 min, make an incision in the skin under the sternum and open the abdominal cavity to the groin to expose the branch point of the vena cava.

6. After 4 min (from phage infusion), inject 150 µL of heparin into the vena cava and close the puncture site with a cotton swab stick. Allow the heparin to circulate for a minute (*see* **Note 18**). During this time, cut through the diaphragm and pericardium to expose the beating heart.

7. Five minutes after the initial infusion (*see* **Note 19**), obtain a blood sample by cardiac puncture before the animal is perfused under physiological pressure with saline, having first moved the cotton swab from the vena cava to provide an exit route for the saline (it may be necessary to enlarge this).

8. Continue perfusion until the perfusate from the vena cava runs clear and the organs appear free from blood (this is most obvious in the lungs and kidneys—*see* **Note 20**). For the first round, it is recommended to harvest as many complete organs (only one lobe of the liver is required) as possible, as this first round is the only one that requires using library phage as the input and so will be the most costly (*see* **Note 21**). Add these organs and tissues to the tubes containing DMEM-PI and place on ice. The tissues can be kept in this buffer for 1–2 h (on ice).

9. Cut the organs (usually into four pieces), and snap-freeze through isopentane (*see* **Note 22**). Once frozen, transfer to labelled tubes and keep at –70°C until tissue extracts are prepared.

3.3. Tissue Extraction

1. Slowly defrost the tissue samples on ice.
2. Weigh the tissue (*see* **Note 23**), and place in a 1.5-mL ribolyzer tube.
3. Add 1 mL of ice-cold DMEM-PI to each tube and ribolyze at 5.5 speed for 45 s in a tissue homogenizer (*see* Note **24**) for three cycles, placing the samples on ice for 10 min (*see* **Note 25**). Repeat the ribolyzing three more times.
4. Transfer the tissue extract to a sterile 2 mL Eppendorf and place on ice.
5. Add a further 500 µL DMEM-PI to the ribolyzer tube and repeat the ribolyzing three more times.
6. Add this 500 µL to the 1 mL in the Eppendorf, add a final 500 µL to the tube and ribolyze again, three times.
7. Add this to the Eppendorf and spin in a bench-top centrifuge for 10 min at 13,000g (4°C).
8. Remove the supernatant to a sterile bijou and place on ice. Wash the remaining pellet with 500 µL of ice cold DMEM-PI. Repeat the centrifuge step. Remove the additional supernatant and add to the bijou. Store the tissue extract in the fridge (< 2 wk) until it is titered and/or amplified to prepare the input for the next round (*see* **Note 26**).

3.4. Phage Amplification

It is at this point that the phage protocols for linear and constrained phage libraries diverge. Amplification of the phage from the tissue of interest is essential to obtain enough phage to go back into the in vivo model for subsequent rounds of biopanning, as only a small proportion of the library input will be localized in the chosen target (*see* **Note 27**).

A major problem in any phage display experiment is contamination with wild-type phage in the amplification step. Wild-type phage can replicate faster than modified phage because they do not face the additional burden of expressing the peptide on the coat protein. Using a phage library, in which the peptides are expressed linearly has a major advantage at the amplification step over a constrained library as linear libraries are at less of a growth disadvantage than constrained libraries compared to wild-type phage. As a result, phage amplification from these two types of library is performed differently.

3.4.1. Linear Library Amplification

For linear libraries, the tissue extract can be amplified directly.

1. Select a single colony of ER2738 from the plate (at the end of the day—*see* **Note 28**), and grow overnight in a light protected Erlenmayer flask with 50 mL LB broth + tetracycline (10 μg/mL), incubating overnight at 37°C with vigorous shaking (180 rpm).
2. Add 49 mL LB broth (do not use tetracycline) to the desired number of Erlenmayer flasks (usually two or more Erlenmayers will be used to amplify each tissue). Add 500 μL of overnight ER2738 culture to each flask. Add a maximum of 500 μL of tissue extract to each Erlenmayer (*see* **Note 29**). Put flasks in an orbital shaker (180 rpm) at 37°C for 4.5–5 h (do not exceed 5 h—*see* **Note 30**).
3. After this time, transfer the culture to 50 mL falcon tubes and spin at 750*g* for 20 min. Transfer the supernatant to a fresh tube and respin at 3800 rpm for 10 min. Carefully remove the top 80% of the supernatant and transfer to a fresh tube (*see* **Note 31**).
4. Add 1/6 vol of PEG/NaCl, invert the tube to mix, and incubate overnight at 4°C to precipitate the phage.
5. Spin down the phage precipitate for 30 min at 750*g* (4°C—*see* **Note 32**). Gently pour off the supernatant and resuspend the pellet in 1 mL TBS. Transfer this to a sterile Eppendorf and add 1/6 vol (167 μL) PEG/NaCl. Mix and place the tube on ice for 60 min.
6. After 60 min, spin the purified phage pellet at 13,000*g* for 10 min (4°C). Remove all the supernatant (do another spin if necessary) and resuspend the pellet in 200 μL TBS/NaN$_3$.
7. Leave at room temperature for 20 min to allow the phage to dissolve. Spin the tube for 2 min at 13,000*g* (4°C) to remove any residual insoluble matter.
8. Transfer the supernatant to a fresh tube.
9. Store this amplified phage solution at 4°C until it is titered and used.

If insufficient phage are recovered following amplification, resulting in titers too low for subsequent rounds of biopanning, further amplifications must be performed from the remaining tissue extract. These can all be combined, reprecipitated at the PEG/NaCl **step 5** under **Subheading 3.4.1.**, and resuspended in a smaller volume. For long-term storage of this amplified phage, it is recommended that the phage be stored in 50% glycerol at –20°C (*see* **Note 33**).

3.4.2. Constrained Library Amplification

To amplify phage displaying the peptide in a constrained manner, serial dilutions of the tissue extract are required such that there are enough well-defined phage plaques to select (100–200 per large plate; 600–700 in total— *see* **Note 34**).

1. As for linear phage amplification, an overnight culture of a single ER2738 colony in 50 mL of LB containing tetracycline is required. From this, 5 mL is added to 500 mL of LB (with no tetracycline). Add 750 μL of this 1:100 ER2738:LB dilution to each well of a 48-well plate.
2. To each well, add a discrete phage plaque, which has been "picked" from the large LB plate using a sterile Pasteur pipet plug (one per plaque).
3. When a sufficient number of plaques have been "picked" (in our experience approx 600), allow the phage to amplify for 4–4.5 h (do not exceed this time— *see* **Note 30**), in an orbital shaker (180 rpm), at 37°C.
4. After this time, pool the contents of each well in falcon tubes and then follow the protocol for linear phage under **Subheading 3.4.1., step 3**.

3.5. Second-Round In Vivo Biopanning

The second round of in vivo biopanning is exactly the same as the first round except that whereas round 1 used library phage as the input, round 2 uses amplified phage isolated from the organ of interest during round 1. The same input phage titer is used for each round. Normally, three rounds of in vivo biopanning are required to demonstrate and identify sequence enrichment; in some cases it may be necessary to do a fourth round.

3.6. Analysis of Phage Peptides

The results of titer analysis between rounds of biopanning can say only so much about what is happening. Although one hopes that the number of phage obtained from the target tissue will increase over several panning rounds, along with a general decrease in nontarget tissue, this may not always occur. We have found that the liver and spleen, for example, showed very little change in phage titers over several rounds even though they were nontarget tissue (*see* **Note 16**). We have found that for this method, the change in diversity of the phage population is more important. To identify this change, it is necessary first to isolate phage found in the tissue, and second, to sequence the peptide expressed by these phage. We choose to archive many phage from the target tissue as well as phage found in nontarget tissue (*see* **Note 35**).

1. Plate out dilutions of the tissue extract, as described under **Subheading 3.1.**
2. Take care to pick single, well-defined plaques from the agar plates (*see* **Note 36**).
3. An overnight culture of a single ER2738 colony in 50 mL of LB containing tetracycline is required. From this, add 500 µL per 49.5 mL of LB (with no tetracycline).
4. Add 750 µL of this to each well of a 48-well plate.
5. Add a discrete blue plaque, which has been "picked" from the LB plate using a sterile Pasteur pipet plug (one per plaque).
6. Place the plates in an orbital shaker (180 cycles/min) for 4–4.5 h (do not exceed this—*see* **Note 30**), at 37°C.
7. Collect the contents of each well separately and place in sterile 1.5-mL Eppendorf tubes.
8. Spin these tubes at 750*g* for 10 min to pellet the bacteria (*see* **Note 30**).
9. Collect the supernatant and split equally between one sterile Eppendorf, which will be used in a PCR reaction, and another containing an equal volume of sterile glycerol.
10. Mix the phage and glycerol by vortexing and store at –20°C (if this is not mixed, the phage will not survive in the freezer—*see* **Note 37**).

From this point, it is at the investigator's discretion to select the most appropriate PCR and sequencing method to determine the peptide sequences expressed by the phage homing to the tissue of interest (*see* **Note 38**).

4. Notes

1. There are advantages and disadvantages in using linear or constrained libraries and in using a library consisting of short peptides rather than long peptides. A random 7-mer library, for example, has greater diversity in a given volume compared to a 20-mer library. Larger peptide libraries and peptides presented in a constrained manner are more likely to fold into short structural elements, which may be of use when the panning target requires structured ligands. Therefore, the user must decide whether to go with a more diverse library or with one that presents the peptide to the panning target in a structurally more useful way, though as a consequence does not display as many possible sequence conformations.
2. The displayed heptapeptides are expressed at the N-terminus of pIII, i.e., the first residue of the mature protein is the first randomized position.
3. Cloning into the pIII protein means that only 1–5 copies of the peptide are expressed per phage, compared to over 200 copies if the peptide is cloned into the pVIII protein. However, using the pIII protein allows larger peptides to be cloned and selects for higher-affinity interactions.
4. Using the lacZα gene in the library and growing the bacteria on X-gal/IPTG plates makes it easier to titer the phage. Recombinant library phage plaques appear blue against the lawn of bacteria. Using this also allows recombinant phage to be distinguished from any contaminating wild-type phage, which appear as clear plaques.

5. M13 can only infect cells expressing the F-factor. The ER2738 *E. coli* host strain supplied with the library contains a mini-transposon within this gene that confers tetracycline resistance. Therefore on a tetracycline plate, all colonies must have this transposon and, consequently, express the F-factor.

6. The plate should be inverted to prevent excess moisture collecting on the surface of the plate. If this occurs, the ER2738 does not grow as isolated colonies but instead forms a lawn. The plate must also be kept in a dark incubator, as tetracycline is inactivated by light.

7. ER2738 cultures for infection can be grown either in LB or LB-tet media. Loss of the F-factor in nonselective media is insignificant provided the cultures are not serially diluted repeatedly.

8. Phage require replicating bacteria for infection. When M13 infects bacteria, it does not lyse them but slows their growth as it utilizes the host cell systems to replicate. If there are insufficient bacteria to infect, the phage will degrade in the culture. After approx 4.5 h, there are not enough bacterial cells for the phage to infect, so the titer starts to fall.

9. A temperature of 45°C is sufficient to keep agarose tops melted but cool enough so that the bacteria are not killed when added to it.

10. Keep agarose tops in 30-mL aliquots in falcon tubes. Melt enough of these in a microwave to allow one per plate.

11. Plating out more than one dilution of each extract allows an accurate determination of the phage titer. It also can identify contamination problems (i.e., if the titers are the same for several dilutions, then contamination has occurred).

12. No phage dilution is added to the control. This tests for contamination of the bacterial culture with any phage.

13. The incubation time allows any phage in the dilution to bind to and enter the bacteria.

14. Plating the control first minimizes the risk of contamination with phage from other dilutions.

15. To do this, simply multiply the number of blue plaques present on the plate by the dilution factor to give the titer per 10 μL. Multiply this number by 100 to give the titer as PFU/mL. An example is that if 10 μL of a 10^{-10} dilution of phage was plated out and yielded 93 plaques, then the titer would be

$$93 \times 10^{10} = 9.3 \times 10^{11} \text{ PFU/10 μL}$$
$$(9.3 \times 10^{11}) \times 100 = 9.3 \times 10^{13} \text{ PFU/mL}$$

16. An input of 2×10^{11} PFU phage will theoretically include approx 70 copies of each sequence in the linear library. Ideally, many copies of each sequence should be infused (the liver and spleen take up phage and destroy them via a nonspecific process that is not attributated to the peptide expressed on their surface but due to the physiological role performed by these tissues in clearing the body of microorganims). Therefore, sufficient phage should be present to first saturate this system, allowing other phage to bind to their target specifically.

17. This buffer protects the phage in the tissue from degradation.

18. Heparin is infused to minimize the risk of blood clots forming during the saline perfusion step. These would prevent blood from clearing from the tissues.
19. Phage are allowed to circulate for 5 min. In this time, many will bind to cells in the target tissues. A longer circulation time may lead to some of these phage being taken up by these cells and destroyed (leading to loss of the peptide sequence).
20. As much blood should be cleared from the organs as possible, to remove phage that may be present within the organ but not bound. If these are not removed, they will be amplified with tissue-binding phage and give false-positive sequence results. Some tissues such as the spleen and liver retain most of the blood, while the lungs and brain perfuse completely.
21. Storing additional organs means that at a later date, other tissues can be examined for targeting phage.
22. Snap-freezing in isopentane consists of partially immersing a plastic beaker containing isopentane in liquid nitrogen until it is chilled. Tissue is then added to this beaker until it has frozen. Snap-freezing helps protect the phage from being destroyed at –70°C.
23. Weighing the tissue means that the phage titers of different tissues can be compared on a gram basis. Also, tissue extract from the liver will have to be diluted more for titering than those from other organs, such as the brain and heart, as they will contain many more phage.
24. We use a Fastprep system (FP120 Cell Disrupter from Qbiogene).
25. The sample temperature must not exceed 55°C, as this will destroy the phage.
26. Longer storage can result in some phage degrading while others persist. This can give a false indication of the diversity of the phage population.
27. A large proportion of the phage input will be taken up by the liver and spleen.
28. ER2738 should not be allowed to grow beyond this stage, as the culture will enter the death phase and will be unsuitable for phage infection.
29. We do not recommend using more than this volume, as proteases in the extract can inhibit phage amplification.
30. After 5 h, the phage will greatly outnumber the available bacteria and will begin to be degraded.
31. Removing only the top supernatant ensures that none of the bacterial pellet is carried through the subsequent purification steps.
32. It is important to ensure from this point onward that the phage be spun at 4°C to reduce the risk of destroying them.
33. Note that diluting the phage in glycerol will reduce the titer per milliliter accordingly. Ideally, the amplification should be retitered at this point.
34. For the constrained library, as many plaques should be picked between rounds (especially between the first and second round) as possible, because the more diverse the library is, the more likely it will be that a specific tissue-binding phage peptide will be found.
35. This allows phage that home to one tissue or more to be identified.
36. It is extremely important to ensure that each plaque is well defined and separate from any others, to avoid the possibility of obtaining mixed clones.

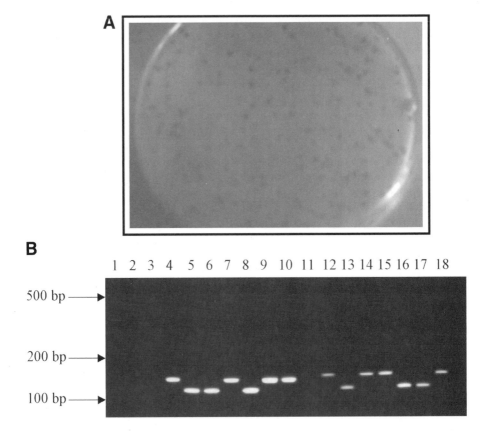

Fig. 2. Methodological illustrations. (**A**) A plate showing the recombinant (blue) phage clones at a suitable dilution for titering or plaque selection to sequence/amplify. The bacterial lawn has been retarded where phage is present, resulting in the color change due to the presence of the LacZ gene in the phage and X-gal/IPTG in the agar plate. (**B**) PCR was carried out across the site of peptide insertion using the primers described (*see* **Note 38**) and product resolved on a 2.5% agarose gel. Lane 1 = 100-bp ladder, lane 2 = PCR control (no phage), lane 3 = empty, lanes 4–10 = PCR products obtained from a linear 7-mer phage pool, lane 11 = empty, lanes 12–18 = PCR products obtained from a constrained phage pool. Note the difference in size of PCR product from phage containing a peptide insert (approx 140 bp) and those without (approx 120 bp). Also, there is a more subtle difference evident between PCR products from the two libraries with those from the constrained possessing an extra 9 bp.

37. The glycerol stock is essential should this phage clone be needed for study at a later date.
38. For our PCR protocol, we use the reverse sequencing primer –96 gIII (5'-CCC TCA TAG TTA GCG TAA CG-3'), which is included in the library kit, and a

forward sequencing primer, which we have designed (5'-GCA ATT CCT TTA GTG GTA CC-3'). These bind downstream and upstream of the 7-mer insert region, respectively, and result in a band of 142 bp when there is a peptide insert present and 121 bp when the phage is insertless. This can be resolved on a 2.5% agarose gel and used as a prescreen before sequencing, thus reducing costs of sequencing phage clones without an insert (**Fig. 2**). Furthermore, the PCR product can be sequenced directly following a clean-up step using exonuclease I and shrimp alkaline phosphatase.

References

1. Rajotte, D., Arap, W., Hagedorn, M., Koivunen, E., Pasqualini, R., and Ruoslahti, E. (1998) Molecular heterogeneity of the vascular endothelium revealed by in vivo phage display. *J. Clin. Invest.* **102**, 430–437.
2. Arap, W., Kolonin, M. G., Trepel, M., et al. (2002) Steps towards mapping the human vasculature by phage display. *Nat. Med.* **8**, 121–127.
3. Work, L. M., Nicklin, S. A., White, S. J., and Baker, A. H. (2002) Use of phage display to identify novel peptides for targeted gene therapy. *Meth. Enzymol.* **346**, 157–176.
4. Nilsson, F., Tarli, L., Viti, F., and Neri, D. (2000) The use of phage display for the development of tumour targeting agents. *Adv. Drug Del. Rev.* **43**, 165–196.
5. Koivunen, E., Arap, W., Rajotte, D., Lahdenranta, J., and Pasqualini, R. (1999) Identification of receptor ligands with phage display peptide libraries. *J. Nuclear Med.* **40**, 883–888.
6. Rodi, D. J. and Makowski, L. (1999) Phage-display technology—finding a needle in a vast molecular haystack. *Curr. Opin. Biotechnol.* **10**, 87–93.
7. Lowman, H. B. (2000) Bacteriophage display and discovery of peptide leads for drug development. *Ann. Rev. Biophys. Biomol. Struct.* **26**, 401–424.
8. Smith, G. P. (1985) Filamentous fusion phage: novel expression vectors that display cloned antigens on the virion surface. *Science* **228**, 1315–1317.
9. Pasqualini, R. and Ruoslahti, E. (1996) Organ targeting in vivo using phage display peptide libraries. *Nature* **380**, 364–366.
10. Ruoslahti, E. and Pierschbacher, M. D. (1987) New perspectives in cell adhesion: RGD and integrins. *Science* **238**, 491–497.
11. Koivunen, E., Gay, D. A., and Ruoslahti, E. (1993) Selection of peptides binding to the $\alpha_5\beta_1$ integrin from phage display library. *J. Biol. Chem.* **268**, 20,205–20,210.
12. Koivunen, E., Wang, B., and Ruoslahti, E. (1995) Phage libraries displaying cyclic peptides with different ring sizes: ligand specificities of the RGD-directed integrins. *Biotechnology (N.Y.)* **13**, 265–270.
13. Pasqualini, R., Koivunen, E., and Ruoslahti, E. (1997) α_v integrins as receptors for tumor targeting by circulating ligands. *Nat. Biotechnol.* **15**, 542–546.
14. Arap, W., Pasqualini, R., and Ruoslahti, E. (1998) Cancer treatment by targeted drug delivery to tumor vasculature in a mouse model. *Science* **279**, 377–380.
15. Nicklin, S. A. and Baker, A. H. (2002) Tropism-modified adenoviral and adeno-associated viral vectors for gene therapy. *Curr. Gene Ther,* **2**, 273–293.

16. Work, L. M., Nicklin, S. A., and Baker, A. H. (2003) Targeting gene therapy vectors to the vascular endothelium. *Curr. Athero. Rep.* **5**, 163–170.

17. Colombo, G., Curnis, F., De Mori, G. M. S., et al. (2002) Structure-activity relationships of linear and cyclic peptides containing the NGR tumor-homing motif. *J. Biol. Chem.* **277**, 47,891–47,897.

18. Pasqualini, R., Koivunen, E., Kain, R., et al. (2000) Aminopeptidase N is a receptor for tumor-homing peptides and a target for inhibiting angiogenesis. *Cancer. Res.* **60**, 722–727.

19. Curnis, F., Arrigoni, G., Sacchi, A., et al. (2002) Differential binding of drugs containing the NGR motif to CD13 isoforms in tumor vessels, epithelia and myeloid cells. *Cancer. Res.* **62**, 867–874.

20. Burg, M. A., Pasqualini, R., Arap, W., Ruoslahti, E., and Stallcup, W. B. (1999) NG2 proteoglycan-binding peptides target tumor neovascualture. *Cancer. Res.* **59**, 2869–2874.

21. Fukuda, M. N., Ohyama, C., Lowitz, K., et al. (2000) A peptide mimic of E-selectin ligand inhibits sialyl Lewis X-dpendent lung colonisation of tumour cells. *Cancer Res.* **60**, 450–456.

22. Koivunen, E., Arap, W., Valtanen, H., et al. (1999) Tumor targeting with a selective gelatinase inhibitor. *Nat. Biotechnol.* **17**, 768–774.

23. Porkka, K., Laakkonen, P., Hoffman, J. A., Bernasconi, M., and Ruoslahti, E. (2002) A fragment of the HMGN2 protein homes to the nuclei of tumor cells and tumor endothelial cells in vivo. *Proc. Natl. Acad. Sci. USA* **99**, 7444–7449.

24. Binetruy-Tournaire, R., Demangel, C., Malavaud, B., et al. (2000) Identification of a peptide blocking vascular endothelial growth factor (VEGF)-mediated angiogenesis. *EMBO J.* **19**, 1525–1533.

25. Hetian, L., Ping, A., Shumei, S., et al. (2002) A novel peptide isolated from phage display library inhibits tumor growth and metastasis by blocking the binding of vascular endothelial growth factor to its kinase domain receptor. *J. Biol. Chem.* **277**, 43,137–43,142.

26. Asai, T., Nagatsuka, M., Kuromi, K., et al. (2002) Suppression of tumor growth by novel peptides homing to tumor-derived new blood vessels. *FEBS Letts.* **510**, 206–210.

27. Oku, N., Asai, T., Watanabe, K., et al. (2002) Anti-neovascular therapy using novel peptides homing to angiogenic vessels. *Oncogene* **21**, 2662–2669.

28. Arap, W., Haedicke, W., Bernascni, M., et al. (2002) Targeting the prostate for desctruction through a vascular address. *Proc. Natl. Acad. Sci. USA* **99**, 1527–1531.

29. Essler, M. and Ruoslahti, E. (2002) Molecular specialization of breast vasculature: A breast-homing phage-displayed peptide binds to aminopeptidase P in breast vasculature. *Proc. Natl. Acad. Sci. USA* **99**, 2252–2257.

30. Lee, L., Buckley, C., Blades, M. C., Panayi, G., George, A. J. T., and Pitzalis, C. (2002) Identification of synovium-specific homing peptides by in vivo phage display selection. *Arth. Rheum.* **46**, 2109–2120.

31. Audige, A., Frick, C., Frey, F. J., Mazzucchelli, L., and Odermatt, A. (2002) Selection of peptide ligands binding to the basolateral cell surface pf proximal convoluted tubules. *Kidney Int.* **61,** 342–348.

32. Michon, I. N., Hauer, A. D., von der Thusen, J. H., et al. (2002) Targeting of peptides to restenotc vascular smooth muscle cells using phage display in vitro and in vivo. *Biochim. Biophys. Acta* **1591,** 87–97.

33. Sambrook, J., Fritsch, E. F. & Maniatis, T. (1989) *Molecular Cloning—A Laboratory Manual,* 2nd ed., vol. 3, Cold Spring Harbor Laboratory Press, Cold Spring Harbor, NY.

34. Pasqualini, R., Arap, W., Rajotte, D., and Ruoslahti, E. (2000) In vivo selection of phage-display libraries. In *Phage Display: A Laboratory Manual* (Barbas, C., Burton, D., Silverman, G., and Scott, J., eds.), Cold Spring Harbor Press, Cold Spring Harbor, NY, pp. 22.1–22.24.

VI

Stem Cells

27

Cardiomyocytes Derived From Embryonic Stem Cells

Kenneth R. Boheler, David G. Crider, Yelena Tarasova, and Victor A. Maltsev

Summary

Self-renewing embryonic stem (ES) cells have been established from early mouse embryos as permanent cell lines. By cultivation in vitro as three-dimensional aggregates called embryoid bodies (EBs), ES cells can differentiate into derivatives of all three primary germ layers, including cardiomyocytes. ES cells thus represent a useful model system for studying cardiomyocyte developmental paradigms. This chapter describes techniques and protocols for the cultivation and maintenance of ES cell lines, and the differentiation of ES cell lines into all specialized cell types of the heart, including atrial-, ventricular-, sinus nodal- and Purkinje-like cardiomyocytes. We also include protocols for the isolation and evaluation (morphological, molecular, and functional) of in vitro-generated cardiomyocytes. We consider these latter techniques to be prerequisites for the successful use of this model system to study cardiomyocyte differentiation. Finally, our objective in writing this chapter is to provide sufficient detail and explanation so that any competent scientist who is new to the field will be able to successfully establish and employ this model system for the analysis of ES cell-derived cardiomyocytes.

Key Words: Embryonic stem cells; embryoid bodies; in vitro differentiation; cardiomyocytes; heart; mouse.

1. Introduction

In 1981, the groups of Evans and Kaufman (*1*) and Martin (*2*) independently isolated embryonic stem (ES) cells from the preimplantation mouse embryo (inner cell mass or epiblast). Later, Wobus (*3*) and Doetschman (*4*) independently observed that ES cells grown in suspension form three-dimensional cell aggregates termed embryoid bodies (EBs) that readily differentiate into recognizable cell types, including cardiomyocytes. Ensuing studies revealed that induction and differentiation of ES cells to cardiomyocytes faithfully recapitulates many of the physical and molecular properties of developing myocardium in vivo (for review, *see* **ref. 5**). This in vitro system generates a heterogeneous population of cells, containing noncardiomyocytes and

From: *Methods in Molecular Medicine, Vol. 108: Hypertension: Methods and Protocols*
Edited by: J. P. Fennell and A. H. Baker © Humana Press Inc., Totowa, NJ

cardiomyocytes with characteristics typical of primary myocardium, atrium, ventricle, sinus node, or the His-Purkinje system *(4,6,7)*. The relative proportion of cardiomyocytes differs with cultivation conditions, but enrichment of cardiomyocyte subtypes can be achieved through addition of exogenous factors *(8)*, FACS sorting *(9)*, or antibiotic selection *(10,11)*. Because ES cells can be readily cultivated, genetically modified (*see* **ref.** *12* for targeting protocols), and examined morphologically and electrophysiologically in vitro, this model system has proven extremely useful in providing insights into cardiomyocyte differentiation and development. More recently, pluripotent human ES cell lines have been generated *(13)*, which are also capable of differentiating into cardiomyocytes. Because human ES cell lines are more laborious to maintain than mouse ES cells, we will only describe the mouse system to illustrate how to cultivate, differentiate and characterize ES cell-derived cardiomyocytes in vitro. The reader is referred to two other publications, which serve as excellent companions to the methods presented here *(12,14)*.

2. Materials

1. Phosphate-buffered saline (PBS), pH 7.2: without Ca^{2+} and Mg^{2+}.
2. Dulbecco's Modified Eagle's medium (DMEM), 4.5 g/L glucose; or Iscove's modified Dulbecco's medium (IMDM), 25 mM HEPES, with Na bicarbonate and GlutaMax™ (*see* **Note 1**).
3. Fetal bovine serum (FBS): ES cell-qualified. Mycoplasma, virus, endotoxin tested (selected batches—*see* **Note 2**).
4. L-Glutamine (200 mM).
5. 100X Penicillin (5000 U/mL)/streptomycin (5000 μg/mL) solution.
6. 100X Nonessential amino acids (10 mM).
7. Leukemia inhibitory factor (LIF): 10 ng/mL LIF.
8. β-mercaptoethanol stock solution: 10 mM β-ME in PBS. Prepare fresh and store at 4°C for 2–3 d.
9. Monothioglycerol (MTG) solution: Prepare a fresh 150 mM stock solution of MTG in IMDM.
10. Trypsin solution: 0.2% trypsin (1:250, Gibco BRL) in PBS.
11. Trypsin:EDTA solution: 0.25% trypsin, 1 mM EDTA-Na(tetrasodium).
12. Gelatin solution: 0.1% gelatin in PBS.
13. Mitomycin C (MC) stock: 0.2 mg/mL Mitomycin C in PBS, filter sterilize. MC is light sensitive and should be prepared weekly.
14. Cultivation medium I: DMEM supplemented with 15% FBS, 50 U penicillin, 50 μg/mL streptomycin.
15. Cultivation medium II: DMEM (4.5 g/L glucose) supplemented with 15% FBS, 2 mM L-Glutamine, 10 μM β-mercaptoethanol, 0.1 mM nonessential amino acids (100X, Gibco BRL, cat. no. 11140-035), 50 U/mL penicillin, 50 μg/mL streptomycin.

16. Differentiation medium: DMEM supplemented with 20% FBS and 2 mM L-Glutamine, 10 μM β-mercaptoethanol, 0.1 mM nonessential amino acids, 50 U/mL penicillin, 50 μg/mL streptomycin.

17. Retinoic acid: Prepare a 10^{-3} M stock solution of all-*trans* retinoic acid in 96% ethanol. Store aliquots at –20°C in the dark and use at once after thawed.

18. Ca^{2+}-free (modified) Hanks solution: 120 mM NaCl, 5.4 mM KCl, 5 mM MgSO$_4$, 5 mM Na-pyruvate, 20 mM glucose, 20 mM taurine, 10 mM HEPES, pH 7.2 (NaOH adjusted), preferably made up in HPLC-grade water (calcium-free).

19. Supplemented low-Ca^{2+} medium: 120 mM NaCl, 5.4 mM KCl, 5 mM MgSO$_4$, 5 mM Na-pyruvate, 20 mM glucose, 20 mM taurine, 10 mM HEPES-NaOH, pH 6.9 at 24°C, supplemented with 1 mg/mL collagenase B (Boehringer Mannheim) and 30 μM CaCl$_2$.

20. KB medium: 85 mM KCl, 30 mM K$_2$HPO$_4$, 5 mM MgSO$_4$, 1 mM EGTA, 5 mM Na-pyruvate, 5 mM creatine, 20 mM taurine, 20 mM glucose, freshly added 2 mM Na$_2$ATP; pH 7.2 at 24°C.

21. RNA lysis buffer: Add 23.6 g of guanidinium thiocyanate to 5 mL of 250 mM Na-citrate, pH 7.0, 2.5 mL of 10% Sarcosyl, and add DEPC-H$_2$O to a total volume of 49.5 mL and mix carefully. Make fresh at monthly intervals. Add 1% β-ME before use.

22. RIPA buffer: 2 mM EDTA, 150 mM NaCl, 1.0% NP-40, 0.5% deoxycholate, 0.1% sodium dodecyl sulfate (SDS), 50 mM TRIS, pH 8.0 (Aliquot and freeze). Add protease inhibitors just before use, i.e., 1 mg/L pepstatin, 1 mg/L leupeptin, 2 mg/L trypsin inhibitor, 0.05 M phenylmethylsulfomyl (PMSF). PMSF is labile in aqueous solution and should be discarded after approx 35 min at 25°C at pH 8.0. Stocks are usually stored at 10 mM or 100 mM stock (1.74 or 17.4 mg/mL) in isopropanol.

23. 2% or 4% Paraformaldehyde (PFA): Dissolve 2 (or 4) g PFA in PBS and adjust to 100 mL with PBS, heat the mixture to 70°C, stir until the solution becomes clear, and cool to room temperature. (The concentration of PFA depends on the primary antibodies and must be tested. PFA is toxic. Work under the hood and prepare fresh solutions weekly.)

24. 10% Goat serum (Sigma, cat. no. G6767) or 1% bovine serum albumin (BSA) in PBS for blocking unspecific binding of antibodies.

25. Mounting medium: Vectashield (Vector, Burlingame, CA, USA, cat. no. H-1000).

3. Methods

3.1. General Considerations

The maintenance of high-quality, pluripotent, and undifferentiated ES cells is critical to in vitro differentiation protocols. Many methods for the cultivation of ES cells have been reported, but several independent parameters consistently influence the differentiation potential of mouse ES cells to cardiomyocytes. These include: (1) the ES cell lines used for cultivation, (2) the medium and its components (FBS, growth factors, and additives), (3) the culture conditions, including the number of cells present in forming EBs, and (4) the EB plating time.

Several mouse ES cell lines or their derivatives have proven highly effective in the formation of cardiomyocytes in vitro: D3, R1, Bl17, AB1, AB2.1, CCE, HM1, and E14.1 *(12)*. Although some ES cell lines are commercially available (e.g., American Type Culture Collection), most can be obtained from the lab of origin. Other ES cell lines are likely to prove effective at generating cardiomyocytes, but the efficiency of differentiation with cultivation conditions must be tested. Mouse ES cell lines generally require inactivated fibroblast feeder layers for good growth and maintenance in an undifferentiated state *(1,2)*. Some ES cell lines require both feeder cells and leukemia inhibitory factor (LIF), and it is advisable to culture ES cells in a manner consistent with the protocol of derivation. Feeder cell-independent growth of ES cells is also possible by cultivation in the presence of LIF or conditioned media, but long-term, these conditions often prove inadequate. Good-quality FBS is also critical for long-term culture and differentiation of ES cells. Not all ES cell-approved lots of FBS are necessarily suitable for ES cell differentiation to cardiomyocytes. Failure to adequately test serum represents one important reason why ES cells may not differentiate efficiently to cardiomyocytes (*see* **Note 2**).

The number of ES cells employed for efficient differentiation to cardiomyocytes varies, and depending on the cultivation medium, EBs formed in suspension (i.e., hanging drops or mass culture) work well; however, EBs generated in mass culture are less efficient (as a percentage) at generating beating cardiomyocytes than those formed through the hanging-drop technique. The timing of EB body plating is a critical factor in cardiomyocyte formation. Within the developing EB, cardiomyocytes develop between an epithelial layer and a basal layer of mesenchymal cells *(15)*, requiring a certain degree of differentiation before plating. Premature plating (insufficient development) or delayed plating (necrosis and other cell death) of EBs may result in heterogeneous cell populations containing very few to no cardiomyocytes.

3.2. Maintenance of ES Cells (see Note 3)

Pluripotent ES cells should be routinely cultivated on monolayers of mitotically inactivated fibroblast feeder cells *(2,4)*. Alternatively, cells can be cultivated on gelatin- or extracellular matrix (ECM)-coated *(16)* tissue culture dishes in the presence of Buffalo rat liver (BRL) cell conditioned medium *(17,18)* and/or in the presence of LIF *(19,20)*. For long-term culture and maintenance, mitotically inactivated feeder layers (mitomycin-C treated or γ-irradiated) are optimal. Primary mouse fetal fibroblasts and STO fibroblast cell lines are commonly employed as feeder layers, but primary feeder layers are preferable to established cell lines (*see* **Note 4**). The technique presented here relies solely on freshly prepared fibroblast feeder layers from CD-1 outbred mice. Although this technique is more labor-intensive than using frozen cells or STO cells, the ES cell lines remain in an undifferentiated, pluripotent state suitable for differentiation to cardiomyocytes.

3.2.1. Preparation and Cultivation of Feeder Cells

1. Every 1–2 wk, kill a pregnant CD-1 (Charles River Laboratories) mouse (fetuses at d approx 14.5 to 17.5 dpc) by cervical dislocation and place the mouse in a beaker containing absolute ethanol.
2. In a laminar flow hood, remove the mouse from the ethanol, pin it to a dissecting board, open the skin along the abdominal midline, and aseptically remove and transfer the uterus (with fetuses) to a Petri dish containing PBS (10 mL).
3. Remove the placenta and fetal membranes. Decapitate the fetuses and transfer the bodies to a Petri dish containing trypsin solution (10 mL at room temperature).
4. Carefully remove the viscera (heart, liver, intestine, etc.) and as much blood as possible. Transfer the carcasses to another Petri dish containing trypsin solution (10 mL) and remove any residual viscera or blood.
5. Transfer the carcasses to a third Petri dish with trypsin (10 mL) and cut up the tissue into small pieces. This takes about 10 min.
6. With a large bore pipet (e.g., disposable 25 mL), transfer the finely minced tissues to an Erlenmeyer flask containing a stir bar, glass beads (5 mm diameter), and 2–3 mL of trypsin solution (prewarmed to 37°C) per fetus.
7. Mix on a magnetic stir plate at room temperature (RT) for 25–30 min. Enzymatic digestion times should be increased when the fetuses are older (i.e., >16.5 dpc).
8. Filter the cell suspension through a sieve or cheesecloth and add an equal volume of cultivation medium I to the filtered suspension. Transfer the contents to a 15-mL centrifuge tube with lid. Centrifuge 5 min at 500g.
9. Carefully remove the supernatant and resuspend the cell pellet in about 3 mL of cultivation medium I. Plate the cells on 10-cm tissue culture plates (about 2×10^6 cells per 10-cm dish) containing 10 mL cultivation medium I.
10. The following morning, remove the medium and wash thoroughly with PBS to remove nonadherent cells and cellular debris. Add 10 mL of fresh cultivation medium I and incubate for an additional 1–2 d.
11. To passage, remove media and rinse once with 10 mL PBS (room temperature) to remove residual FBS (α1-antitrypsin, present in FBS, inhibits trypsin activity).
12. Add 3–6 mL of warm (37°C) trypsin solution. Leave the solution on the cells for 45–60 s (less time as passage number increases) before aspirating.
13. As the cells begin to loosen from the plate surface, add 3 mL cultivation medium I. Dissociate the cells by trituration and split 1:3 to 1:4 on 10-cm tissue culture plates. Add 10 mL of cultivation medium I.
14. Passage the primary mouse embryonic fibroblasts every 2–3 d. Embryonic fibroblasts at passages 2–4 are optimal for cultivation of undifferentiated ES cells. At passages 5 or 6, passage the cells 1:2 or 1:3. After passage 6, discard the feeder layers (**Fig. 1A**).

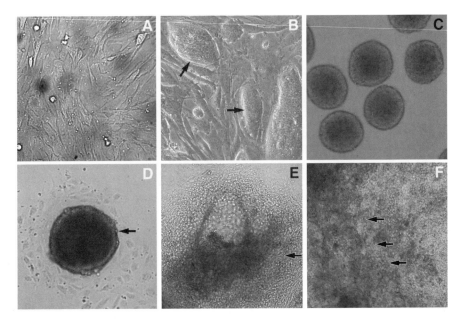

Fig. 1. (**A**) Mouse embryonic feeder cells at passage 2 in culture. (**B**) R1 embryonic stem (ES) cells growing on feeder cells under optimal conditions. ES cells cultivated under these conditions grow as compact colonies and have smooth edges. Individual cells within the colonies should have a high nucleus-to-cytoplasmic ratio. When the cells are not growing optimally, the nucleus-to-cytoplasmic ratio decreases, the colonies begin to flatten and spread, and the colony edges are no longer smooth. These latter cells are inappropriate for differentiation to cardiomyocytes. (**C**) Aggregated R1 ES cells form uniformly sized embryoid bodies (EBs) via the hanging-drop method when grown in suspension for 5 d. (**D**) Embryoid body plated at d 7 on gelatin-coated culture dishes, shown at d 7 + 1. The arrow points to an overlaying area of developing endoderm, beneath which can be seen an internal layer of ectodermal cells. (**E**) Embryoid body differentiating into a cardiomyocyte, shown at d 7 + 3 (3 d after plating), arrow shows a region of contracting cells. (**F**) Terminally differentiated cardiomyocytes eminating from an EB body, 14 d after plating (7 + 14). The arrows point to a large area of contracting cells, where multiple subtypes of cardiomyocytes can be found.

3.2.2. Inactivation of Embryonic Feeder Cells

We use mitomycin C to inactivate primary mouse embryonic feeder layers (*see* **Note 5**). Alternatively, γ-irradiation at 6000–10,000 rad can be employed to inhibit proliferation, but equipment is required that may not be available to all labs.

1. Treat a confluent 10-cm plate of feeder cells with 0.01 mg/mL mitomycin C (MC) for 2.5 h (2–3 h range).

2. Remove the MC-containing solution and wash the cells 3× with 10 mL PBS.
3. Add 3–5 mL trypsin solution (37°C) to the MC-treated feeder cells and remove almost immediately. As the cells begin to dislodge from the plate, add 1 mL of cultivation medium I and triturate to break up the cell aggregates.
4. Passage the cells onto 6-cm gelatin-coated tissue-culture plates containing cultivation medium I. Tissue culture dishes should be gelatinized for 0.5–1 h (or 24 h in advance and stored at 4°C) before plating of the MC-treated feeder cells. Early-passage (2–4) feeder cells can be split 1:5 to 1:6 after treatment, but late passages should be split 1:3 to 1:4.
5. Swirl plates in a "figure 8" motion several times to obtain a uniform distribution of cells. Transfer the cells to an incubator and allow cells to attach >3 h before co-culture with ES cells. Plating 1 d prior to co-culture is optimal.

3.3. Expansion, Culture, and Freezing of Mouse ES Cells

The culture conditions described in this section are employed routinely in the lab for mouse R1 and D3 embryonic stem cells. These protocols are designed to maintain ES cells in an undifferentiated, pluripotent state suitable for differentiation to cardiomyocytes. It is important to routinely passage ES cells cultivated on feeder layers every 18–48 h, depending on colony number and size. Although high dilutions of the ES cells can delay passaging for up to 4–5 d, this is not recommended for routine cultures. At high densities, ES cells start to differentiate, lose pluripotentiality, or die. Under optimal conditions, ES cells should grow as small clusters or mounds (**Fig. 1B**). If the conditions are suboptimal, differentiated derivatives will appear: ES cell clusters will start to flatten, and individual cells will become more distinct. ES cells maintained in conditioned medium and grown on gelatin or feeder layer derived extracellular matrix also have a flattened morphology, but remain pluripotent.

3.3.1. Cultivation of Undifferentiated Mouse ES Cells

1. Thaw 1 mL (1–1.5 × 10^6 cells) of frozen ES cells rapidly at 37°C. Swab the outside of the freezing vial with ethanol and transfer to a laminar-flow hood.
2. Transfer the cells to a 15-mL centrifuge tube containing 10 mL of cultivation medium II, centrifuge at 300*g* for 3–5 min, and remove supernatant.
3. Resuspend the cell pellet in 1 mL of cultivation medium II and transfer the cells to 6-cm tissue culture plates containing either (*see* **Note 6**).
   a. A monolayer of MC-treated feeder cells containing 2–3 mL of cultivation medium II (ideal conditions)
   or
   b. 3 mL of BRL-CM + LIF, BRL-CM, or cultivation medium II + 10 ng/mL LIF (*see* **Note 7**). These plates should either be gelatinized or coated with a feeder layer-derived extracellular matrix (*16*).
4. Change the medium the following morning to remove dead cells.
5. Before passaging, change the medium 1–2 h before trypsinization. Passage the ES cells every 18–48 h. Ideally, ES cells should be passaged at least one time on feeder layers after thawing, and a second time before preparation of EBs.

6. Remove the medium, and wash with PBS (3 mL). Add 0.5–0.75 mL of prewarmed (37°C) trypsin/EDTA and incubate at room temperature for 30 to 60 s. Add 1.0–0.75 mL cultivation medium II.
7. Disperse the cell suspension by pipetting (10–15 times) through the narrow bore of a 2-mL glass Pasteur pipet. It is very important to triturate the cells adequately to get a good suspension of single cells. Centrifuge (300*g*) and passage, freeze (*see* **Subheading 3.3.2.**) or proceed to in vitro differentiation (*see* **Subheading 3.4.**).
8. If passaging, resuspend the cells in cultivation medium II and passage 1:3 to 1:10 onto MC-treated (6-cm) feeder cells (as in **step 3a**) or passage 1:3 to 1:6 onto ECM- or gelatin-coated plates (6-cm) (as in **step 3b**) (**Fig. 1B**).

3.3.2. Freezing of Embryonic Stem Cells

1. ES cell cultures should be growing in log phase prior to freezing.
2. Follow **steps 5–7** under **Subheading 3.3.1.**, but resuspend the cell pellet (from **step 7**, **Subheading 3.3.1.**) in freezing medium. The freezing medium is similar to cultivation medium II except that it contains 20% FBS and 8% dimethyl sulfoxide (DMSO, Sigma).
3. One milliliter of medium should contain from $1–1.5 \times 10^6$ ES cells, which should be aliquoted into 1-mL sterile freezing vials (Nunc) with a screw cap and rubber seal. (Make sure to label the cells and note the passage number in a cell log.)
4. Place the vials in a cryofreezing container that achieves a rate of cooling of approx –1°C/min at –70°C. Place the container in a –70°C freezer overnight, followed by transfer to a liquid nitrogen container for long-term storage.

3.4. Differentiation of Mouse ES Cells to Cardiomyocytes

For differentiation to cardiomyocytes, ES cells must be cultivated as three-dimensional aggregates termed embryoid bodies, primarily by the hanging-drop method or by mass culture. The hanging-drop method generates EBs of a defined cell number and size. Mass cultures of EBs may be used for generation of a large number of differentiated cells. For mass culture, 5×10^5 to 2×10^6 cells (depending on the ES cell line) are plated into bacteriological Petri dishes containing either cultivation medium or differentiation medium, depending on the cell line. Once EBs have formed, the cells should be cultured in differentiation or cultivation medium until the time of plating. Spinner flasks can also be employed for the generation of very large numbers of cardiomyocytes *(21)*. The mass culture technique is less efficient than the hanging-drop technique, but the technique is less labor-intensive and many EBs can be produced rapidly.

3.4.1. Hanging-Drop Method

1. From **step 7** (**Subheading 3.3.1.**), resuspend the cells in differentiation medium and count the cells with a hemocytometer. (ES cells are small and round, whereas contaminating feeder cells are generally much larger in size.)
2. Count the cells (20 µL cell suspension + 10 µL Trypan Blue + 20 µL medium),

and dilute the cell suspension to 400–1000 (600 is optimal) ES cells per 20 µL of differentiation medium (*see* **Note 8**).

3. Place 20-µL drops (*n* = 50–60) of the ES cell suspension on the lids of 10-cm bacteriological Petri dishes containing 5–10 mL PBS. For rapid preparation of hanging drops, we employ a multichannel pipetter.

4. Incubate the ES cells in hanging drops for 2 d. The cells will aggregate and form one EB per drop. Do not disturb the developing EB during this period.

5. Rinse the EBs carefully from the lids with 2 mL of cultivation medium II and transfer EBs into a 60-mm suspension culture dish containing 2–3 mL of cultivation medium II.

6. Cultivate the EBs in suspension for 2–5 d until the desired time of plating or assay. (*see* **Note 9** and **Fig. 1C**). (To enhance the development of ventricular-cardiomyocytes *[8]*, add retinoic acid [10^{-9} *M*] between d 5 and d 15 of culture.)

7. To plate, gelatinize 24-well microwell plates, 6- or 10-cm tissue culture dishes for 1–24 h at 4°C. Remove the gelatin solution and add cultivation medium II.

8. Transfer a single EB into each well of gelatinized 24 well plates for morphological analysis, 20–40 EBs per dish onto 6-cm tissue culture dishes containing 4 cover slips (10 × 10 mm) for immunofluorescence, or 15–20 EBs onto 6-cm dishes for reverse-transcription polymerase chain reaction (RT-PCR) analysis or dissections of EB outgrowths.

9. For the investigation of early cardiac stages, plate EBs at d 4–5, but otherwise, plate on d 6–7. The first beating clusters can be seen in d 7–8 EBs, but maximal cardiac differentiation is achieved after plating (**Fig. 1D–F**).

10. Change the medium every second or third day. Count the number of EBs with beating areas (from at least 24 wells) to calculate the percentage of EBs that differentiates to cardiomyocytes. We routinely obtain >90% with this technique.

3.4.2. Mass Culture Procedure

1. From **step 7**, **Subheading 3.3.1.**, add 500,000 R1 ES cells to a 10-cm bacteriological Petri dish containing 10 mL differentiation medium.

2. After 2 d, remove the differentiation media and replace with 10 mL of cultivation medium II.

3. From this point on, change the medium every second day, but add 1/2 vol of cultivation medium (5 mL) on the intervening alternate days.

4. On d 7 or 8, plate the EBs on two or three tissue culture plates (10 cm), and maintain in cultivation medium II. Spontaneously beating cardiomyocytes should be visible within 1–2 d after plating. Because of the large number of EBs that can be plated, it is essential to change the medium regularly, because changes in pH will adversely affect the longevity of the ES cell-derived cardiomyocytes.

3.5. Isolation and Examination of ES Cell-Derived Cardiomyocytes

ES cell-generated cardiomyocytes can be examined within an EB (pharmacological measurements, protein, RNA) or as single cells (immunofluorescence, electrophysiological).

The choice of analysis is left up to the investigator; however, we provide several common methods for analyzing ES cell-derived cardiomyocytes either within EBs or as isolated cells (*see* **Note 10**).

3.5.1. Cardiomyocytes in Embryoid Bodies

3.5.1.1. PREPARATION OF CELL EXTRACTS: RNA

1. Cultivate EBs in suspension or plate the EBs in microwell plates or tissue culture dishes as described under **Subheading 3.4.**
2. At specified (predetermined) times, EBs in suspension culture should be pelleted by centrifugation in a 15-mL centrifuge tube (300g), followed by washing in PBS and recentrifugation. Plated EBs should be washed 1X with PBS.
3. For RNA preparation, the washed EBs should be lysed with RNA lysis solution. Guanidine is a chaotropic agent that inactivates ribonucleases and yields good-quality RNA for subsequent analyses.
4. Process the lysed cells for the preparation of total RNA, using any standard RNA protocol. Total RNA can then be employed for RT-PCR analyses or Northern blotting (*12*). A useful set of "cardiac primers" for RT-PCR is given in **Table 1**.

3.5.1.2. PREPARATION OF CELL EXTRACTS: PROTEIN

1. Cultivate EBs in suspension or plate in microwell plates or tissue culture dishes as described under **Subheading 3.4.**
2. At specified time points, pool the EBs by centrifugation (if in suspension) and wash with PBS. Discard the PBS.
3. For plated EBs, wash in PBS and discard. Add 1 mL PBS and scrape the cells. Transfer to a 15-mL centrifuge tube and spin at 400g for 5 min. Discard the supernatant (unless secreted proteins are to be analyzed). Fifty to several hundred EBs may be needed to prepare adequate quantities of protein for some analyses.
4. Lyse the cells in RIPA buffer (50 µL or as needed), vortex, and incubate on ice for 30 min. Sheer the cells through a 27-gage needle. (Large quantities of cells may require homogenization.)
5. Calculate the amount of protein using a standard protocol (e.g., Lowry assay). Ideally, the protein should be at approx 5 mg/mL. Store on ice or long-term in a freezer.
6. Proteins can be assayed by Western blots on 5–20% Tris-HCl gels using 5–40 µg of protein extract.

3.5.1.3. RATE MEASUREMENTS IN EBs

1. Cultivate EBs in 24-well microwell plates until >90% of the EBs contain clusters of beating cardiomyocytes. Beating cardiomyocytes should comprise at least 5–30% of the EB outgrowths area. One day before measurements, change the medium and add exactly 1 mL of medium per well.
2. Place the 24-well microwell plate on the inverted microscope equipped with a 37°C heating plate and a CO_2 incubation chamber. Localize independent beating areas ($n = 20$) and measure the spontaneous beating frequency (*see* **Note 11**).

Table 1
Useful Primers for RT-PCR Analysis of Mouse ES Cell-Derived Cardiomyocytes

Cell type	Genes	Primer sequences (5'–3') (12,24)	Size (bp)	Annealing temperature (°C)
Cardiac cells	Cardiac α-MHC	CTGCTGGAGAGAGGTTATTCCTCG GGAAGAGTGAGCGGCGCATCAAGG	302	64
	Cardiac β-MHC	TGCAAAGGCTCCAGGTCTGAGGGC	205	64
		GCCAACACCAACCTGTCCAAGTTC TGTGGGTCACCTGAGGCTGTGGTTCAG	189	60
	MLC-2V	GAAGGCTGACTATGTCCGGGAGATGC CAGACCTGAAGGAGACCT	286	52
	MLC-2A	GTCAGCGTAAAACAGTTGC TGATAGATGAAGGCAGGAAGCCGC	203	64
	ANF	AGGATTGGAGCCCAGAGTGGACTAGG GAGTGTGTCAATTGTGGGGCCATGT	242	60
	GATA-4	CCGCAGGCATTACATACAGGCTCA ACCATCACCATCACCCGACCTACT	409	60
	GATA-6	CACCCTCAGCATTTCTACGCCATA CGACGGAAGCCACGCGTGCT	181	60
	Nkx 2.5	CCGCTGTCGCTTGCACTTG	317	60
Internal standard	β-tubulin	GGAACATAGCCGTAAACTGC TCACTGTGCCTGAACTTACC		

3. The spontaneous beating frequency can be measured visually or optimally with a video camera system (a Crescent Electronics Video Edge Detector, model VED-104, Sandy, UT, and a Panasonic TV Camera, model VW-1100A, Matsushita Communication Industrial Co., Japan). Rate data should be analyzed in real time using a threshold-crossing criterion, and averaged every 5 s *(22)*.

4. To test the effects of drugs on rate, add various concentrations (e.g., 10^{-9} to 10^{-4} M) of a test substance and measure beating frequencies (*see* **Note 12**).

5. Calculate the mean values (± standard error of the mean) of beats per minute for each data point in the presence and absence of test drugs. Test for significance and calculate dose–response curves.

3.5.2. Individual Cardiomyocytes

For many assays (immunofluorescence, electrophysiology [EP], single-cell RT-PCR), isolated cardiomyocytes are required. Optimization of the isolation technique, however, can be difficult because the batch (and activity[*]) of collagenase, the duration of collagenase treatment[*], and Ca^{2+} concentration[*] can all adversely affect the isolation process. A successful isolation balances effective digestion of the connective (collagen) tissue with minimized membrane damage to the cells. Increasing any of the three parameters ([*]) promotes digestion, but concomitantly leads to more cell membrane damage.

3.5.2.1. ISOLATION

1. Isolate the beating areas of EBs ($n = 10$–20) mechanically using a pulled-glass Pasteur pipet with a beveled end and fitted with a cotton-plugged tube and mouthpiece or with a microscalpel under an inverted microscope. Dissect as close to the outer edges of the beating cells as possible to minimize noncardiomyocyte contamination. During dissections, spontaneous contractions often cease.

2. Once the beating region is dissected free from the EB, transfer it to a 15-mL polypropylene centrifuge tube containing approx 12 mL Ca^{2+}-free Hank's solution at room temperature. If a microscalpel is employed, transfer the cells with a sterile pipet (such as a 10-µL tip on a Gilson Pipetman) (*see* **Note 13**).

3. Leave the cells in the calcium-free solution for at least 20 min (up to 60 min for terminally differentiated cells) and centrifuge at 300g for 1 min. Remove the supernatant.

4. Add 1 mL of low-Ca^{2+} (10–30 µM) solution supplemented with collagenase B (1 mg/mL). Incubate the pellet in collagenase B-supplemented low-Ca^{2+} medium at 37°C for 25–45 min depending on the collagenase activity. For the isolation of cardiac clusters, shorten the incubation time to 10–20 min. The collagenase solution can be prepared in advance, but should not be kept longer than 3–4 d.

5. Centrifuge the dissociated cells at 300g for 2 min and remove the enzyme solution. Resuspend the cell pellet in 0.8–1.0 mL of KB medium and incubate at 37°C (or 24°C) for 30–60 min with gentle periodic shaking.

6. Transfer the cell suspension into tissue culture plates containing gelatin-coated slides (or MatTek dishes) and incubate the cells in cultivation medium II (KB medium should be diluted at least 1:10) at 37°C. (*see* **Note 14**).

7. The next morning, change the medium to cultivation medium II. Cardiomyocytes begin beating rapidly thereafter and within a few hours can be employed for electrophysiological measurements (up to 24 h after plating) (*see* **Subheading 3.5.2.3.**). A 24-h recovery time is necessary for immunostaining (*see* **Subheading 3.5.2.2.**).

3.5.2.2. IMMUNOFLUORESCENCE (**FIG. 2**)

The presence of cardiac-associated proteins in the EB outgrowths can be analyzed by immunofluorescence with a fluorescence microscope or a confocal microscope. For characterization of ES cell-differentiated phenotypes, monoclonal and some polyclonal antibodies (mAbs) against tissue-specific intermediate filament proteins or sarcomeric proteins are suitable.

1. Rinse cover slips or MatTek (MatTek corporation) dishes (35 mm, 14-mm microwell) containing EB outgrowths twice with PBS.

2. Fix the cells with methanol/acetone (7/3), methanol/acetone/H_2O (50/20/30%) at –20°C for 10 min, or with 2% paraformaldehyde in PBS at RT for 10 min (*see* **Note 15**).

3. Rinse cover slips twice with PBS at RT for 10 min.

4. Incubate the cells with 10% goat serum/PBS or 1% BSA in PBS in a humidified chamber at RT for 60 min to prevent nonspecific immunostaining.

5. Incubate with the primary antibody at 37°C for 30–60 min, or at 4°C overnight (final concentration according to manufacturers' instructions) in wash buffer.

6. Rinse cover slips with PBS 3–5 × at RT for 10 min.

7. Incubate with the secondary antibody (i.e., dilute goat anti-mouse IgG 1:100 in PBS or prepare goat anti-rat IgG, at 12 µg protein/mL final concentration, depending on the primary antibody) in a humidified chamber at 37°C for 45–60 min.

8. Rinse cover slips 3–5 × with PBS at RT for 5 min.

9. Embed cover slips in mounting medium and analyze immunolabeled cells with a conventional fluorescence microscope or a confocal laser-scanning microscope.

3.5.2.3. ELECTROPHYSIOLOGICAL MEASUREMENTS IN ES CELL-DERIVED CARDIAC CELLS

1. Transfer glass fragments with cells to the recording chamber with fine-tip forceps and wash with Ca^{2+} containing (1.8 m*M*) Hank's solution.

2. Observe the cells by phase contrast. The cardiac cells attached to the glass slips are distinguished by their morphology and/or by their contractile activity in Ca^{2+} containing Hank's solution. In the absence of contractions, it may be difficult to identify cardiomyocytes (*see* **Note 16**).

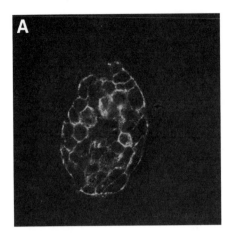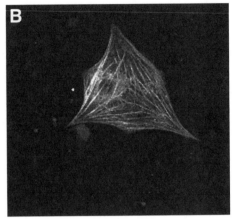

Fig. 2. **(A)** Localization of mouse STAT3 protein along the cell membrane in undifferentiated R1 ES cells. The ES cells were fixed in 2% paraformaldehyde, and immunofluorescence performed using the protocols described in the text. Visual analyses were performed by confocal microscopy, 18 h after passaging onto gelatinized coverslips. The cells were incubated overnight with anti-phospho-STAT3 (1:1000), followed by a secondary antibody to Alexa Fluor 568-labeled goat anti-rabbit IgG (1:1000). **(B)** Indirect immunofluorescence performed on isolated ES cell-derived cardiomyocytes. Isolated cells were fixed with methanol/acetone/H_2O (50/30/20%). Tissues were rehydrated and blocked with 10% goat serum. Anti-troponin T (JLT-12) or anti-α-sarcomeric actin (5C5) (Sigma) were used as primary antibodies with a goat anti-mouse IgG-FITC or IgM-FITC (Zymed) secondary antibody, respectively. In this image, only fluorescence to troponin T is shown.

3. A tight seal ("Giga-Ω" seal *[23]*) can be formed with ES cell-derived cardiomyocytes by a slight touch of the pipet to the cell surface or after application of slight suction of about 5–10 cm (negative) of water. Once a tight seal is formed, perforated patch-clamp recordings or cell-attached single-channel recordings can begin. For whole-cell recordings, the patch in the tip of the pipet should be disrupted by suction. (*see* **Note 17**).

4. Voltage-clamp recordings can be performed on isolated ES cell-derived cardiomyocytes held with an Axopatch 200-A amplifier (Axon Instruments, Foster City, CA) in the voltage-clamp mode (*see* **Note 18** and **Fig. 3B**).

5. Action potential (AP) data can be acquired on isolated cardiomyocytes with an Axopatch-1D patch clamp amplifier (Axon Instruments, Foster City, CA) in the current-clamp mode using a perforated patch-clamp technique to record spontaneous APs. For the evaluation of the resting membrane potential, the minimal diastolic potential can be taken and the action potential duration (APD) estimated.

6. For confocal Ca^{2+} imaging, ES cell-derived cardiomyocytes can be loaded with 5 μM of fluo-3 AM (or fluo-4 AM) directly in the recording chamber for 10–20 min (**Fig. 3A**).

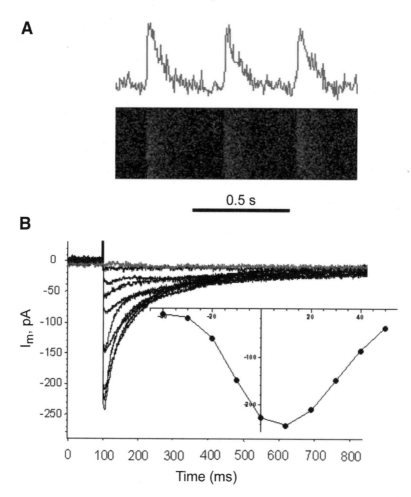

Fig. 3. **(A)** Example of a Ca^{2+} transient in an isolated ES-derived cardiomyocyte measured by confocal microscopy in the line-scan mode. The data shown are: F/Fo curve (above) and imaged calcium signal (below) seen in the respective cell loaded with fluo-4. **(B)** An IV curve for L-type Ca^{2+} currents in an isolated ES cell-derived cardiomyocyte (traces and plot, whole-cell configuration).

4. Notes

1. Either Dulbecco's modified Eagles medium (DMEM) or Iscove's modified Dulbecco's medium (IMDM) can be employed for cultivation of undifferenti-ated ES cells. Differentiation with IMDM may require fewer starting cells than differentiation with DMEM, but this tendency is sometimes subtle. In general, and when starting with the same number of starting cells, IMDM promotes cardiomyocyte formation and differentiation more rapidly than DMEM.

2. FBS testing: The most convenient tests for sera include (a) comparative plating efficiencies at 10, 15, and 30% serum concentrations, (b) alkaline phosphatase activity in undifferentiated ES cells, and (c) in vitro differentiation capacity of ES cells to cardiomyocytes after five passages in selected batches of serum. The latter is essential for studies of cardiomyocyte differentiation.

3. All tissue culture manipulations should be performed in a laminar-flow cabinet and cells/EBs incubated in a humidified incubator (37°C, 5% CO_2). Both cultivation of ES cells and differentiation of ES cells to cardiomyocytes can be adversely affected by mycoplasm, yeast or bacterial contaminations, changes in CO_2 levels and cellular pH, inadequate feeding or passaging of ES cells. Ideally, ES cell lines are cultivated without antibiotics, but the addition of penicillin and streptomycin to the culture generally proves useful.

4. Previously frozen primary fibroblast feeder cells are inferior to freshly cultivated feeder layers, and the reliability of different STO cell lines to maintain optimal ES growth conditions varies considerably. We find that feeder cells produced with CD-1 mice last longer in culture than those produced with inbred lines of mice (e.g., C57Bl/6, MTK-neo^R). The NMRI strain in Europe is also very good for making feeder cells. A major disadvantage of primary fibroblasts is their relatively short lifespan. After about 15–20 divisions (2 wk in culture with passaging), these cells senesce, go into "crisis," and are no longer suitable for the maintenance of ES cell cultures.

5. Mitomycin C is a DNA cross-linker and a suspected carcinogen. Both mitomycin C and γ-irradiation treatments cause the fibroblasts to accumulate in the G2 phase of the cell cycle, preventing further division.

6. We do not routinely add LIF to R1 or D3 mouse ES cell lines grown on MC-treated feeder layers, except for when the feeder cells were previously frozen.

7. ES cells can be maintained in an undifferentiated state by cultivation in the presence of Buffalo rat liver conditioned medium (BRL-CM) or in the presence of LIF. The active factor secreted by BRL cells is identical to LIF, but we find that differentiation to cardiomyocytes is improved when ES cell cultures are grown in the presence of both BRL-CM and LIF. We always add LIF to ES cells grown on ECM- or gelatin-coated dishes. BRL-conditioned media (BRL-CM) contains DMEM (or IMDM) supplemented with BRL stock (60 mL stock per 100 mL total), 15% FBS (9 mL/100 mL). The BRL stock contains 10% FBS, 0.01 mg/mL transferrin, 2 mM L-Glutamine, 10 μM β-mercaptoethanol, 0.1 mM nonessential amino acids, 50 U/mL penicillin, 50 μg/mL streptomycin. (If IMDM is used, replace β-mercaptoethanol with 450 μM MTG). The preparation of BRL-CM and stock is described in **ref. 14**.

8. The number of starting cells varies among ES cell lines, but 400–800 cells/hanging drop work very well for both D3 and R1 ES cell lines. Importantly, ES cells cultured on feeder layers should contain >100-fold more ES cells than fibroblasts, because contaminating fibroblasts in the developing EBs can adversely affect cardiomyocyte differentiation.

9. "Good" culture dishes for EB suspension cultures can be purchased from Kord Products Inc. (Ontario, Canada, cat. no. 901).

10. In general, analyses should be performed only on plated EBs containing a very high percentage of beating cardiomyocytes/EB (i.e., >90%). Low percentages of beating cells/EB may give misleading results and are indicative of problems with the differentiation procedure.

11. If a CO_2 chamber is unavailable, measurements can only be made for short periods of time, and failure to maintain the temperature will adversely affect measurements.

12. Positive chronotropic (BayK 8644 serves as a positive control) or negative chronotropic drugs (Diltiazem serves as a positive control) should be added for only about 3 min before recording beating rates. Other drugs, such as thapsigargin (TG, 1 μM) or ryanodine (Rya, 10 μM), may require incubation times of 30 min or more to be fully effective. Make sure that the temperature of the cells stays constant. Variations in temperature dramatically affect beating rates.

13. The tubing and mouthpiece attached to the beveled dissecting pipet allow rapid transfer of isolated cell clusters from the plate to the Hank's solution. Isolation of 10–20 beating areas takes about 20 min.

14. For electrophysiological analyses, the dish should contain small glass fragments (5 × 7 mm) cut to fit the recording chamber. The glass can be cut with a wolfram/diamond cutter from standard glass slides (e.g., 24 × 40 mm) used for light microscopy. Cut glass should be cleaned with ethanol and autoclaved.

15. The method of fixation depends on the primary antibody. We routinely fix cells with all three techniques to test primary antibodies with which we have no previous experience. Alternatively, employ conditions that have been previously published. If cells are fixed in PFA, cells should be washed with 100 mM glycine/PBS for 15 min and then be permeabilized with Triton X-100 (0.1% in PBS) for 20 min.

16. Cardiomyocytes isolated from EBs tend to form small clusters. Some of the isolated cells may maintain electrical coupling with nearby cells, even when the cells are separated by up to 100 μm.

17. For voltage-clamp measurements, it is important to identify single cells and form a tight electric seal. When cells are coupled, the ion current (evoked by a depolarization voltage step) usually displays an artifact in the form of a delayed and reversed action potential. The presence of these artifacts is an indication that cardiac cells are coupled and cannot be used for voltage-clamp examination. Data can be acquired at a sampling rate of 10 kHz and filtered at 1 or 2 kHz.

18. The most important requirement for a successful voltage-clamp experiment is formation of a tight seal ("Giga-Ω" seal) between the patch pipet and plasma membrane *(23)*. It is important to apply suction almost immediately after contact to avoid hard "pushing" of the pipet tip toward the cell (resulting in punching and damaging the cell). The pressure in the pipet should be set to 0 before contact. When moving the patch pipet toward the cell, use caution and watch for pipet resistance changes. The pipet resistance should change only slightly after contact, e.g., from 3 mΩ to 3.5 mΩ. The part of the cell for "successful" patch clamping is the bulkiest part of the cell (usually in the geometric center of the cell), where there is "room" (along the vertical, Z axis) for contact. Sometimes it is

helpful to drop the holding potential from 0 to about –60 mV after the initial contact and suction for tight seal formation.

Acknowledgments

We are grateful to Dan Riordon for expert technical assistance and for reviewing sections of the text to ensure the accuracy of the procedures.

References

1. Evans, M. J. and Kaufman, M. H. (1981) Establishment in culture of pluripotential cells from mouse embryos. *Nature* **292,** 154–156.
2. Martin, G. R. (1981) Isolation of a pluripotent cell line from early mouse embryos cultured in medium conditioned by teratocarcinoma stem cells. *Proc. Natl. Acad. Sci. USA* **78,** 7634–7638.
3. Wobus, A. M., Holzhausen, H., Jakel, P., and Schoneich, J. (1984) Characterization of a pluripotent stem cell line derived from a mouse embryo. *Exp. Cell Res.* **152,** 212–219.
4. Doetschman, T. C., Eistetter, H., Katz, M., Schmidt, W., and Kemler, R. (1985) The in vitro development of blastocyst-derived embryonic stem cell lines: formation of visceral yolk sac, blood islands and myocardium. *J. Embryol. Exp. Morphol.* **87,** 27–45.
5. Boheler, K. R., Czyz, J., Tweedie, D., Yang, H. T., Anisimov, S. V., and Wobus, A. M. (2002) Differentiation of pluripotent embryonic stem cells into cardiomyocytes. *Circ. Res.* **91,** 189–201.
6. Wobus, A. M., Wallukat, G., and Hescheler, J. (1991) Pluripotent mouse embryonic stem cells are able to differentiate into cardiomyocytes expressing chronotropic responses to adrenergic and cholinergic agents and Ca^{2+} channel blockers. *Differentiation* **48,** 173–182.
7. Maltsev, V. A., Rohwedel, J., Hescheler, J., and Wobus, A. M. (1993) Embryonic stem cells differentiate in vitro into cardiomyocytes representing sinusnodal, atrial and ventricular cell types. *Mech. Dev.* **44,** 41–50.
8. Wobus, A. M., Guan, K., Jin, S., et al. (1997) Retinoic acid accelerates embryonic stem cell-derived cardiac differentiation and enhances development of ventricular cardiomyocytes. *J. Mol. Cell. Cardiol.* **29,** 1525–1539.
9. Muller, M., Fleischmann, B. K., Selbert, S., et al. (2000) Selection of ventricular-like cardiomyocytes from ES cells in vitro. *FASEB J.* **14,** 2540–2548.
10. Klug, M. G., Soonpaa, M. H., Koh, G. Y., and Field, L. J. (1996) Genetically selected cardiomyocytes from differentiating embronic stem cells form stable intracardiac grafts. *J. Clin. Invest.* **98,** 216–224.
11. Ventura, C., Zinellu, E., Maninchedda, E., Fadda, M., and Maioli, M. (2003) Protein kinase C signaling transduces endorphin-primed cardiogenesis in GTR1 embryonic stem cells. *Circ. Res.* **92,** 617–622.

12. Wobus, A. M., Guan, K., Yang, H. -T., and Boheler, K. R. (2002) Embryonic stem cells as a model to study cardiac, skeletal muscle and vascular smooth muscle cell differentiation. In *Methods in Molecular Biology, Vol. 185* Turksen, K. ed. Humana Press, Totowa, NJ, pp. 127–156.

13. Thomson, J. A., Itskovitz-Eldor, J., Shapiro, S. S., et al. (1998) Embryonic stem cell lines derived from human blastocysts. *Science* **282,** 1145–1147.

14. Boheler, K. R. (2003) ES Cell differentiation to the cardiac lineage. Keller, G. and Wassarman, P. M. eds. *Methods Enzymol.* **365,** 228–241. Academic Press, San Diego, CA, in press.

15. Hescheler, J., Fleischmann, B. K., Lentini, S., et al. (1997) Embryonic stem cells: a model to study structural and functional properties in cardiomyogenesis. *Cardiovasc. Res.* **36,** 149–162.

16. Abbondanzo, S. J., Gadi, I., and Stewart, C. S. (1993) Derivation of embryonic stem cell lines. In *Guide to Techniques in Mouse Development, Vol. 225,* Wassarman, P. M., and DePamphilis, M. L. eds. Academic Press, San Diego, CA, pp. 803–822.

17. Smith, A. G. and Hooper, M. L. (1987) Buffalo rat liver cells produce a diffusible activity which inhibits the differentiation of murine embryonal carcinoma and embryonic stem cells. *Dev. Biol.* **121,** 1–9.

18. Anisimov, S. V., Tarasov, K. V., Tweedie, D., Stern, M. D., Wobus, A. M., and Boheler, K. R. (2002) SAGE identification of gene transcripts with profiles unique to pluripotent mouse R1 embryonic stem cells. *Genomics* **79,** 169–176.

19. Smith, A. G., Heath, J. K., Donaldson, D. D., et al. (1988) Inhibition of pluripotential embryonic stem cell differentiation by purified polypeptides. *Nature* **336,** 688–690.

20. Williams, R. L., Hilton, D. J., Pease, S., et al. (1988) Myeloid leukaemia inhibitory factor maintains the developmental potential of embryonic stem cells. *Nature* **336,** 684–687.

21. Hescheler, J., Wartenberg, M., Fleischmann, B. K., Banach, K., Acker, H., and Sauer, H. (2002) Embryonic stem cells as a model for the physiological analysis of the cardiovascular system. *Meth. Mol. Biol.* **185,** 169–87.

22. Yang, H. T., Tweedie, D., Wang, S., et al. (2002) The ryanodine receptor modulates the spontaneous beating rate of cardiomyocytes during development. *Proc. Natl. Acad. Sci. USA* **99,** 9225–9230.

23. Hamill, O. P., Marty, A., Neher, E., Sakmann, B., and Sigworth, F. J. (1981) Improved patch-clamp techniques for high-resolution current recording from cells and cell-free membrane patches. *Pflugers Arch.* **391,** 85–100.

24. Anisimov, S. V., Tarasov, K. V., Riordon, D., Wobus, A. M., and Boheler, K. R. (2002) SAGE identification of differentiation responsive genes in P19 embryonic cells induced to form cardiomyocytes in vitro. *Mech. Dev.* **202,** 25–74.

VII

BIOINFORMATICS

28

In Silico and Wet-Bench Identification of Nuclear Matrix Attachment Regions

Stephen A. Krawetz, Sorin Draghici, Robert Goodrich, Zhandong Liu, and G. Charles Ostermeier

Summary

Chromatin loops are tethered at discrete regions that are approx 100–1000 bp in length. These regions of attachment serve as specific sequence landmarks, anchoring the DNA to the fibers of the chromosomal scaffold. It has been estimated that our genome contains 70,000 nuclear matrix attachment sites that serve as a dynamic nuclear organizer in both the interphase and metaphase cell. Approximately 30,000–40,000 matrix attachment regions (MARs) serve as origins of replication. MARs can also be associated with chromosomal segments densely populated with transcription factor-binding sites. This may facilitate transcription that is initiated within the region of the chromosome coincident with the surface of the nuclear matrix. Assuming an average somatic loop size of 100 kb, it is reasonable to propose that each cell utilizes 30,000 MARs to anchor each of the approx 20,000 active genic domains. This is sufficient to encompass the 30,000 functional genes in our genome that exist as members of single or multigenic families, each constituting a single chromatin domain.

With the sequencing phase of various genome projects complete, *in silico* tools are being developed to identify the long-range control elements that modulate gene expression. This information is necessary to specifically target the time-intensive wet-bench verification and expression experiments that will provide a unified understanding of gene regulation. In this chapter we review some of the *in silico* strategies that are currently available and a new in vivo method based on the real-time polymerase chain reaction, to assess regions of matrix association.

Key Words: Ensemble; *in silico*; MAR; MarFinder; MarScan; matrix attachment region; PCR; real-time; SMARTest.

1. Introduction

Like its structure, the nuclear matrix field is dynamic. The concepts and actions of its components continue to evolve *(1–3)*. Current thoughts consider this structure as a dynamic nuclear organizer serving different functions in both

From: *Methods in Molecular Medicine, Vol. 108: Hypertension: Methods and Protocols*
Edited by: J. P. Fennell and A. H. Baker © Humana Press Inc., Totowa, NJ

the interphase and metaphase cell. For example, the association with genes and the purification of transcription factors from the nuclear matrix *(4)* has been clearly demonstrated within the nucleus of the interphase cell *(5)*. In contrast, in the metaphase cell, regions of attachment to the nuclear matrix can serve as origins of replication *(6)*. The nuclear matrix may also provide the backbone for chromosome territories, where again it displays a dynamic structure *(7)*. While its structure has not been clearly defined, several *in silico* and wet-bench methods that permit its identification have been developed *(8–12)*. In this chapter we will review some of the *in silico* strategies that are currently available. It must be remembered that these *in silico* methods are only predictions, and each must be biologically verified. Thus, we also describe a new in vivo method based on the real-time polymerase chain reaction (PCR), to assess regions of matrix association.

2. Materials

1. 5 *M* NaCl.
2. 1 *M* TRIS.
3. 2 *M* Sucrose.
4. 5 *M* $MgCl_2$.
5. 0.5 *M* EDTA.
6. 1 *M* Dithiothreitol (DTT).
7. 100 mg/mL bovine serum albumin (BSA).
8. Phosphate-buffered saline (PBS): 4.3 m*M* Na_2HPO_4, 137 m*M* NaCl, 2.7 m*M* KCl, 1.5 m*M* KH_2PO_4. (20X PBS: dissolve 6.104 g Na_2HPO_4, 80.063 g NaCl, 2 g KCl, and 2 g KH_2PO_4 in 500 mL H_2O.)
9. Nuclei buffer: 10 m*M* Tris-HCl, pH 7.7, buffer containing 100 m*M* NaCl, 300 m*M*, sucrose, 3 m*M* $MgCl_2$, 0.5% Triton-X 100. Note that Triton X-100 is added after autoclaving.
10. Halo buffer: 10 m*M* Tris-HCl, pH 7.7, buffer containing 10 m*M* EDTA, 2 *M* NaCl, 1 m*M* DTT. Note that DTT is added just before use.
11. Frozen storage buffer (FSB): 50 m*M* HEPES, 10 m*M* NaCl, 5 m*M* MgOAC, 25% glycerol; pH 7.5.
12. Restriction buffer: 50 m*M* Tris-HCl, pH 8.0, buffer containing 10 m*M* MgCl, pH 8.0, (20X restriction buffer stock: Dissolve 4.44 g Tris-HCl, 2.65 g TRIS base, 2.033 g MgCl in 50 mL H_2O.)
13. Proteinase K buffer: 50 m*M* Tris-HCl, pH 8.0, buffer containing 50 m*M* NaCl, 25 m*M* EDTA, 0.5% SDS. Note: SDS is added after autoclaving.
14. TE buffer: 10 m*M* Tris-HCl, 1 m*M* EDTA, pH 7.5.

The above reagents and buffers are prepared, autoclaved except where indicated, then stored at 4°C (*see* **Note 1**). All pH values are at room temperature and are adjusted with HCl or NaOH as required (*see* **Note 2**).

15. Complete proteinase inhibitor (Roche Biochemicals, Indianapolis, IN).
16. Prep-a-Gene (Bio-Rad Laboratories, Hercules, CA).

17. PicoGreen (Molecular Probes, Eugene, OR).
18. DAPI Counterstain (Downers Grove, IL).
19. SYBR-Green (Molecular Probes, Eugene, OR).
20. HotStar *Taq* polymerase system (Qiagen, Valencia, CA).
21. Cytospin 2 (Thermo Shandon, Pittsburgh, PA).
22. Typhoon 9210 (Amersham Biosciences, Piscataway, NJ).
23. Microplate wells (flat-bottomed Costar model 2592 microtiter plate).
24. DNA Engine Opticon (MJ Research, Waltham, MA).

The following are computer programs (*see* **Note 3**).

1. ENSEMBL: www.ensembl.org.
2. SMARTEST: www.genomatix.de/cgi-bin/smartestpd/smartest.pl.
3. MAR-WIZ (MARFINDER): www.futuresoft.org/MarFinder.
4. MARSCAN: www.hgmp.mrc.ac.uk/Software/EMBOSS.
5. WEBCUTTER: www.firstmarket.com/cutter/cut2.html
6. DS Gene: www.accelrys.com/dstudio/dsgene/index.html.
7. OLIGO: www.oligo.net.
8. TAQ-Software: vortex.cs.wayne.edu/Projects.html.

3. Methods

We will use the human β-actin gene as an example. The β-actin gene is ubiquitously expressed in every cell. Accordingly, this gene must always be available for transcription and should provide a clear example of a region that contains a constitutively utilized matrix attachment region (MAR). Before we can proceed to the analysis we must retrieve the corresponding sequence of interest from the appropriate genomic database. In this example we will use the ENSEMBL server at www.ensembl.org. This site is packed with useful tools and annotations that are updated on a regular basis. At the time of writing, the genomes from human, mouse, rat, fugu, zebrafish, mosquito, *Drosophila*, *C. elegans*, and *C. briggsae* were available. This list has been expanded. In general, it is always a good practice to recover your genomic sequence of interest flanked on either side by 50,000 bp regions. This ensures that the statistical analytical routines that are employed by most algorithms described below operate at optimum capacity. The following steps will retrieve the human β-actin gene sequence.

3.1. Sequence Retrieval

1. Logon to the ensembl site at www.ensembl.org.
2. Select Human from the ENSEMBL species list.
   Enter beta actin, next to Search for Anything, and then click Lookup. This will retrieve several sequences. Find the highlighted BETA-ACTIN sequence, then click on the ENSEMBL GENE: ENSG00000075624.

3. Click on Genomic Location 5211155 - 5214605 bp (5.2 Mb). This will take you to a view of the specific region of human chromosome 7 containing the human β-actin gene. Notice that the gene only extends 3.45 kb. The exact distance is shown above, as part of the jump to chromosome 7 bp 5211155 to 5214605 field. Remember you want to recover this sequence with approx 50 kb on each side. We can use the Zoom feature to zoom out to cover a region that extends from 5162880 to 5262880 or we can enter bp 5161155 to 5264605 in the Jump to Chromosome 7 box, then click Refresh. Notice that when using the Jump command, the view has expanded to 103.45 kb with the actin gene centered. For this example we will use the sequence that extends from 5162880 to 5262880 that was recovered with the Zoom function.

5. Click the Export button on the display, then select FASTA. This is a standard default sequence file format that most programs accept. You will be taken to another page. Make sure the Text option is marked in the Select Output Format section and then click Export.

6. The file will appear in a browser window. Simply save the sequence text file as actinlocus to your hard drive.

3.2. In Silico *Detection of MAR Candidates*

Currently, two different strategies have been applied to the *in silico* detection of MARs. The first relies on pattern matching *(8,10,11)*. The second employs a biophysical approach that calculates the relative helix destabilization potential at each nucleotide base *(12,13)*. The pattern-matching MAR detection programs are freely available and can be accessed using the World Wide Web. Some do require that you register. MARFINDER, now known as MARWIZ, was the first MAR detection algorithm to be released *(8)*. It utilizes a predefined series of sequence specific patterns that have been previously defined as a MAR. Using a sliding window approach, the representation of each pattern is calculated as a weighted function of the probability that each pattern occurred by chance. The results are presented in both graphical and tabular form. Similarly, SMARTest *(11)* uses a series of precalculated weight matrices derived from the S/MAR database *(14)*. Using a similar sliding window strategy, the co-occurrence of weighted matrix patterns is considered. Once a threshold value is exceeded, a candidate list of MARs is reported. In contrast, the MARSCAN program outputs a list of the locations of the 8–16 bp bipartite candidate MAR sequence element pairs that occur within a 200-bp span *(15)*. The following outlines the use of MARWIZ, MARSCAN, and SMARTest (*see* **Notes 4** and **5**).

3.2.1. MARWIZ

1. Logon to the MARWIZ site at www.futuresoft.org/MarFinder.

2. Click MAR Search from the left menu. You will be prompted for your user name and password. Registration and use is free.
3. To process sequences as large as 500,000 bp, click on the MAR-Wiz 1.5 applet button.
4. When using a PC, always upload your files. Do not cut and paste. Click on the Upload a Sequence File. Click Browse on the next screen. Select actinlocus, then upload the file named actinlocus.
5. The default settings can be modified once you have gained experience. Click on the FINDMAR button to run the program. When the calculation is complete, a graph will appear. Click on Summary Report to view a detailed synopsis of the analysis which lists the patterns identified and their location as shown in **Fig. 1**.

3.2.2. MARSCAN

1. Logon to MARSCAN using EMBOSS at bioinfo.pbi.nrc.ca:8090/EMBOSS.
2. Scroll down the left side to the program section Nucleic Gene Finding, then click on MARSCAN.
3. Use the browse button to select the file that you want to upload, i.e., actinlocus.
4. Click the Run button.
5. A list of coordinates of each bipartite element will appear.
6. The candidate MAR will extend the length of the bipartite pair, as shown in **Fig. 2**.

3.2.3. SMARTest

1. Logon to SMARTest at www.genomatix.de/cgi-in/smartest_pd/smartest.pl.
2. Scroll down and use the browse button to select the file that you want to upload, i.e., actinlocus.
3. If you would like the results E-mailed to your account, enter your E-mail address.
4. Click the Start SMARTest button.
5. A link to your results will appear. Click on the link, and the start and ending positions of the MAR candidates will be displayed as shown in **Fig. 3**.

3.3. Analysis of the Results

It is wise to view a collective summary of the results from MARWIZ, SMARTest, and MARSCAN. This facilitates developing an appropriate srategy for the next task. As shown below, a strategy graph can be produced with DS Gene, www.accelrys.com/dstudio/ds_gene/index.html, that can be used to develop a plan to test the candidates as shown in **Fig 4A**.

As discussed, the above only contains a listing of potential MAR candidates. Each candidate must be assessed for biological activity in the cell type of interest. This is accomplished by first developing a restriction site map, then selecting the appropriate PCR primer pairs. Several restriction map programs are available. WEBCUTTER is very flexible, and the output can be adjusted.

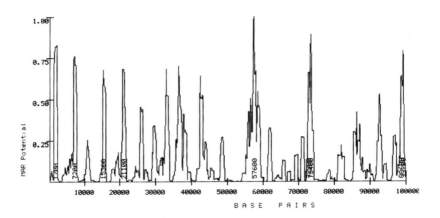

MAR-Analysis Summary Report

Sequence Description:
Sequence Length: 100000
Maximum and Minimum Potential = [0.00292924 .. 37.3244]

High Scoring Regions with threshold = 0.6		
Region	**Average Strength**	**Integrated Strength**
1200 ... 2100	0.780474	703.207
6800 ... 7600	0.704673	564.443
15200 ... 15400	0.621741	124.97
20800 ... 21300	0.660168	330.744
57100 ... 58000	0.743002	669.445
72700 ... 73100	0.640315	256.766
73300 ... 73500	0.781422	157.066
99100 ... 99300	0.728347	146.398

Fig. 1. MAR-WIZ analysis of the human β-actin gene locus. The 5162880–5262880 region surrounding the human β-actin locus was analyzed by the MAR-WIZ program. The upper panel shows the relative location and confidence level for each candidate MAR region. The lower panel shows the corresponding nucleotide coordinates. Note: Eight candidate MAR regions were detected.

The program is available at www.firstmarket.com/cutter/cut2.html, and its use is outlined below.

3.4. WEBCUTTER

1. As before, upload your sequence using the Browse and Upload functions.
2. Scroll down to the section "Please indicate which enzymes to include in the analysis."

MARSCAN: OUTPUT

OUTPUT FILE: **outf** [RIGHT CLICK TO SAVE]

```
##gff-version 2.0
## ## date 2003-02-12
##Type DNA HUMAN

HUMAN     marscan     misc_signal  63822  63844  0.000  +  .     Sequence "HUMAN.1" ; note "MAR/SAR
recognition site (MRS). 8bp pattern=63822..63829. 16bp pattern = 63829..63844"

HUMAN     marscan     misc_signal  72993  73009  0.000  +  .     Sequence "HUMAN.2" ; note "MAR/SAR
recognition site (MRS). 8bp pattern=72993..73000. 16bp pattern = 72994..73009"

HUMAN     marscan     misc_signal  78363  78410  0.000  +  .     Sequence "HUMAN.3" ; note "MAR/SAR
recognition site (MRS). 8bp pattern=78363..78370. 16bp pattern = 78395..78410"

HUMAN     marscan     misc_signal  96407  96423  0.000  +  .     Sequence "HUMAN.4" ; note "MAR/SAR
recognition site (MRS). 8bp pattern=96416..96423. 16bp pattern = 96407..96422"
```

[home]

Fig. 2. MARSCAN analysis of the human β-actin gene locus. The 5162880–5262880 region surrounding the human β-actin locus was analyzed by the MARSCAN program. A listing of the coordinates of the bipartite MAR signal are summarized. Note: Four candidate MAR regions were detected.

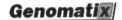

Genomatix   License Agreement   Your Comments   ***SMARTest***

| **SMARTest Release 2.2 October 2001** | **Wed Feb 12 23:03:46 2003** |

Solution parameters:

Sequence file: FASTAhuman_beta_actin.seq (100000 bps)
Library: SMARTest Matrix Library Version 3.0 August 2002

Regions of potential S/MARs:

Inspecting sequence HUMAN (1 - 100000):

[HUMAN BETA ACTIN Untitled5 - Nucleotide Sequence]

Start	End	Length in bp
69811	70425	615

Total length of S/MAR regions in sequence: 615 bp (0.6 %)

Statistics:

Number of sequences containing S/MARs: 1
Number of sequences containing no S/MARs: 0
Overall content of S/MARs: 0.6%
Total number of predicted S/MARs: 1

A total of 1 sequences were inspected by SMARTest (100000 bp)

Fig. 3. SMARTest analysis of the human β-actin gene locus. The 5162880–5262880 region surrounding the human β-actin locus was analyzed by the SMARTest program. A single candidate MAR region was detected.

3. Click only on the Following Enzymes button.
4. While holding down the ctrl key, select Bam HI, Eco R1, and Hind III.
5. Click on the Analyze Sequence button.

The restriction sites will be indicated on the sequence and the results will also be presented in tabular form. This data can then be incorporated into the strategy graph of **Fig. 4B**. The next task is to select a series of primers that will cover each restriction fragment that contains a candidate MAR. For example, digestion of genomic DNA with *EcoRI* and *BamHI* will yield an approx 20-kb *Bam*HI fragment containing six candidate MARs and an approx 4-kb *EcoRI BamHI* fragment containing a single candidate MAR. PCR primers can be designed to any region within each of these fragments using the following criteria. The amplicons should range in size from 200 to 500 bp. The region to be amplified should be free of repetitive DNA sequences. For ease of identification, it is optimal to ensure that the amplicons are of different size. To design primers we typically utilize the Oligo program *(16)*. It is commercially available at www.oligo.net, and therefore the operation of this program will not be discussed. Freeware programs such as eprimer3 are available at bioinfo.pbi.nrc.ca:8090/EMBOSS, and its use is outlined below.

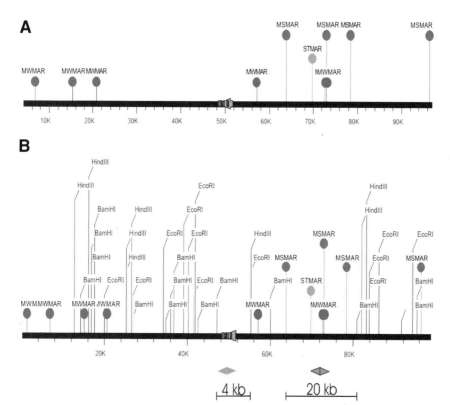

Fig. 4. MAR Strategy. (**A**) The location of each candidate MAR predicted by MAR-WIZ, MWMAR; MARSCAN, MSMAR; SMARTest, STMAR is shown. Note the relative level of similarity among the predictions. (**B**) The strategy map is then overlayed with a restriction map. The locations of the PCR primers designed to amplify the 4-kb and 20-kb fragments to test the predictions are indicated.

3.5. Eprimer 3

1. Logon to eprimer 3 using EMBOSS at bioinfo.pbi.nrc.ca:8090/EMBOSS.
2. Scroll down the left side to the program section Nucleic primers, then click on eprimer 3.
3. Use the Browse button to select the file that you would like to upload, i.e., actinlocus.
4. Scroll down to Sequence opt section.
5. Under Included region(s), the region from which oligonucleotides are to be selected, enter the base-pair coordinates separated by a dash. This should correspond to the location of the approx 20-kb *Bam*HI fragment.
6. Scroll down to the end of the page and click Run eprimer 3.
7. A list of PCR primer pairs will appear.
8. Repeat **steps 4–7** for the approx 4-kb Eco RI Bam HI fragment.

9. Compare the product lengths to make sure they are different, and the primer melting temperatures to ensure they are compatible.

3.6. PCR Optimization

The optimal annealing temperature for quantitative real-time PCR is identified by carrying out a series of PCR reactions in duplicate over a range of six different temperatures. The annealing temperature gradient typically spans 10°C and starts approx 5°C less than the predicted optimal annealing temperature. The fluorescence of 0.25 X SYBR-Green (Molecular Probes, Eugene, OR) is measured during each amplification step.

1. Perform 60 cycles of PCR with HotStar *Taq* polymerase system (Qiagen, Valencia, CA) using the primer pairs shown in **Table 1**.
2. Generate a melting curve for each reaction to verify appropriate product accumulation and to determine an optimal plate read temperature.
3. Verify the appropriately sized product by agarose gel electrophoresis and the product is corroborated with the melting-curve data. This positive control standard is utilized in all subsequent analyses.
4. Select the highest annealing temperature that produced a fluorescent amplification curve yielding a product of appropriate size and melting curve.
5. Determine the optimum plate read temperature *(17)* by comparing the ratio of the fluorescent melting curve profile of the product to that of the blank.
6. Select the point of maximum difference, i.e., signal to noise as the plate read temperature.

3.7. Preparation of HeLa Cell Nuclear Matrix

3.7.1. Halos on Slides

Prior to the in vivo determination of matrix attachment, an optimal time for nuclear protein extraction for each cell type must be resolved. This begins by isolating nuclei from intact cells. They are subsequently attached to slides, then treated with halo buffer for varying times. Each halo preparation is then fixed, stained with DAPI counterstain (Vysis, Downers Grove, IL), then visualized. The time required for nuclear protein extraction is determined as a function of the distance from the edge of the nuclear matrix to the perimeter of the extracted DNA. The minimum time required to reach maximum halo diameter is considered optimal. The protocol is described below for use with previously collected cells stored frozen at –80°C in Frozen Storage Buffer (FSB).

1. Gently thaw previously collected cells stored in FSB (1.25×10^6 cells in 1 mL FSB). Wash the FSB thawed cells by adding approx 2 mL PBS pH 7.4 buffer, supplemented with 1-mg/mL BSA to which Roche Biochemicals complete proteinase inhibitor was added just prior to use (*see* **Note 6**). Centrifuge the resulting mixture at 200*g* for 7 min at 4°C.

Table 1
PCR Primer Information

Amplicon	Primer sequence	TA predicted	TA used	TM predicted	Plate read
20 kb	(f) gat cag gcc tcc cag cta aca	59.5	60	89.7	87.4
20 kb	(r) cag ccctgc ggtcct c				
4 kb	(f) aac acc cca gcc atg tac g	60.1	59.8	90.7	87
4 kb	(r) atg tca cgc acg att tcc c				

TA, annealing temperature; TM, product melting temperature; Plate read, temperature used to eliminate spurious PCR products.

2. Resuspend the cell pellet in approx 2 mL of PBS pH 7.4 buffer, supplemented with Roche Biochemicals complete proteinase inhibitor, then centrifuge at 200g for 7 min at 4°C.
3. Resuspend the washed cells in 2 mL nuclei buffer supplemented with fresh Roche Biochemicals complete proteinase inhibitor, then incubate on ice for 15 min.
4. Centrifuge at 200g for 7 min at 4°C then remove the supernatant.
5. Resuspend the cell pellet in approx 2 mL of PBS pH 7.4 buffer, supplemented with Roche Biochemicals complete proteinase inhibitor added just prior to use, then centrifuge at 200g for 7 min at 4°C.
6. Adjust the concentration of nuclei to 1.5 × 10^5/mL with PBS pH 7.4 buffer, supplemented with Roche Biochemicals complete proteinase inhibitor.
7. Place 100 µL of nuclei solution into each cytospin funnel. Attach the nuclei onto slides by centrifugation in a Cytospin 2 cytofuge (Thermo Shandon, Pittsburgh, PA) for 5 min at 200g.
8. Remove the slides and place face up on a bed of ice. To determine optimal extraction time, overlay nuclei with 50 µL of 2 M NaCl containing halo buffer and incubate for varying times. These typically range from 1 to 10 min.
9. Stop the reaction by washing the slide. Each slide is washed for 1 min in each of a graded series of ice-cold 10X, 5X, 2X, and 1X PBS pH 7.4 buffer by placing the slides in a Coplin jar filled with washing solution. (Note: The pH of each dilution of PBS must be adjusted to 7.4.)
10. Similarly, the washed slides are dehydrated using a series of 1-min washes in 50%, 70%, 95%, and 100% graded ice-cold ethanol baths.
11. Fix the nucleic acid to the slide by baking for 2 h at 70°C. Fixed specimens may be stored at –20°C for extended periods of time.

As shown in **Fig. 5A**, this HeLa nuclear matrix preparation yielded a maximum-sized halo within 3 min.

3.7.2. Halos in Solution

Nuclear halos can be prepared in solution once the time required for nuclear protein extraction is determined. Similar to the above, and as outlined below and in **Fig. 5B**, nuclei isolated from intact cells are treated with 2 M NaCl. At this juncture, the halo preparations are quite fragile. Utmost care should be taken not to collapse the structure using either forceful centrifugation or creating excessive circulatory force when adding the restriction digestion buffer. The extraction of nuclear proteins is terminated by adjusting the salt concentration by dilution to 100 mM in preparation for restriction endonuclease digestion. The matrix-associated and loop-enriched fractions are then separated by restriction enzyme digestion as described below. Once obtained, the matrix associated and loop enriched DNA must be purified and the sample concentrations equalized before interrogation with real time PCR. The protocols are outlined below.

1. Gently thaw the previously collected cells stored in FSB (1.25×10^6 cells in 1 mL FSB). Wash the FSB thawed cells by adding approx 2 mL PBS pH 7.4 buffer, supplemented with 1-mg/mL BSA and Roche Biochemicals complete proteinase inhibitor added just before use (*see* **Note 6**). The resulting mixture is then centrifuged at 200g for 7 min at 4°C.
2. Resuspend the cell pellet in approx 2 mL of PBS pH 7.4 buffer, supplemented with Roche Biochemicals complete proteinase inhibitor that was added just before use, then centrifuge at 200g for 7 min at 4°C.
3. Resuspend the washed cells in 2 mL nuclei buffer supplemented with fresh Roche Biochemicals complete proteinase inhibitor, then incubate on ice for 15 min.
4. Centrifuge at 200g for 7 min at 4°C, then remove the supernatant.
5. Resuspend the cell pellet in approx 2 mL of PBS pH 7.4 buffer, supplemented with Roche Biochemicals complete proteinase inhibitor added just before use, then centrifuge at 200g for 7 min at 4°C.
6. Resuspend nuclei in 2 mL halo buffer supplemented with Roche Biochemicals complete proteinase inhibitor, added just before use, then incubate on ice for the appropriate period (3 min) as determined using the Halos on slides protocol.
7. Stop the reaction by adjusting the volume of the nuclear extract to 40 mL with 1X restriction buffer (*see* **Notes 7** and **8**).
8. Centrifuge at 200g for 7 min at 4°C. Remove the majority of the supernatant, leaving approx 1 mL of restriction buffer to cover the pellet.
9. To the mixture add 100 U each of *Eco*RI and *Bam*HI, then incubate for 4 h at 37°C.

Fig. 5. In vitro determination of MARs. (**A**) Nuclei are prepared, attached to slides, and treated with 2 M NaCl for varying lengths of time, as indicated in the upper right corner of each image. Measuring the nuclear halo length and identifying the shortest time associated with the maximum halo span determines the optimal time for nuclear protein extraction. (**B**) To ascertain nuclear matrix association, nuclear matrix- and loop-associated DNA fractions should be prepared and interrogated as outlined. (1) Starting with permeabilized cells, nuclear proteins are extracted with 2 M NaCl. (2) Restriction enzymes are then used to digest the DNA, freeing loop-associated regions

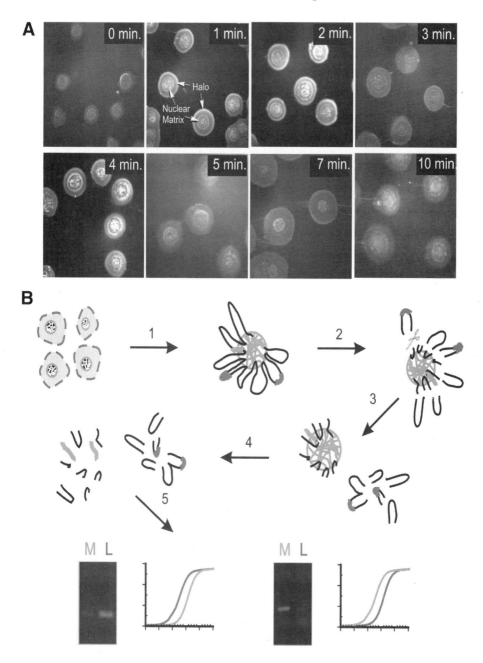

Fig. 5. (*continued*) from the nuclear matrix. (3) Matrix-associated and loop-enriched DNA fractions are obtained following centrifugation. (4) To establish the location of specific DNA regions, the loop (L) and matrix (M) DNA can be interrogated using standard PCR or quantitative real-time PCR.

10. Subsequent to resticiton digestion, pellet the matrix fraction by centrifugation at 16,000g for 5 min at 4°C, remove the supernatant fraction that contains the loop and place in a clean reaction vessel.

11. Wash the matrix-containing pellet 3× with the addition of 1 mL of restriction buffer, then centrifuge at 16,000g for 5 min at 4°C. After each wash, remove the supernatant and discard.

12. Add 300 μL of proteinase K buffer separately to a final concentration of 1X to the pellet and loop fraction.

13. Digest both fractions overnight with approx 120 μg of proteinase K.

14. Purify DNA from both fractions using either phenol/chloroform extraction or a nucleic acid-based affinity matrix (18). One can expect to recover 30–40% of the nucleic acid in the nuclear matrix fraction and 60–70% in the loop fraction.

3.7.3. Determining Concentrations of Loop and Matrix DNA

Densitometry and ultraviolet spectrophotometric quantitation are routinely employed to determine DNA concentration. However, fluorescent assays are rapidly becoming the method of choice, owing to their increased sensitivity and reduced interference by contaminates (19). Several fluorescent dyes are available for nucleic acid quantitation, although many are hindered by their range of detection (20–23). PicoGreen demonstrates a broad range of sensitivity, exhibits a strong resistance to contaminant interference (24), and is used routinely. The method (38) of quantitation is outlined below.

1. Dilute picoGreen 200-fold in TE buffer.

2. Dilute λ DNA standard (Invitrogen) in TE buffer creating a series of known concentrations ranging from 500 to 7.81 pg/μL. A blank containing only the fluorescent dye reagent and TE buffer must be prepared for global background subtraction.

3. The unknown samples are serially diluted in TE so that one or two of the dilutions may fall within the range of the prepared standards.

4. Equal volumes (50 μL) of 1X PicoGreen reagent and TE buffer containing the nucleic acid are added to individual microplate wells (flat-bottomed Costar model 2592 microtiter plate).

5. Mix the samples, then incubate for 5 min at room temperature while protected from light. An aluminum foil cover works well.

6. Remove each 8-well strip containing the standard or samples from the microplate carrier, then scan using a Typhoon 9210 (Amersham Biosciences, Piscataway, NJ). Removal of the 8-well strips cannot be overlooked. Results are inconsistent if the strips remain in the microplate carrier when scanned (*see* **Note 9**).

7. Once the results are obtained, the DNA concentrations of the loop and matrix fractions should be adjusted to approx 150 pg/μL with H_2O.

3.8. Determining Regions of Matrix Association

Matrix association has been assessed using Southern hybridization (25), reassociation (26,27), and standard PCR assays. These techniques are not as amenable to the rapid genome-wide analysis afforded by real-time PCR. With real-time PCR, product accumulation is measured with each amplification cycle *(28,29)*. Two real-time PCR quantification methods, absolute and relative, have been adopted, to analyze differences in the amount of starting template. Absolute quantification allows the determination of the original number of target molecules within a reaction *(30)*, whereas relative quantification describes the change in the number of target molecules with respect to a reference *(31)*.

Relative differences in the number of target molecules are usually assessed by the $2^{\Delta\Delta}ct$ method *(31)*. Using this approach, the difference in the number of cycles required for the reference and test samples to surpass an arbitrarily selected threshold *(ct)* is determined. Assuming optimum amplification efficiency, the calculated cycle difference ($\Delta\Delta ct$) is used as the exponent in the $2^{\Delta\Delta}ct$ equation to approximate the fold discrepancy in the amount of starting template between the two reactions. For example, if the matrix fraction crosses the *ct* at 3 cycles before the loop fraction, there is an approximate 2^3 or 8-fold difference between the fractions. Using Eq. 1 and solving for *X*, it can be estimated that the loop fraction contains 11% while the matrix fraction contains 89% of the amplicon of interest.

$$X + 2^{\Delta\Delta}ct(X) = 100\% \quad (1)$$

The validity of the $2^{\Delta\Delta}ct$ method requires that the amplification efficiencies of both the target and reference PCR reactions be within 5% of one another *(31)*. Unfortunately, this is not usually observed.

To alleviate the necessity of similar amplification efficiencies, a log-linear regression *(32)* has been implemented in the TAQ-software (http://vortex.cs.wayne.edu/Projects.html). This approach uses a log transformation of the fluorescent amplification curve data to fit a line to the linear portion of the curve. Considering amplification efficiency, the software solves the linear equation to calculate the fluorescent intensity that is directly proportional to the initial amount of template. The percent enrichment can then be determined if one assumes that the combined loop and matrix factions contain 100% of the original amplicon that was present in the nucleus. For example, if the TAQ software estimates that 1.03×10^{-13} and 3×10^{-13} fluorescent units are associated with the initial matrix and loop fractions, respectively, there is $[1.03 \times 10^{-13}/(1.03 \times 10^{-13} + 3 \times 10^{-13})]$ or 26% of the amplicon in the matrix and 74% in the loop fraction. The method utilized by the TAQ-software offers several advantages compared to the $2^{\Delta\Delta}ct$ method. First, it eliminates the deceptive discrepancies introduced by different amplification efficiencies that are often observed between experiments. Second, the user is not required to select an arbitrary threshold. The threshold is calculated from the data and is therefore consistent among experiments. Third, the amplification efficiency is calculated for each reaction, providing the user with invaluable information regarding the "quality" of the PCR and facilitating the optimization of laboratory procedures.

To ascertain matrix association of the 4-kb β-actin and 20-kb β-actin candidate MAR regions shown in **Fig. 4B**, quadruplicate parallel real-time PCR assays are carried out on the matrix-associated and loop-enriched DNA samples using the MJ Research Opticon Monitor (MJ Research, Waltham, MA). An example of the PCR reaction parameters for the 4-kb β-actin and 20-kb β-actin MAR primer pairs is shown in **Table 1**. This includes the specified annealing (*TA*) and plate-read temperatures using 300 pg of template per 20 μL reaction. The results obtained utilizing the TAQ-software are summarized in **Table 2**. They clearly reiterate the necessity of biologically verifying the MAR predictions. In this example, all prediction programs tested highlighted the 20-kb β-actin region as a likely position for nuclear matrix attachment. However, only 42.5% of the amplicon was observed within the matrix associated DNA fraction. In contrast, 59.1% of the 4-kb β-actin region that was not predicted to contain a MAR was found within the matrix-associated fraction.

3.9. Future Prospects

Individual chromosomes occupy distinct territories within the cell nucleus *(33–35)*. This arrangement protects the genome while providing a primary control point regulating gene expression. The mechanism organizing chromatin within the cell nucleus provides a rich source of complexity and scientific debate. The nuclear matrix acts as an organizer providing a framework for the transcription machinery and the environment for active genes to intermingle *(5,18)*. While this would suggest a dynamic nature, some DNA regions that anchor the chromatin to the nuclear matrix act as boundary elements that shield specific domains from neighboring enhancers and the silencing effects of heterochromatin *(36,37)*. Although these and other roles of nuclear matrix-DNA interaction have been scrutinized *(1)*, the exact nature of their association and the role provided by the nuclear matrix remains to be fully characterized. In this chapter we have provided some necessary tools to systematically study and characterize the structure and association of DNA to the nuclear matrix.

4. Notes

1. Always add the detergent after any reagent has been autoclaved.
2. Always verify and adjust the PBS buffer to pH 7.4 when necessary.
3. The various parameters of each program discussed in the chapter can be adjusted. This is best carried out once you have familiarized yourself with the program.
4. Remember, most computer programs that identify biological function only yield estimates or best guesses. These predictions always require confirmation in the wet-bench.

Table 2
β-Actin MAR Analysis Results

Fraction	y-intercept	Efficiency	Percent enriched	Fraction	y-intercept	Efficiency	Percent enriched
4-kb loop	2.29E-09	0.857430		20-kb loop	7.77E-14	0.963544	
4-kb loop	7.30E-10	0.973768		20-kb loop	2.66E-13	0.847417	
4-kb loop	1.04E-09	0.942354		20-kb loop	1.07E-13	0.972535	
4-kb loop	1.21E-09	0.906002		20-kb loop	1.26E-12	0.884681	
Average	1.32E-09		40.9	Average	4.27E-13		57.5
4-kb matrix	1.62E-09	0.916485		20-kb matrix	3.44E-13	0.894340	
4-kb matrix	1.55E-09	0.912035		20-kb matrix	3.98E-13	0.918440	
4-kb matrix	2.78E-09	0.869781		20-kb matrix	1.69E-13	0.960597	
4-kb matrix	1.67E-09	0.913150		20-kb matrix	3.51E-13	0.944101	
Average	1.91E-09		59.1	Average	3.16E-13		42.5

Average, mean of quadruplicates; Percent enriched, percent of amplicon found within the specified fraction.

5. When possible, it is best to compare the results obtained from several different algorithms.
6. The Roche Biochemicals complete proteinase inhibitor is always freshly added just before use.
7. Once nuclear halos are formed in solution, they are quite fragile. Thus, extreme care should be taken so as not to collapse the structure.
8. When stopping the nuclear protein extraction, the halo structures may be observed sticking to the side of the reaction vessel. If this is the case, restriction digestion can be done by slowly rocking and rotating the reaction vessel in a hybridization oven. This will effectively wash the restriction buffer and enzymes over the halo structures, freeing the loop-enriched DNA.
9. To determine DNA concentration, the 8-well strips must be removed from the microplate carrier, as inconsistent data are obtained if the strips are not removed prior to scanning.

References

1. Bode, J., Benham, C., Knopp, A., and Mielke, C. (2000) Transcriptional augmentation: Modulation of gene expression by Scaffold/Matrix-Attached regions (S/MAR elements). *Crit. Rev. Eukaryot. Gene Expression* **10(1),** 73–90.
2. Hancock, R. (2000) A new look at the nuclear matrix. *Chromosoma* **109(4),** 219–225.
3. Heng, H. H. Q., Krawetz, S. A., Lu, W., Bremer, S., Liu, G. and Ye, C. J. (2001) Redefining the chromatin loop domain. *Cytogenet. Cell Genet.* **93(3–4),** 155–161.
4. Kramer, J. A. and Krawetz, S. A. (1996) Nuclear matrix interactions within the sperm genome. *J. Biol. Chem.* **271(20),** 11,619–11,622.
5. Yasui, D., Miyano, M., Cai, S. T., Varga-Weisz, P., and Kohwi-Shigematsu, T. (2002) SATB1 targets chromatin remodelling to regulate genes over long distances. *Nature* **419(6907),** 641–645.
6. Jackson, D. A., Bartlett, J., and Cook, P. R. (1996) Sequences attaching loops of nuclear and mitochondrial DNA to underlying structures in human cells: The role of transcription units. *Nucleic Acids Res.* **24(7),** 1212–1219.
7. Mahy, N. L., Perry, P. E., and Bickmore, W. A. (2002) Gene density and transcription influence the localization of chromatin outside of chromosome territories detectable by FISH. *J. Cell Biol.* **159(5),** 753–763.
8. Singh, G. B., Kramer, J. A., and Krawetz, S. A. (1997) Mathematical model to predict regions of chromatin attachment to the nuclear matrix. *Nucleic Acids Res.* **25(7),** 1419–1425.
9. Jackson, D. A. (1998) Analyzing the structure and function of mammalian nuclei, in vitro. In *Chromosome Structure: A Practical Approach* (Bickmore, W., ed.) Oxford University Press, New York, NY, pp. 147–166.
10. Rice, P., Longden, I., and Bleasby, A. (2000) EMBOSS: The European Molecular Biology Open Software Suite. *Trends Genet.* **16(6),** 276–277.

11. Frisch, M., Frech, K., Klingenhoff, A., Cartharius, K., Liebich, I., and Werner, T. (2002) *In silico* prediction of scaffold/matrix attachment regions in large genomic sequences. *Genome Res.* **12(2),** 349–354.

12. Goetze, S., Gluch, A., Benham, C., and Bode, J. (2003) Computational and in vitro analysis of destabilized DNA regions in the interferon gene cluster: Potential of predicting functional gene domains. *Biochemistry* **42(1),** 154–166.

13. Benham, C., KohwiShigematsu, T., and Bode, J. (1997) Stress-induced duplex DNA destabilization in scaffold/matrix attachment regions. *J. Mol. Biol.* **274(2),** 181–196.

14. Liebich, I., Bode, J., Reuter, I., and Wingender, E. (2002) Evaluation of sequence motifs found in scaffold/matrix-attached regions (S/MARs). *Nucleic Acids Res.* **30(15),** 3433–3442.

15. van Drunen, C. M., Sewalt, R., Oosterling, R. W., Weisbeek, P. J., Smeekens, S. C .M., and van Driel, R. (1999) A bipartite sequence element associated with matrix/scaffold attachment regions. *Nucleic Acids Res.* **27(14),** 2924–2930.

16. Offerman, J. D. and Rychlik, W. (2003) *OLIGO Primer Analysis Software.* Humana Press, Totowa, NJ.

17. Morrison, T. B., Weis, J. J., and Wittwer, C. T. (1998) Quantification of low-copy transcripts by continuous SYBR Green I monitoring during amplification. *Biotechniques* **24,** 954–962.

18. Kramer, J. A. and Krawetz, S. A. (1997) PCR-based assay to determine nuclear matrix association. *Biotechniques* **22(5),** 826–828.

19. Jones, L. J., Yue, S. T., Cheung, C., and Singer, V. L. (1998) RNA quantitation by fluorescence-based solution assay: RiboGreen reagent characterization. *Anal. Biochem.* **265,** 368–374.

20. Le Pecq, J. B. and Paoletti, C. (1966) A new fluorometric method for RNA and DNA determination. *Anal. Biochem.* **17,** 100–107.

21. Labarca, C. and Paigen, K. (1980) A simple, rapid, and sensitive DNA assay procedure. *Anal. Biochem.* **102,** 344–352.

22. Markovitz, J., Roques, B. P., and Le Pecq, J. B. (1979) Ethidium dimer: A new reagent for the fluorimetric determination of nucleic acids. *Anal. Biochem.* **94,** 259–264.

23. Rye, H. S., Dabora, J. M., Quesada, M. A., Mathies, R. A., and Glazer, A. N. (1993) Fluorometric assay using dimeric dyes for double- and single-stranded DNA and RNA with picogram sensitivity. *Anal. Biochem.* **208,** 144–150.

24. Singer, V. L., Jones, L. J., Yue, S. T., and Haugland, R. P. (1997) Characterization of PicoGreen reagent and development of a fluorescence-based solution assay for double-stranded DNA quantitation. *Anal. Biochem.* **249,** 228–38.

25. Lauber, A. H., Barrett, T. J., Subramaniam, M., Schuchard, M., and Spelsberg, T. C. (1997) A DNA-binding element for a steroid receptor-binding factor is flanked by dual nuclear matrix DNA attachment sites in the c-myc gene promoter. *J. Biol. Chem.* **272(39),** 24,657–24,665.

26. Mirkovitch, J., Mirault, M. E., and Laemmli, U. K. (1984) Organization of the higher-order chromatin loop: specific DNA attachment sites on nuclear scaffold. *Cell* **39(1),** 223–232.
27. Mielke, C., Christensen, M. O., Westergaard, O., Bode, J., Benham, C. J., and Breindl, M. (2002) Multiple collagen I gene regulatory elements have sites of stress-induced DNA duplex destabilization and nuclear scaffold/matrix association potential. *J. Cell Biochem.* **84(3),** 484–496.
28. Winer, J., Jung, C. K., Shackel, I., and Williams, P. M. (1999) Development and validation of real-time quantitative reverse transcriptase-polymerase chain reaction for monitoring gene expression in cardiac myocytes in vitro. *Anal. Biochem.* **270(1),** 41–49.
29. Heid, C. A., Stevens, J., Livak, K. J., and Williams, P. M. (1996) Real-time quantitative PCR. *Genome Res.* **6(10),** 986–994.
30. Bustin, S. A. (2000) Absolute quantification of mRNA using real-time reverse transcription polymerase chain reaction assays. *J. Mol. Endocrinol.* **25(2),** 169–193.
31. Livak, K. J. and Schmittgen, T. D. (2001) Analysis of relative gene expression data using real-time quantitative PCR and the 2(-Delta Delta C(T)) Method. *Methods* **25(4),** 402–408.
32. Wiesner, R. J. (1992) Direct quantification of picomolar concentrations of mRNAs by mathematical analysis of a reverse transcription/exponential polymerase chain reaction assay. *Nucleic Acids Res.* **20(21),** 5863–5864.
33. Jackson, D. A. (2000) Features of nuclear architecture that influence gene expression in higher eukaryotes: confronting the enigma of epigenetics. *J. Cell Biochem. Suppl.* **35,** 69–77.
34. Dundr, M. and Misteli, T. (2001) Functional architecture in the cell nucleus. *Biochem. J.* **356(Pt 2),** 297–310.
35. Wolffe, A. P. and Hansen, J. C. (2001) Nuclear visions: functional flexibility from structural instability. *Cell* **104(5),** 631–634.
36. Namciu, S. J., Blochlinger, K. B., and Fournier, R. E. (1998) Human matrix attachment regions insulate transgene expression from chromosomal position effects in Drosophila melanogaster. *Mol. Cell Biol.* **18(4),** 2382–2391.
37. McKnight, R. A., Shamay, A., Lakshmanan, S., Wall, R. J., and Hennighausen, L. (1992) Matrix-attachment regions can impart position-independent regulation of a tissue-specific gene in transgenic mice. *Proc. Natl. Acad. Sci. USA* **89,** 6943–6947.
38. Goodrich, R. J., Ostermeier, G. C., and Krawetz, S. A. (2003) Multitasking with molecular dynamics typhoon: quantifying nucleic acids and autoradiographs. *Biotechnol. Lett.* **25,** 1061–1065.

29

Biomedical Informatics Methods in Pharmacogenomics

Qing Yan

Summary

Pharmacogenomics is the study of the genetic basis of individual variation in response to therapeutic agents. Pharmacogenomics may potentially affect on every step of health care and every drug treatment protocol. The optimal approach to pharmacogenomics in hypertension requires the integration of different disciplines, in which biomedical informatics plays an essential role. This chapter describes biomedical informatics methods used in dealing with key issues in pharmacogenomics. These key issues include the association between structure and function, the interaction between gene and drug, and the correlation between genotype and phenotype. Heterogeneous resources, including web sites, databases, and software analysis tools, are selected, organized, and integrated in practical methods to support these studies. Bioinformatics methods described in this chapter include genetic sequence searching, comparison, structural modeling, functional analysis, and systems biology studies, with emphasis on single-nucleotide polymorphism (SNP) analysis. Medical informatics methods such as disease and drug information and clinical terminology are also embraced in this chapter. This combination of both biological and medical informatics provides comprehensive methodologies to resolve complex problems in pharmacogenomics.

Key Words: Biomedical informatics; bioinformatics; pharmacogenomics; single-nucleotide polymorphism (SNP); database; software; genotype; phenotype; structure; function; disease; drug.

1. Introduction
1.1. Pharmacogenomics

Pharmacogenomics is considered the future of drug therapy. This emerging area has advanced rapidly in recent years. Pharmacogenomics studies the genetic basis of individual variation in response to therapeutic agents *(1)*. The understanding of genetic sequence diversity in humans can make it possible to tailor optimal drug prescription to avoid adverse drug events and to achieve personalized medicine. Although it has been used interchangeably with phar-

From: *Methods in Molecular Medicine, Vol. 108: Hypertension: Methods and Protocols*
Edited by: J. P. Fennell and A. H. Baker © Humana Press Inc., Totowa, NJ

macogenetics, the term "pharmacogenomics" usually represents the entire spectrum of genes that are associated with drug behavior and sensitivity *(1)* (*see* Chapter 17 for a discussion of this terminology).

Pharmacogenomics may potentially affect every step of health care, from diagnosis to drug prescription, and from drug design to clinical trials. For example, the application of pharmacogenomics in diagnostic tests can help predict a patient's response to a particular drug based on the patient's genetic profile. Such diagnostic tests may empower physicians to make decisions and choose the right dose of the right drug for the right disease and the right patient.

For the drug development industry, pharmacogenomics can be applied to identify drug targets for certain patient populations to achieve optimized drug efficacy. In November 2003, the US Food and Drug Administration (FDA) published Guidance for Industry Pharmacogenomic Data Submissions, which provides guidelines on using genetic data to make better and safer drugs *(2)*.

The application of pharmacogenomics has the potential to influence almost every drug treatment protocol including those for cardiovascular diseases *(3–5)*, neurological diseases *(6,7)*, cancer *(8–10)*, pain management *(11)*, and infectious diseases *(12)*. In cardiovascular diseases, genetic variants have been shown to have important pharmacodynamic effects on antiarrhythmic, renin-angiotensin, β-blocker, lipid-lowering, and antithrombotic drugs *(5)*. Genetic variations that are linked to cardiovascular risk include glutathion-*S*-transferase (GSH-T), CYP450 phase I and II enzymes, and drug transporters *(3–5)*. The C825T polymorphism in the gene GNB3 has been found to be a potential marker that differentiates drug responders and nonresponders, which could make it an excellent candidate gene in cardiovascular pharmacogenomics *(13)*. In the treatment of hypertension, polymorphisms in angiotensin-converting enzyme have been shown to be helpful in predicting responses to the inhibition of this enzyme *(14)*.

Pharmacogenomics is multidisciplinary, and includes structural genomics, functional genomics, proteomics, disease pathogenesis, pharmacology, and toxicology *(1)*. The correct approach to pharmacogenomics in hypertension requires the integration of these different disciplines *(15)*. Before we can achieve the ultimate goal of pharmacogenomics, the key issues to be solved include elucidating the association between structure and function, the interaction between gene and drug, and the correlation between genotype and phenotype *(1)*. These three issues are critical in dissecting complex problems in pharmacogenomics. The clarification of these issues can facilitate the integration of different disciplines from various aspects.

For example, the longer TA repeat unit in the promoter of the atrial natriuretic peptide receptor (Npr1) regulates the transcription of the *Npr1* gene, with consequences on diastolic blood pressure *(16)*. This finding explains the association between the promoter structure of the *Npr*1 gene and its functional effects on transcription and gene expression. This example also indicates the correlation between the genotypic feature and the blood pressure phenotype. Another example linking genotypes with altered phenotypes is that single-nucleotide polymorphisms (SNPs) in the kidney-specific human urea transporter-2 (HUT2) open reading frame (ORF) are associated with variation in blood pressure *(17)*. In addition, the identification of several SNP-genotypes that may be used as predictors of blood pressure reduction after antihypertensive treatment, reveals the interaction between genetic features and drug responses *(18)*.

As shown in the above examples, the key issues are interlinked *(1)*. The association between genetic structure and observable normal functions represents normal phenotypes. Altered genetic structure can cause malfunction and disorders that are disease phenotypes. Varied genetic structure and altered functions may influence the interaction between genes and drugs, which ultimately affects drug-response phenotypes. Among these three issues, the correlation between genotype and drug-response phenotype is the most comprehensive one to be investigated.

Various technologies have been developed to address these issues, such as techniques for single SNP detection and genetic profiling. SNPs are genetic sequence variations that occur when a single nucleotide in the genome sequence is altered. SNPs are the most frequent cases of sequence variation. They are useful markers for mapping and discovering associations between genes and diseases, and between genes and drug responses. Laboratory technologies that have been used for SNP genotyping include polymerase chain reaction (PCR), capillary electrophoresis, allele-specific hybridization, microarray, and mass spectrometry (*see* Chapters 11–13).

An alternative method to these laboratory methods is *in silico* discovery, for example, using computer resources to mine databases to identify polymorphisms. Biomedical informatics methods are indispensable for every process in pharmacogenomics, from high-throughput data collection to clinical decision support. In this chapter, we focus on the application of biomedical informatics methods in the study of pharmacogenomics.

1.2. Biomedical Informatics Methods in Pharmacogenomics

Here biomedical informatics refers to using computational approaches to solve biological and clinical problems, and to improve the communication, understanding, and management of biomedical information. In pharmacogenomics, the major challenge for biomedical informatics is to help solve the key issues mentioned above, i.e., the correlations in structure–function, gene–drug, and genotype–phenotype. Although many biomedical data and informatics resources are available, difficulties exist in how to integrate these data and resources, and how to make the best use of them. Data integration is the process of transforming data into information, then into useful knowledge *(19)*. In this chapter we select, organize, and integrate various bioinformatics resources for practical studies of the three correlations so that readers can find materials easily and apply methods they need readily (*see* **Note 1**).

Bioinformatics has extensive applications in pharmacogenomics to help elucidate the relationship between genetic structure and function. Sequence comparison algorithms and tools such as Basic Local Alignment Search Tool (BLAST) (*see* **Subheading 3.1.2.**) and CLUSTAL W (*see* **Subheading 3.1.3.**) are important in identifying genetic variations and evolutionary relationships. The Human Genome Variation Database (HGVbase) contains information on physical and functional relationships between sequence variations and neighbor genes (*see* **Subheading 3.1.8.1.**). Pattern analysis using PROSITE and Pfam databases can help correlate sequence structure to functional motifs such as phosphorylation sites (*see* **Subheading 3.1.6.**). The database Protein Data Bank (PDB) and the program CPHmodels are useful for protein structure three-dimensional (3-D) modeling (*see* **Subheading 3.1.7.**).

As more features of genetic sequences are being discovered, the next question is how those genetic molecules interact with each other in their network structure. This system-level understanding of biology is the aim of the emerging systems biology field *(20)*. Such understanding is required in order to explore what roles biological molecules play in the underlying mechanisms of diseases, and how such information can be used to transform drug development to better medicine. For pharmacogenomics, systems biology studies are fundamental for insight into the associations between genetic structure and function, gene and drug, and genotype and phenotype. Informatics tools, such as databases describing protein–protein interaction and pathways, provide clues for understanding the genetic information at systematic levels (*see* **Subheading 3.1.9.**).

The essential gene–drug interaction composes the central theme of pharmacogenomics, as it studies genetic mechanisms and the functional pharmacological context, in association with clinical medicine *(1)*. Biomedical informatics helps approach the problem from various aspects. Some web sites and databases have been established for studying specific genetic molecules responding to drugs, such as receptors and transporters (*see* **Table 7**). Various software tools are available to characterize pharmacokinetic (PK) and pharmacodynamic (PD) profiles (*see* **Table 3**). Some databases provide information on genetic alteration that affect drug efficacy through the process of uptake, binding, biotransformation, and excretion (*see* **Subheading 3.2.1.**).

Biomedical informatics plays an essential role in exploring the correlation between genotype and phenotype, which is crucial in translating pharmacogenomics into clinical medicine. Databases and other software can be used in the design and data interpretation of genotyping tests, such as microarray tests. Various SNP databases, such as dbSNP (*see* **Subheading 3.1.8.1.**), can be used to search for individual genotype data. Some databases provide direct linkages between sequence variation genotype and disease phenotype, such as the Online Mendelian Inheritance in Man (OMIM) database.

The following sections will describe what, when, and how to apply biomedical informatics methods in pharmacogenomics studies.

2. Materials

In this part, we introduce biomedical informatics resources that can be used for pharmacogenomics studies. These resources include web sites, databases, and software tools. For convenient and worldwide access, most of the resources listed are freely available online with Universal Resource Locators (URLs) provided (*see* **Note 2**). The details on how to use these resources are discussed under **Subheading 3.**

2.1. Web Sources

The web sources listed here collect relevant information on certain projects, programs, or topics. These web sites are usually hosted by governments, research institutions, or industry. Many of these comprehensive sites have links to relevant databases, software programs, and other sites (*see* **Note 3**). Some individual databases and tools that are contained in these web sites will be discussed specifically under **Subheadings 2.2.** and **2.3.**

Table 1 summarizes web sources that are useful for bioinformatics research. These sources are categorized into different aspects, including general bioinformatics sites, sites specific for genomic research, and sites about microarrays. In the following, each category will be discussed with some web sites as examples.

Most bioinformatics sites listed here are comprehensive sites or portals that contain databases and tools for genomic, proteomic, and functional analysis. For example, the site of the National Center for Biotechnology Information (NCBI) was established as a US national resource for biological information. The NCBI hosts databases such as GenBank and genetic tools such as BLAST. With the advances of new knowledge and technology, the contents at these sites are updated quite frequently.

Table 1
Relevant Bioinformatics Sites for Pharmacogenomics Research

Category	Name	URL	Description
Relevant bioinformatics sites	NCBI	www.ncbi.nlm.nih.gov	Updated databases and tools
	European Bioinformatics Institute (EBI)	www.ebi.ac.uk/	Databases and software
	Weizmann Institute	http://bip.weizmann.ac.il/ index.html	Databases and tools
Genomic research	Human Genome Project (HGP)	www.ornl.gov/ TechResources /Human_Genome /home.html	Information about Human Genome Project
	Complete Genomes	www-nbrf.georgetown. edu/pir/genome.html	Genome sequences
	Ensembl	www.ensembl.org	Automatic annotation on genomes
	UCSC Genome Bioinformatics	http://genome.ucsc.edu	Browse, search, analyze, view maps
	Stanford University Genome Resources	www-genome.stanford. edu/index.html	Links to databases, knowledgebase, and tools
	VISTA Genome Browser	http://pipeline.lbl.gov/ index.html	Browse whole-genome alignments
	Genome Channel	http://compbio.ornl.gov/ channel	Search of genomes
Microarray	NHGRI Microarray Project	http://research.nhgri. nih.gov/microarray/ main.html	Protocols, databases and tools
	Microarray Informatics at EBI	www.ebi.ac.uk/microarray	Microarray data management, storage, and analysis
	Bibliography on Microarray Data Analysis	www.nslij-genetics.org/ microarray	Links and publications related to data analysis

Table 2
Web Site for Sequence Variation Research

Category	Name	URL	Description
Sequence variation (SNP and mutation)	The SNP Consortium (TSC)	http://snp.cshl.org	Database, linkage map
	The Human Genome Variation Society (HGVS)	www.genomic.unimelb.edu.au/mdi	Links to variation databases and relevant information
	The Environmental Genome Project (EGP)	www.niehs.nih.gov/envgenom	SNP database and research platform
	The UW-FHCRC Variation Discovery Resource (SeattleSNPs)	http://pga.mbt.washington.edu/welcome.html	Gene resources, data download, software, pathways, protocols

Many sites focus on genome information. The sites listed in **Table 1** are some commonly used ones. For example, the site of the Human Genome Project (HGP) provides information relevant to the US and worldwide Human Genome Project. The HGP describes goals, progress, history and relevant information about research, education, medicine, as well as ethical, legal, and social issues.

Microarray is an important technology in pharmacogenomics studies *(21)*. Some web sites provide protocols, databases, and tools for data analysis, such as the site of the National Human Genome Research Institute (NHGRI) Microarray Project. The site of Microarray Informatics at the European Bioinformatics Institute (EBI) provides resources for microarray data management, storage, and analysis.

Some web sites contain information exclusively about genomic variations, such as the SNP Consortium (TSC) and the site of the Human Genome Variation Society (HGVS) (*see* **Table 2**). The TSC site provides data searching, linkage maps, and data download for SNPs. The HGVS site contains links to different genetic variation databases, publications, and other relevant inform-ation.

Table 3
Web Sites for Disease and Pharmacological Information

Category	Name	URL	Description
Disease	American Society of Hypertension (ASH)	www.ash-us.org/ about_hypertension/index.htm	Information about hypertension
	World Hypertension League	www.mco.edu/whl/index.html	Hypertension information resource
Drug	FDA Drug Information	www.fda.gov/cder/drug/ default.htm	Products the FDA regulates
PK/PD	Pharmacokinetic and Pharmacodynamic Resources	www.boomer.org/pkin	Searchable site with links to software and other relevant resources
	PK/PD software links	www3.usal.es/~galenica/clinpkin/ software.htm	A collection of links to software
	Stanford PK/PD Software Server	http://anesthesia.stanford. edu/pkpd	Software and relevant resources

Web sites about disease and drug information are collected in **Table 3**. The site of the American Society of Hypertension (ASH) contains a multitude of information about hypertension, including publications and a collection of links to other relevant sites. The FDA Drug Information site contains information about products that it regulates, including new prescription drug approvals, detailed information about drugs, drug safety and side effects, clinical trials, public health alerts, and relevant reports and publications.

Pharmacological information composes a critical part of the multidisciplinary pharmacogenomics. Several web sites about PK/PD are listed in **Table 3**. For example, the Pharmacokinetic and Pharmacodynamic Resources site provides links to relevant software, courses, textbooks, and journals.

Table 4 lists sites about standardization and terminology issues in biomedical informatics relevant to pharmacogenomics. Standardization is important for data integration and communication improvement, as it facilitates mutual understanding of data and terms from heterogeneous resources. Contents in **Table 4** include web resources for terminology in genetics such as the Gene Ontology (GO) Consortium, and standardized terminology in clinical use such as International Classification of Diseases (ICD).

Table 4
Web Sites About Standardization and Terminology in Biomedical Informatics

Category	Name	URL	Description
Terminology— genetics	Gene Ontology(GO) Consortium	www.geneontology.org/	A controlled vocabulary that can be applied to all organisms
	Glossary of Genetic Terms (NHGRI)	www.genome.gov/ 10002096	Help understand the terms and concepts used in genetic research
	GeneCards	http://bioinformatics. weizmann.ac.il/ cards/index.html	Integrated site of human genes, products, and involvement in diseases
Terminology— clinical	International Classification of Diseases (ICD)	www.cdc.gov/nchs/about/ otheract/icd9/ abticd10.htm	Classification for coding diagnoses
	Systematized Nomenclature of Medicine (SNOMED)	www.snomed.org	Clinical terminology for encoding the medical record
	Current Procedural Terminology (CPT)	www.ama-assn.org/ama/ pub/category/3113.html	For coding clinical procedures

2.2. Databases

Unlike web sites in the previous section, databases collected in **Tables 5–7** are mostly about individual topics, so that readers would know which database to use directly for their objectives. Databases listed here are categorized similarly to the last section. **Table 5** summarizes some general bioinformatics databases and search engines. Frequently used databases for sequence variation are collected in **Table 6**. **Table 7** lists some databases useful for studying gene–drug and genotype–phenotype correlations. Many of the databases here provide search tools and maps to facilitate data access and representation. The detailed application of some databases will be described under **Subheading 3.**

Table 5
Relevant Bioinformatics Databases
and Search Engines for Pharmacogenomic Studies

Category	Name	URL	Description
General bioinformatics	Entrez	www.ncbi.nlm.nih.gov Entrez/index.html	Search engine for various databases
	dbEST	www.ncbi.nlm.nih.gov/dbEST	Expressed sequence tags (EST) database
	UniGene	www.ncbi.nlm.nih.gov/entrez/ query.fcgi?db=unigene	Gene-oriented clusters
	The Genome Database (GDB)	www.gdb.org	Genomic information
	GeneLoc (UDB)	http://genecards.weizmann.ac.il/ geneloc	An integrated map for chromosomes
	PROSITE	http://us.expasy.org/prosite	Protein families and domains
	Pfam	www.sanger.ac.uk/ Software/Pfam	Protein families database of hidden Markov models (HMMs)
	Protein Data Bank (PDB)	www.rcsb.org/pdb	Biological macromolecular structure data
	The Cambridge Structural Database	www.ccdc.cam.ac.uk/ products/csd	Small-molecule crystal structures
Systems biology —pathways	KEGG	www.genome.ad.jp/ kegg/kegg2.html	Pathway maps, ortholog group tables, catalogs
	Cell Signaling Networks Database (CSNDB)	http://geo.nihs.go.jp/csndb	Signaling pathways of human cells

(continued)

Table 5 (*Continued*)
Relevant Bioinformatics Databases
and Search Engines for Pharmacogenomic Studies

Category	Name	URL	Description
Systems biology —interactions	Database of Interacting Proteins (DIP)	http://dip.doe-mbi.ucla.edu	Interactions between proteins
	Biomolecular Interaction Network Database (BIND)	www.blueprint.org/bind/ bind.php	Interactions and pathways
Microarray and gene expression	Stanford Microarray Database	http://genome-www5. stanford.edu	Microarray database and analysis tools
	Gene Expression Omnibus	www.ncbi.nlm.nih.gov/geo	Gene expression and array database
Literature searching	PubMed	www.ncbi.nlm.nih.gov/ PubMed	Searchable citations from journals

Table 6
Databases About Sequence Variation

Category	Name	URL	Description
SNP	dbSNP	www.ncbi.nlm.nih.gov/SNP	The database of SNPs by NCBI
	Human SNP Database	www.broad.mit.edu/snp/human	Database map by several institutions
	Human Chromosome 21 cSNP Database and MAP	http://csnp.unige.ch	Human Chromo-some 21 SNPs
	Japanese Single Nucleotide Polymorphisms (JSNP)	http://snp.ims.u-tokyo.ac.jp	Developed by Japan

(*continued*)

Table 6 (*Continued*)
Databases About Sequence Variation

Category	Name	URL	Description
	GeneSNPs	www.genome.utah.edu/genesnps	Annotated gene models, pathways
	Human Genome Variation Database (HGVbase)	http://hgvbase.cgb.ki.se	Curated and annotated database with search tools
	MASC SNP DB	www.mpiz-koeln.mpg.de/masc/ search_masc_snps.php	Search tool for polymorphic sites
	The PCR and SNP primer(s) Database	http://las.perkinelmer.com/ content/forms/SNPDatabase/ welcome.asp	Based on human SNPs
	The Mouse SNP Database	http://mousesnp.roche.com/ cgi-bin/msnp.pl	A SNP database of mouse
	Mouse SNP Data	www.broad.mit.edu/snp/mouse	Mouse SNPs
Mutation	Human Gene Mutation Database (HGMD)	http://archive.uwcm.ac.uk/ ucwm/mg/hgmd0.html	Gene lesions responsible for inherited disease
	Mammalian Gene Mutation Database (MGMD)	http://lisntweb.swan.ac.uk/ cmgt/index.htm	Mutagen-induced gene mutations in mammalian tissues
	Mutation Spectra Database at Yale University	http://info.med.yale.edu/ mutbase	Mutations in various species
	Ribosomal RNA (rRNA) Mutation Database	www.fandm.edu/Departments/ Biology/Databases/ RNA.html	rRNA alterations from *E. coli* and other organisms
Population	ALFRED—Allele Frequency Database	http://alfred.med.yale.edu/ alfred/index.asp	Gene frequency data on human populations
	The Distribution of the Human DNA—PCR polymorphisms	www.uniduesseldorf.de/www/ MedFak/Serology/ database.html	Population polymorphisms

Table 7
Databases to Study Genotype–Phenotype, and Gene–Drug Correlations

Category	Name	URL	Description
Disease	Online Mendelian Inheritance in Man (OMIM)	www3.ncbi.nlm.nih.gov/omim	A catalog of human genes and genetic disorders
	GeneDis Human Genetic Disease Database	http://life2.tau.ac.il/GeneDis	Disease-related genetic mutations and analysis tools
	Frequency of Inherited Disorders Database (FIDD)	http://archive.uwcm.ac.uk/ uwcm/mg/fidd/ introduction.html	For medical and epidemiological studies
	Hypertension Candidate Gene SNPs	http://cmbi.bjmu.edu.cn/ genome/candidates/ snps.html	SNPs of hypertension candidate genes
Specific molecules	Human Cytochrome P450 (*CYP*) Allele Nomenclature	www.imm.ki.se/cypalleles	Data for the human polymorphic *CYP* genes
	Low density lipoprotein receptor (LDLR) gene in familial hypercholes-terolemia	www.ucl.ac.uk/fh	Database and map of variations, primers and oligonucleotides of LDLR
	GRAP Mutant Databases	www-grap.fagmed.uit.no/ GRAP/homepage.html	G-protein coupled receptors (GPCRs)
	Androgen Receptor (AR) Mutation Database	http://ww2.mcgill.ca/ androgendb/data.htm	Mutations and phenotypes of AR

(*continued*)

Table 7 (*Continued*)
Databases to Study Genotype–Phenotype, and Gene–Drug Correlations

Category	Name	URL	Description
	Human Membrane Transporter Database	http://lab.digibench.net/ transporter	For transporter pharmaco- genomics
	The international ImMunoGene Tics informa- tion system (IMGT) Databases	http://imgt.cines.fr/	Sequences, structures, tools about proteins of the immune system
Drug	RxList	www.rxlist.com	Drug index
	AdvancePCS Drug List	www.druglist.com	Drug list
Adverse drug events (ADEs)	FDA Adverse Event Reporting System (AERs)	www.fda.gov/cder/ aers/default.htm	Safety reports
Gene–drug interaction	Drug ADME Associated Protein Database	http://xin.cz3.nus.edu.sg/ group/admeap/ admeap.asp	Drug ADME- associated proteins

2.3. Analysis Tools

Table 8 shows bioinformatics analysis tools that can be used for pharmacogenomics. These tools are categorized according to their applications. Some tools specific for SNP studies are listed in **Table 9**. Methods of using these tools will be discussed under **Subheading 3.**

3. Methods

In this section we discuss biomedical informatics methods for pharmacogenomics based on database and software examples with emphasis on those that are specific for pharmacogenomics research, such as methods for SNP studies.

Table 8
Bioinformatics Tools for Pharmacogenomics

Category	Name	URL	Description
Genomics—Sequence similarity searching	Basic Local Alignment Search Tool (BLAST)	www.ncbi.nlm.nih.gov/BLAST	To compare novel sequences with known genes
Sequence alignment	CLUSTAL W	www.ebi.ac.uk/clustalw	Align sequences for their identities, similarities and differences
Gene prediction and sequence annotation	GenScan	http://genes.mit.edu/GENSCAN.html	Predict genes in genomic sequences
Contig assembling	CAP EST Assembler	http://bio.ifom-firc.it/ASSEMBLY/assemble.html	Assemble DNA fragments
Pattern and motif analysis	MotifScan	http://hits.isb-sib.ch/cgi-bin/PFSCAN	Find motifs in a sequence
Secondary structure (2-D)—RNA	GeneBee	www.genebee.msu.su/services/rna2_reduced.html	Predict RNA secondary structure
2-D—Protein	PredictProtein	http://cubic.bioc.columbia.edu/predictprotein/submit_def.html	Predict protein secondary structure
Tertiary structure (3-D)—Protein	CPHmodels	www.cbs.dtu.dk/services/CPHmodels	Homology modeling for protein 3-D
Systems biology—protein localization in cells	PSORT	http://psort.nibb.ac.jp	Prediction of protein localization sites in cells
Systems biology—protein interactions	Protein–Protein Interaction Server	www.biochem.ucl.ac.uk/bsm/PP/server/index.html	Analyze the protein–protein interface

(continued)

Table 8 (*Continued*)
Bioinformatics Tools for Pharmacogenomics

Category	Name	URL	Description
	Protein annotation diagram oriented analysis (PANDORA)	www.pandora.cs.huji.ac.il	Analysis of protein sets by integration of annotation sources

Table 9
Tools for SNPs Studies

Category	Name	URL	Description
SNP—homology and similarity searching	SNP-Fasta	www.ebi.ac.uk/snpfasta3	Search SNPs with the Fasta server for homology and similarity
SNP—Identification	DIFFSEQ	http://bioweb.pasteur.fr/seqanal/ interfaces/diffseq.html	Find SNPs between nearly identical sequences
SNP—annotation	HNP-Human Nucleotide Polymor-phisms	http://batman. embl-heidelberg.de/HNP/	Annotate human nucleotide polymor-phisms
SNP—visualization	SNP Maps	http://gai.nci.nih.gov/html-snp/ imagemaps.html	Genetic and physical locations of SNPs
	Gene Viewer	http://gai.nci.nih.gov/cgi-bin/ GeneViewer.cgi	View SNPs in the context of transcripts, ORFs and motifs
	Expression-Based SNP Imagemaps	http://gai.nci.nih.gov/html-snp/ ts.html	SNPs based on chromosome, tissue, and histology

(*continued*)

Table 9 (*Continued*)
Tools for SNPs Studies

Category	Name	URL	Description
	SNPview	www.gnf.org/SNP	Compare SNP distributions in the mouse genome
SNP/Mutation— functional impact	PolyPhen	www.bork.embl-heidelberg.de/ PolyPhen	Predicts structural and functional effect of SNPs
	rSNP_Guide	wwwmgs.bionet.nsc.ru/ mgs/systems/rsnp	The influence of mutations in regulatory regions onto interactions with nuclear proteins

3.1. Methods to Study the Structure–Function Association

3.1.1. Sequence Searching

To perform genomic analysis, one of the first steps is searching and retrieving sequences of interest. One such searching system is NCBI's Entrez system (*see* **Table 5**). The updated Entrez system has cross-database searching function. The system can be searched for several linked databases, including the GenBank nucleotide sequence database, protein sequence database, the genome database, and other relevant databases such as the structure database.

Users can query the Entrez system through keyword searching (*see* **Note 4**). Sequences, the full gene definition, accession number, source, organism, and references are provided on nucleotide or protein pages. Entrez Gene is a new query environment inside the Entrez system that provides relevant information about the gene in the NCBI's Map Viewer. Entrez Gene can be queried on names, symbols, accessions, publications, chromosome numbers, and other features associated with genes. The Entrez Genome database contains maps for chromosomes, genes, and relevant links and descriptions.

For gene discovery and gene mapping, an important and frequently used sequence database in the NCBI is dbEST (*see* **Table 5**). Expressed sequence tags (ESTs) are cDNA fragments useful for gene prediction and gene expression studies. Another system for gene discovery is UniGene (*see* **Table 5**). UniGene collects subsets of related sequences that represent a unique gene through clustering sequences including ESTs. SNP sequence searching will be discussed separately under **Subheading 3.1.8.**

3.1.2. Sequence Similarity/Homology Searching

In genomic research, a common problem is to identify whether a gene sequence from an experiment has been found before, what the relationship is between the new sequence and those genes already known, and what functions the new gene may have. Programs in BLAST can help solve these problems through comparing novel sequences with known genes that are already in genetic databases (*see* **Table 8** and **Note 5**). BLAST provides similarity search for both nucleotide and protein sequences. The alignment of the query sequence with those known sequences in the BLAST output can help users deduce functional and evolutionary information for their query sequences.

3.1.3. Sequence Comparison/Alignment, Phylogenetic Analysis

Sequence comparison is especially meaningful for the structure–function analysis. This is because those regions that are better conserved than others during evolution are generally important for the function of a protein, and for maintaining its 3-D structure. Sequence comparison composes the foundation of many other analyses that are based on homology search, such as the construction of protein family databases.

For genetic sequence comparison, multiple alignment tools such as Clustal W (*see* **Table 8**) can be used to find conserved regions, to track sequence alterations, and to trace evolutionary relationships. Users can paste or upload sequences that interest them into the program. Regions with conserved or varied sequences are highlighted in different colors in the output page. Evolutionary relationships are represented in phylogenetic tree diagrams.

3.1.4. Contig Assembly

Contig, from the term "contiguous," means a contiguous sequence that can be obtained through assembling several overlapping DNA fragments, such as EST clusters. The program CAP EST Assembler can be used for contig assembly (*see* **Table 8**).

3.1.5. Gene Finding and Annotation

To identify and annotate genes in genomic DNA sequences, the program GenScan can be used (*see* **Table 8**). Users can paste or upload their query sequences to the program. GenScan will predict exons, poly A signals, and the peptide sequence. The annotation of the sequence is shown in a diagrammatic PDF format.

3.1.6. Pattern and Motif Analysis

Besides BLAST, alignment tools, and phylogenetic trees, functional information of genetic sequences can be extracted through analyzing *patterns* in protein sequences. *Patterns* are common features of a protein family, usually a short but characteristic motif. For example, a pattern in the format [GV]-x(3)-{AE} represents [Gly or Val]-any-any-any-{any but Ala or Glu}, and might have certain functional meanings. Proteins or protein domains in a particular family that are originally from a common ancestor usually share functional attributes.

The program MotifScan (*see* **Table 8**) can be used to search for all known motifs that occur in a query sequence. This work is done by examining similarities between the query sequence and motifs in databases such as PROSITE and Pfam (*see* **Table 5**). The program helps identify the known protein family that the query sequence belongs.

3.1.7. Secondary and Tertiary Structure Prediction

To understand how RNA secondary structure influences diverse functional activities, programs such as the one in GeneBee can be used to predict RNA secondary structure (*see* **Table 8**). The program predicts graphical structure models and describes local stack zones.

For protein secondary structure modeling, the program PredictProtein can be used (*see* **Table 8**). The program uses sequence similarity search and neural network algorithms. The output of PredictProtein includes the predicted secondary structure and solvent accessibility, possible transmembrane helices, and the expected accuracy of prediction methods.

For the prediction of 3-D structure, tools such as CPHmodels can be used (*see* **Table 8**). 3-D modeling programs usually use protein domains available in PDB (*see* **Table 5**) as templates. The output of the program includes the template being used, the alignment between the query sequence and the template, and the predicted 3-D model.

3.1.8. Sequence Variation Analysis

3.1.8.1. SEQUENCE VARIATION DATABASES

The identification of associations between a disease and genetic variations in a population plays a crucial role in pharmacogenomics. The database dbSNP contains information about not only SNPs, but also microsatellite repeats and small insertion/deletion polymorphisms (*see* **Table 6**). The database can be searched using keywords and database IDs such as GenBank accession numbers. The output contains FASTA sequences, integrated maps including chro-

A

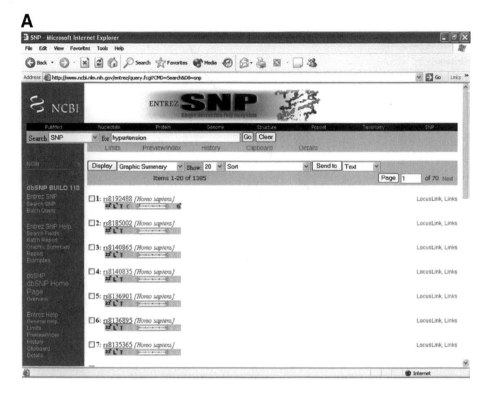

Fig. 1. **(A)** Query results of dbSNP using the keyword "hypertension." **(B)** Detailed information about the SNP rs1838105.

mosome maps, variation summaries, and links to other databases. **Figure 1A** shows a screen shot of the query result page of dbSNP with a search using the keyword "hypertension." The search retrieves more than 1000 entries. **Figure 1B** is a sample page showing detailed information of one entry, rs1838105.

HGVbase is a curated database (*see* **Table 6**). It is a comprehensive catalog of known human gene and genome variation with nonredundant records. The database provides details on how sequence variations are physically and functionally related to their closest neighbor genes. HGVbase can be searched through sequences, chromosome regions, and text. The output of the database contains the varied sequences, features of the gene, links to other databases and records, population frequency information, chromosome positions, assay methods, and source information.

To get allele frequency data on an anthropologically defined human population, the Allele Frequency Database (ALFRED) can be used (*see* **Table 6**). The output of the database includes population name, locus name, polymorphism name, population sample size, allele symbol, and frequency.

B

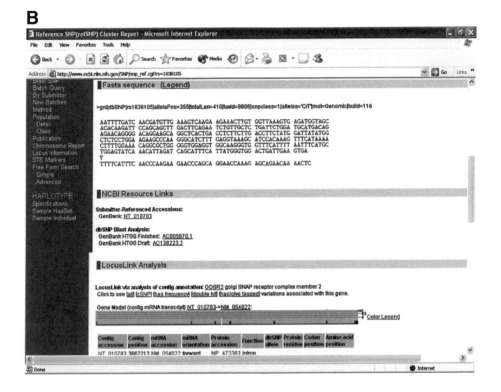

3.1.8.2. SNP ANALYSIS

Many tools can be used for SNP identification, annotation, visualization, and functional impact analysis. To identify SNPs with homology and similarity searching, the program SNP-FASTA can be used (*see* **Table 9**). Users can paste their sequences or upload their sequence files as input to the program. The program compares query sequences against sequence variation databases and returns a result similar to general BLAST searches, including sequence alignments. Another program for SNP annotation is Human Nucleotide Polymorphisms (HNP) (*see* **Table 9**). The program performs BLAST search against several databases, identifies and annotates possible variations in query sequences, and provides links to source databases.

SNP Maps (*see* **Table 9**) is developed by the Cancer Genome Anatomy Project (CGAP) at the National Cancer Institute (NCI). SNP Maps displays SNP information in diagrammatic maps with links, and contains some visualization tools for viewing SNPs in chromosomes. The program Gene Viewer allows users to view SNPs in the context of transcripts, ORFs, and motifs (*see* **Table 9**). Users can query the program through gene names, mRNA accession numbers, protein motif names, or sequences. The output of the program con-

A

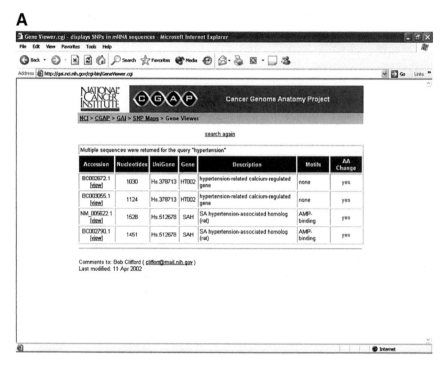

Fig. 2. **(A)** Sample output page of Gene Viewer with the query keyword "hypertension." **(B)** Detailed information of "NM_005622.1" from **Fig. 2A**. **(C)** More detailed information about the significant SNPs plot, motifs, and links to 3D structure.

tains predicted significant SNPs, protein sequence alignments, relevant motifs, statistics about how SNPs affect the fit of protein domains to motif models and 3D structures of motifs if they are known.

Figure 2A is a sample screen image of the result table if we make a query in Gene Viewer using the keyword "hypertension." **Figure 2B** shows the detailed information of the sequence "NM_005622.1" from the table in **Fig. 2A**. **Figure 2C** is a screen capture of the page linked from **Fig. 2B**, which contains more detailed information about cytogenetic location, significant SNPs and the SNP plot, the map of motifs, and links to the 3-D structure.

The Expression-Based SNP Imagemaps (*see* **Table 9**) can be searched by chromosome, tissue, and histology. **Figure 3** shows a sample output map of SNPs in chromosome 9 for normal heart tissue. This diagram illustrates the distribution of SNPs, the genetic map, reference markers, the physical map, and the chromosome 9 ideogram. Each detailed part of the diagram provides links to relevant data.

B

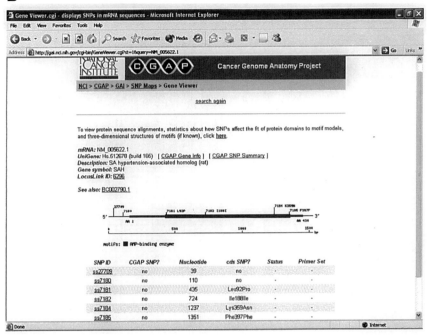

C

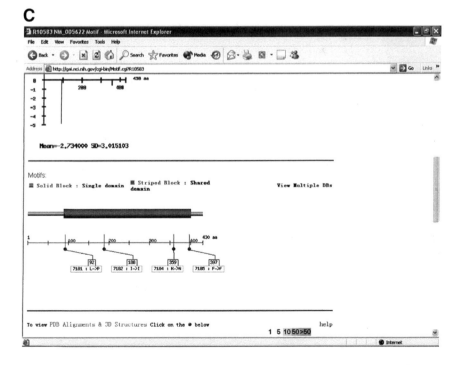

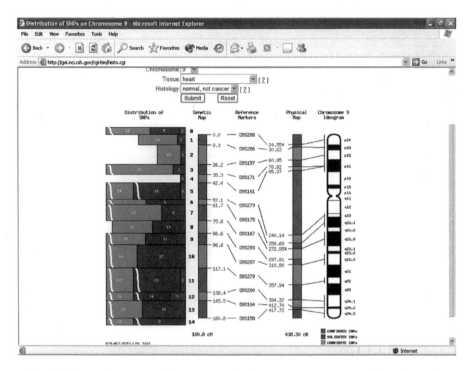

Fig. 3. A sample output of Imagemaps for SNPs in chromosome 9 for normal heart tissue.

To predict the possible impact that SNPs may have on the structure and function of a human protein, the program PolyPhen can be used (*see* **Table 9**). The prediction is based on sequence annotation, multiple alignment, and structure information. The program predicts possible effects on the structure and function for amino acid substitutions in an input sequence. Effects on the structure include probably damaging influences on buried sites such as hydrophobicity disruption and overpacking, and effects on bond formation such as hydrogen bonds. Possible substitution effects on function include probably damaging ligand-binding sites or protein-interaction sites.

3.1.9. Systems Biology Studies

Methods and tools for systems biology studies are emerging. The study of pathways and protein–protein interactions can help us understand how these molecules interact with each other and function at a system-level. Abnormal changes in these pathways and interactions may cause diseases. Such information can be useful for finding drug targets and designing effective drugs.

The pathway database of Kyoto Encyclopedia of Genes and Genomes (KEGG) contains information of metabolic pathways and regulatory pathways (*see* **Table 5**). The database provides graphical pathway maps, ortholog group tables, and molecular catalogs. Cell Signaling Networks Database (CSNDB) is a database for signaling pathways of human cells (*see* **Table 5**). The database collects information on biological molecules, sequences, structures, functions, and biological reactions that transfer cellular signals.

The Database of Interacting Proteins (DIP) collects experimentally determined interactions between proteins (*see* **Table 5**). The database can be searched using protein sequences, motifs, and keywords. Another database, Biomolecular Interaction Network Database (BIND), documents interactions between molecules, molecular complexes, and pathways (*see* **Table 5**). Protein-Protein Interaction Server is a program that analyzes the protein-protein interface of any protein complex (*see* **Table 8**). Through inputting the coordinates of a protein structure, users can get tables describing the nature of the protein-protein interface as the output.

To predict protein sorting signals and localization sites in cells, a program called PSORT can be used (*see* **Table 8**). The input of the program can be amino acid sequences. The program reports the possibility of localization sites for the input protein.

3.2. Methods to Study the Gene–Drug Interaction

Drug information is critical in understanding the gene–drug interaction. Some drug databases are available on the web, such as RxList, an internet drug index (*see* **Table 7**). Information provided in this database includes side effects, drug interactions, and full prescribing information. The database can be searched using drug names, keywords, pill id, imprint codes, and medical terminology.

When drugs enter the human body, they are processed through uptake, binding, distribution, biotransformation, and excretion. A database to study the interaction between proteins and drugs during these processes is the Drug Absorption, Distribution, Metabolism, and Excretion (ADME) Associated Protein Database (*see* **Table 7**). The database collects information about relevant proteins, functions, similarities, substrates, tissue distributions, and other features of targets.

Databases about specific molecules such as CYP450, receptors, and transporters, can also be used (*see* **Table 7**). Some of these databases contain information about SNP effects, tissue distribution, and interacting substrates. To study PK/PD features, resources are available on the web as listed in **Table 3** (*see* **Note 6**).

3.3. Methods to Study the Genotype–Phenotype Correlation

The correlation between genotype and phenotype is the most comprehensive one in the three key issues we have discussed, encompassing the whole biomedical process of drug therapy *(1)*. To study this correlation, many of the above methods and tools can be used. A database that provides direct connections between genotype and phenotype is OMIM (*see* **Table 7**). The database contains textual information about genetic disorders, allelic variants, biochemical and clinical features, clinical diagnosis, inheritance information, genomic mapping, genotype/phenotype research, population genetics, and references. OMIM provides links to other databases including DNA and protein databases, Gen Map, GDB, and MEDLINE.

The database Hypertension Candidate Gene SNPs directly correlates SNP information with the hypertension phenotype (*see* **Table 7**). The database can be browsed through gene symbols or gene functional classes such as apolipoproteins. The database contains information including map location and genetic interval, heterozygosity class, type of change, OMIM number, sequence data, and expression data for each gene.

For genetic profiling associated with certain phenotypes such as hypertension, microarrays are often used. **Table 5** lists some public databases for microarray studies, such as Gene Expression Omnibus for gene expression and array information (*see* **Note 7**). To study specific phenotypes or drug responses such as adverse drug events, web resources such as the Adverse Event Reporting System (AERS) of FDA can be used (*see* **Table 7**). This system collects adverse drug reaction reports for all approved drug and therapeutic biologic products.

4. Notes

1. An important informatics method that is beyond the scope of the chapter is data mining, including analysis at different levels such as data clustering, artificial neural network, decision trees, genetic algorithm, rule induction, and data visualization.

2. Some free or commercial bioinformatics packages contain or combine various databases and software tools together. An example is the open-source package, The European Molecular Biology Open Software Suite (EMBOSS) (http://emboss.org).

3. Many of these sites contain redundant information, so we try to differentiate them based on objectives and features of these sites. Because of the space limitation, we discuss only a few examples here. Readers can learn the most recent advances in the field through browsing these sites regularly, as new databases, tools, or other features are added regularly.

4. To access different information about genetic loci at one single query interface, users can go to NCBI's LocusLink (www.ncbi.nlm.nih.gov/LocusLink/), which presents information on official nomenclature, aliases, sequence accessions, phenotypes, UniGene clusters, homology, map locations, and related web sites.

5. Users need to select the correct BLAST program for the analysis of their nucleotide or amino acid sequences. The program selection guide is available at http://www.ncbi.nlm.nih.gov/BLAST/producttable.shtml.

6. PK/PD data analysis methods are beyond the scope of this chapter and are not described in detail here. Commonly used PK/PD tools can be found on web sites listed in **Table 3**, such as the program NONMEM.

7. Detailed discussion of microarray data analysis methods is beyond the scope and length limit of this chapter. These methods include comparison analysis and clustering analysis such as hierarchical clustering, k-means clustering, and self-organization maps *(22)*. Commonly used microarray data analysis tools include Spotfire, GeneSpring, Cluster and TreeView, dChip, and GenMapp *(22)*.

References

1. Yan, Q. (2003) Pharmacogenomics of membrane transporters: an overview, in: *Membrane Transporters: Methods and Protocols* (Yan, Q., ed.), Methods in Molecular Biology, Humana, Totowa, NJ, pp.1–20.

2. Guidance for Industry Pharmacogenomic Data Submissions. US Department of Health and Human Services, Food and Drug Administration, http://www.fda.gov/cder/guidance/5900dft.pdf.

3. Mukherjee, D. and Topol, E.J. (2003) Pharmacogenomics in cardiovascular diseases. *Curr. Probl. Cardiol.* **28**, 317–347.

4. Siest, G., Ferrari, L., Accaoui, M. J., Batt, A. M., and Visvikis, S. (2003) Pharmacogenomics of drugs affecting the cardiovascular system. *Clin. Chem. Lab. Med.* **41**, 590–599.

5. Anderson, J. L., Carlquist, J. F., Horne, B. D., and Muhlestein, J. B. (2003) Cardiovascular pharmacogenomics: current status, future prospects. *J. Cardiovasc. Pharmacol. Ther.* **8**, 71–83.

6. Rogers, K. L., Lea, R.A., and Griffiths, L. R. (2003) Molecular mechanisms of migraine: prospects for pharmacogenomics. *Am. J. Pharmacogenomics* **3**, 329–343.

7. Tafti, M. and Dauvilliers, Y. (2003) Pharmacogenomics in the treatment of narcolepsy. *Pharmacogenomics* **4**, 23–33.

8. McLeod, H. L. and Yu, J. (2003) Cancer pharmacogenomics: SNPs, chips, and the individual patient. *Cancer Invest.* **21**, 630–640.

9. Lenz, H.J. (2003) Pharmacogenomics in colorectal cancer. *Semin. Oncol.* **30**, 47–53.

10. Toffoli, G. and Cecchin, E. (2003) Pharmacogenetics of stomach cancer. *Suppl. Tumori.* **2**, S19–S22.

11. Flores, C. M. and Mogil, J. S. (2001) The pharmacogenetics of analgesia: toward a genetically-based approach to pain management. *Pharmacogenomics* **2**, 177–194.

12. Hayney, M. S. (2002) Pharmacogenomics and infectious diseases: impact on drug response and applications to disease management. *Am. J. Health Syst. Pharm.* **59,** 1626–1631.

13. Siffert, W. (2003) Cardiovascular pharmacogenetics: on the way toward individually tailored drug therapy. *Kidney Int. Suppl.* **84,** S168–S171.

14. Cadman, P. E. and O'Connor, D. T. (2003) Pharmacogenomics of hypertension. *Curr. Opin. Nephrol. Hypertens.* **12,** 61–70.

15. Bianchi, G., Staessen, J. A., and Patrizia, F. (2003) Pharmacogenomics of primary hypertension—the lessons from the past to look toward the future. *Pharmacogenomics* **4,** 279–296.

16. Tremblay, J., Hum, D. H., Sanchez, R., et al. (2003) TA repeat variation, Npr1 expression, and blood pressure: impact of the Ace locus. *Hypertension* **41,** 16–24.

17. Ranade, K., Wu, K. D., and Hwu, C. M., et al. (2001) Genetic variation in the human urea transporter-2 is associated with variation in blood pressure. *Hum. Mol. Genet.* **10,** 2157–2164.

18. Liljedahl, U., Karlsson, J., Melhus, H., et al. (2003) A microarray minisequencing system for pharmacogenetic profiling of antihypertensive drug response. *Pharmacogenetics* **13,** 7–17.

19. Yan, Q. (2003) Bioinformatics and data integration in membrane transporter studies. In *Membrane Transporters: Methods and Protocols* (Yan, Q., ed.), Methods in Molecular Biology, Humana, Totowa, NJ, pp.37–60.

20. Kitano, H. (2002) Systems biology: a brief overview. *Science* **295,** 1662–1664.

21. Jain, K. K. (2000) Applications of biochip and microarray systems in pharmacogenomics. *Pharmacogenomics* **1,** 289–307.

22. Hu, D. (2003) Microarray data analysis in studies of membrane transporters. In *Membrane Transporters: Methods and Protocols* (Yan, Q., ed.), Methods in Molecular Biology, Humana, Totowa, NJ, pp. 71–84.

Index